Student praise

Reading the last book was a great eye opener for me as a child and family practitioner, I honestly believe that every person working with children should use this book as a resource for engagement and practice. It allowed me to focus on the child as an individual and to realise that often times we label or diagnose children whose behaviours are the result, not of organic deficit, but of poor attachment, early trauma and low levels of empathy and resilience. I especially loved the emphasis on . . . how experiences during childhood shape the development of emotions and impact on every aspect of a child's life. This allowed me in practice to challenge other professionals who were too ready to label, diagnose and medicate children and to advocate for a more holistic approach to servicing the children.

Susan Williams

Just wanted to say thank you. Your book was unbelievable. I'm planning on buying your new book as well. I have almost finished my course, but as a result of this subject I have quit my full time job and have started working at a disability childcare centre. I needed to find some direction with this degree and this subject has certainly done it.

Mitchell Bagou

I enjoy very much the easy-reading style of your book. . . . I am employed by the Department of Community Services so find it extremely interesting and relevant for work.

Jenni Nielsens

Your book is excellent and this is actually the first time that I'm reading an academic book without constantly looking for a dictionary to find meanings for words. English is my sixth language I come from a different culture, a lot different from the Western culture and way of life.

Gabby K

I just finished the book The Emotional Life of Children and I must say I wish I had read it a long time ago . . . not only can I see and understand children's emotions better but I can also understand myself better!!

Shannon Yanez

Understanding Emotional Development

Understanding Emotional Development provides an insightful and comprehensive account of the development and impact of our emotions through infancy, childhood and adolescence. The book covers a number of key topics, including:

- the nature and diversity of emotion and its role in our lives
- differences between basic emotions which we are all born with, and secondary social emotions which develop during early social interactions
- the role of attachment and other factors that determine a child's emotional history and consequential emotional wellbeing or difficulties
- analysing, understanding and empathising with children experiencing emotional difficulties.

Drawing on research from neuroscience, psychology, education and social welfare, the book offers an integrated overview of recent research on the development of emotion. The chapters also consider child welfare in clinical and educational practice, presenting case studies of individual children to illustrate the practical relevance of theory and research.

Written in an engaging and accessible style, the book includes a number of useful pedagogical features to assist student learning, including chapter summaries, discussion questions and suggested reading. *Understanding Emotional Development* will provide valuable reading for students and professionals in the fields of psychology, social work, education, medicine, law and health.

Robert Lewis Wilson has almost 50 years' experience as a practising child psychologist and academic at Charles Sturt University, Australia.

Rachel Wilson has degrees in psychology, audiology and education. After seven years of clinical work with children she moved into research and is currently a senior lecturer at the University of Sydney, Australia.

Understanding Emotional Development

Providing insight into human lives

■ Robert Lewis Wilson and Rachel Wilson

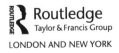
Routledge
Taylor & Francis Group

LONDON AND NEW YORK

First published 2015
by Routledge
27 Church Road, Hove, East Sussex BN3 2FA

and by Routledge
711 Third Avenue, New York, NY 10017

Routledge is an imprint of the Taylor & Francis Group, an informa business

British Library Cataloguing in Publication Data
A catalogue record for this book is available from the British Library

Library of Congress Cataloging in Publication Data
Wilson, Robert Lewis, 1941–
Understanding emotional development : providing insight into human lives
/ Robert Lewis Wilson and Rachel Wilson.
pages cm
Includes bibliographical references and index.
1. Emotions.   2. Emotions in infants.   3. Emotions in children.
4. Emotions in adolescence.   5. Child development.   I. Wilson, Rachel,
1969–   II. Title.
BF531.W55 2015
152.4–dc23

2014024145

ISBN: 978-1-84872-303-0 (hbk)
ISBN: 978-1-84872-304-7 (pbk)
ISBN: 978-1-315-84933-1 (ebk)

Typeset in Sabon
by RefineCatch Limited, Bungay, Suffolk

Contents

List of figures   xi
Preface   xiii

1 The importance of emotion   1
Emotion and psychology   2
Emotion, learning and decision making   4
Emotion and personal success   5
Emotions, social relationships and development   6
Emotion and moral behaviour   7
Emotional development in adverse circumstances   8

2 What is emotion?   11
What then is emotion?   13
Elements of emotion   14
The relationship between these elements of emotion   20
Variation in emotion   21
Understanding emotion   26
The neurology of emotion   27
Theories of emotion   31
Basic and secondary emotions   37

3 The basis of development   41
Early neurological development   44
Implications for child development?   50

4 Emotional development in infancy   59
Dependency needs   61
Dependency, care and the earliest emotional expressions   63
The growth and importance of awareness   64
Emotions in the first year of life   66

Dual coding of mental events: positive and negative emotions   67
Early bases for emotional development   68
The usual course of emotional development in the first year   72
When things go right   76
When things go wrong   76
The first year summarised   78

5 Emotional development in toddlerhood   81
The sense of self   83
The reciprocal relationship   84
The secondary self-conscious emotions   93
The ontogeny of emotion in toddlerhood   94
The importance of love   104
When things go right   105
When things go wrong   105
The early years summarised   106

6 Dependency, attachment and temperament   109
Dependency   110
Dependency as a key concept   114
Attachment   115
Attachment and dependency needs   117
Attachment as a key to development   120
Temperament   121
Temperament and attachment   127
Overview of psychological dynamics   129

7 Parenting, care and the development of secondary emotions   131
The nature of parenting   133
When parenting is not good-enough   135
Intergenerational influences on parenting   138
Parenting styles   140
Is parenting important in child development?   142
Summary of parenting and emotional development   146
A cautionary note   149

8 Emotional development in early and middle childhood   151
Early childhood: the pre-school stage   152
Middle childhood   160
When things go wrong in early and middle childhood   164

9 Oppositional behaviour, aggression and anxious behaviour 169

Oppositional behaviour 170
Aggression 174
Anxiety 183

10 Emotional development in adolescence 193

The importance of adolescence in emotional development 195
How adolescents feel about themselves 199
Adolescent brains, risky behaviour and addiction 201
Adolescence and dependency 203
Adolescence and emotional development 203
When things go wrong: adolescents from adversity 205

11 Understanding children in social/emotional difficulty 209

Interpretation of emotional development 210
A classification of children with social/emotional difficulty 211
Making inferences 215
The case of Jake Smith 215
The case of Jo Lee 217
Further case studies 222
The case of Michael 222
The case of Nik 224
The case of Eve 226
Concluding thoughts 229

Answers to chapter questions 233

References 249
Index 261

List of figures

2.1 The amygdala and projection of the limbic systems to the
     frontal cortex   16
2.2 The limbic system   28
2.3 Myelination   30
3.1 Axonal and dendritic connections   46
3.2 Neuronal density and connectivity in development   47
3.3 Normative versus individual growth   55
4.1 Dependency needs from Maslow   62
4.2 Guide to emotional development in year one   73
5.1 Emotional development in toddlerhood   95

Preface

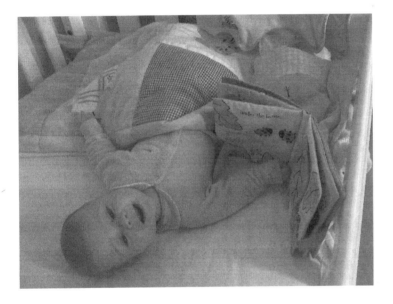

It is a strange fact, that in our quest to understand ourselves we often neglect to look to the emotions at the core of our being. The history of modern psychology has, until fairly recently, tended to focus on how we think and how we behave rather than how we feel. Of course we all ask ourselves questions about emotions like happiness – but to answer them you may find yourself examining ancient Greek philosophy. It seems that modern life concerns itself with what we do and who we are and offers us relatively few resources with which to reflect upon how we feel.

This is perplexing given the powerful, indeed dominant, role our emotions play in life. Understanding emotion holds the key to understanding all that we do, from how we develop personal relationships to how the world economy operates, yet few child development books devote substantial attention to it. In this book we take a different perspective.

Our perspective is that emotional development is at the centre of all development. Understanding emotional development can provide insight into our own lives and our children's lives. Despite the historical neglect of emotion in psychology and other areas of study, in recent years the world of research has turned its focus to discovering the mechanisms and drivers of emotion. There is much to be shared here from the field of neuroscience and we also draw on social work, education and social welfare research. We combine this knowledge with years of experience as practising and research psychologists in writing a guide to the development of emotion. We hope it will provide you with some insight.

What follows is a guide to the emotional development of children in general; it is written to help social workers, teachers, psychologists, nurses and other professionals deal more appropriately with children in emotional difficulties. Throughout this book emphasis is laid on the great variation in human beings and the importance of individual differences. We cover the general emotional development of children and adolescents but with regular emphases on understanding people who experience different emotional development in response to their personal circumstances and events. It is important we try to understand the feelings of such individuals, whose experience may be very different to our own, if we are to provide appropriate support, education and care. This emphasis on diversity is augmented by an expansion of our knowledge from the latest findings in infant neurology. These show that, in addition to variation from genetic sources, the early environment of the infant will influence the child's subsequent emotional development. Thus variations from both environmental and genetic influences are highlighted.

This book also focuses on gaining an understanding of the emotions of children from adverse environments who are experiencing emotional difficulties. In these environments loving nurturance has often been absent or in short supply and this is what leads to persistent problems. Many of the later chapters in this book are written with a distinct orientation towards child welfare in educational and clinical practice, both for children with short term difficulties and for those whose problems are more persistent. To cover such a range of children our description of emotional development must not be narrow but must take into account the familial, social and cultural conditions in which all children live and develop.

Where children suffer from abuse and deprivation the social conditions which make it necessary for child welfare authorities to be involved in their wellbeing have been fully documented many times. Much less attention has been devoted to the feelings and emotions developed by children who live in these adverse and depriving conditions. Yet these emotions should be of great significance when welfare or educational action is taken, be it support or intervention. Our account of emotional development therefore includes, from time to time, a special consideration of the emotions of children and adolescents who come from conditions of deprivation. The unsocialised survival reactions and adaptations of children and adolescents who live in adverse circumstances are often interpreted as behavioural or psychiatric disorders by experts. Our account intends to challenge these interpretations and give the reader an understanding of how such children and young people feel and why they act as they do.

By considering case studies we show how the emotional developmental history of a child is important in explaining his or her current behaviour whether it be in a regular or a depriving or abusive environment. We show how the interventions and support that are implemented to prevent unfavourable emotional reactions or to counteract insensitivity, deprivation or abuse, are best understood and operated if the feelings of the child or young person are kept strongly in mind. These feelings are a product of the child's emotional development and relate closely to the child's sense of happiness and adjustment. Any system of parenting, child welfare or education should regard how a child or young person feels as of central and crucial importance for a positive outcome. Parenting, support or intervention that increases a child's or adolescent's sense of unhappiness is obviously not desirable. By gaining insight into these children's emotional plight we will be better able to help them.

What is insight? Insight is what our students talk of when they complete a course on emotional development – we have drawn the term from them. Many have written of how this different perspective on development has profoundly changed their personal and professional lives. They write of new understanding and empathy for the children they work with. They write of how it has helped them come to terms with their own nature, their own parenting experiences, and frequently, their own childhood experiences. One student wrote of how she used the emotional perspective to learn to understand her once estranged father.

This reported insight is why we have written this book. It is interesting and useful to understand emotional development, not only from a personal perspective. It can also be enormously helpful in terms of working with others, particularly the disadvantaged and vulnerable. However, this understanding does not offer a quick fix. On the contrary, it may provide insight that uncovers new complexity and variation in individual development. Such understanding is more likely to deter us from the sleekly marketed quick fixes of the pharmaceutical world and the false promises of ideologues in the world of therapy. It serves merely to guide us in the complex and difficult paths of parenting, education, therapy, therapeutic environments and rehabilitation.

When child and adolescent development is orientated around emotional development it means that students, professionals, parents and all readers of this book, are encouraged to look beyond the child who is aggressive or a child who is depressed, to ask questions about the personal emotional history that has brought the child to that point. Reading this book should lead to an analysis of the drivers of emotional development. By such analysis we gain insight into the child through a deeper understanding of the path of development. It is not insignificant that in doing so, we are usually compelled to reflect on our own childhoods.

What is the value of a concentration on a deeper understanding of emotion and its development in children? We can only speculate here but a common theme in feedback from students is that there is new empathy and a sense of connectedness with the child. Some have reported a new sense of engagement in their work with disturbed children. While the nurturing of children is always a difficult task we can use understanding and insight to improve things. Even when the path of improvement is not clear, when we are faced with children and young adults for whom there may be no remission in suffering, a sense of insight provides empathy and compassion and stands against ignorance. For this reason the primary objective of this book, and our perspective on child development, is to put emotions at centre stage. It is about a different perspective.

To start writing this book we posed some questions:

- What is emotion?
- Are there different types of emotion?
- Do we all share the same emotions?
- How does emotional development start?
- How do emotions develop over time?
- What are the core drivers of healthy emotional development?
- What are the core stumblers to emotional development?
- Can we change the course of our emotions?

Throughout the book we answer these questions and also pose some more to guide your understanding. We hope this makes understanding emotional development easier and that you enjoy the book.

Chapter 1

The importance of emotion

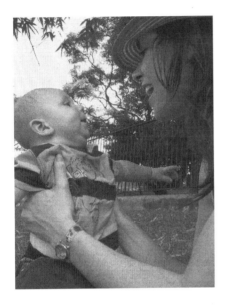

- How we feel is of utmost importance – it determines what we can learn and how decisions are made.
- Psychology has taken a long time to make this realisation and shift focus from cognition (how we think) and behaviour (how we act) towards emotions (how we feel).
- Emotions are not only important givens in life (basic emotions) but many of them are a product of the very social interactions that they serve (secondary/social emotions).
- Healthy emotional development has been shown to predict success in personal and professional life.

> • Understanding emotional development and how it is affected by adverse situations is often the key to helping children who end up failing in education and/or breaking the law.

WHAT IS OF ULTIMATE importance to children in any situation is how they feel. Children are usually not concerned to any degree with how they think or with what has motivated them. They are, like most of us, preoccupied with how they feel in any situation. They are concerned with the emotions that they experience. This concentration on emotion is general in human beings and to give it emphasis is not a new idea.

Following a tradition that stretches back to the Jewish philosopher David Hume and earlier still to Saint Augustine, Jon Elster in his book *Alchemies of the Mind: Rationality and the Emotions* (1999), claimed that:

> emotions matter because if we did not have them nothing else would matter . . . emotions are the stuff of life. (p. 403)

Emotion and psychology

Emotion is undoubtedly a prime factor in human life. Most of human life is involved with emotion. William James recognised the importance of emotion early in the history of modern psychology (1884), yet for most of the twentieth century, psychology, the science of the mind, did not regarded emotion as an important area of study. This was despite the fact that every human mind has probably been continually subject to mood or emotion in some form since the beginnings of history.

Though the origins of psychology late in the nineteenth century involved an introspective analysis of emotion, for the first seven decades of the last century, the focus of psychology was not on emotion; rather it was first on behaviour, and later on cognition. Because an introspective analysis of mental events could not be seen as objective, and therefore not scientific, all introspective views of emotion were cast aside during the middle part of the twentieth century. There are some exceptions to this trend, including Freudian psychology, arising from psychiatry, which was more concerned with unconscious motivation than with conscious emotional experience. Gendron and Barrett (2009) provide a detailed account of this history.

Behaviourism gained a significant hold and emotion was seen as disruptive of human processes. It was best dealt with by eliminating its influence. Thus, although some researchers maintained their interest in emotion, it was largely ignored as a human experience or as a factor in psychological experiments. The problem was that inner states of mind including emotion were deemed unobservable and uncontrollable, and could not therefore be considered as part of scientific psychology.

Even in the late 1980s Skinner, the leading behaviourist, continued to maintain that it was difficult to do much with feeling and states of mind because of their inaccessibility (Skinner, 1989). It seems that the discipline of psychology took delight in spurning the influence of emotional processes, because by doing so matters could be considered rationally, and the discipline could lay claim to an objective scientific approach. Yet what was scientific about leaving out processes that so profoundly affected human beings, the objects of psychological theory and experiment? Emotional processes affect people at every level of their functioning, from the physiological, to the cognitive, to the social and the spiritual.

The behaviourist stance, that inner mental processes should be ignored, took a fatal blow in the 1960s once it was realised that computers could 'think'. It became apparent that inner states of mind were explanatory elements in human affairs as well and could be inferred from observations. This led to the 'cognitive revolution' in psychology whereby many human actions and developments were explained on the basis of very complicated cognitive structures (indeed at this time psychology was often referred to as cognitive science). Many of the theories supporting such cognitive structures and the complex development that they entailed had little foundation either in experiment or in observable neurology. Emotion as a factor in its own right in human affairs was still largely ignored, and was relegated to a very minor aspect of human functioning under the control of cognition (Denham, 1998; Gendron and Barrett, 2009).

When psychologists were forced to consider emotion they called it by a name not normally used in common speech. They called it *affect*. The use of a word not normally understood by ordinary people tended to mystify psychological statements. It also reduced the influence of emotion on psychological explanations. In this way psychologists could avoid the undesirable associations of the word emotion. These associations were of the uncontrollable, the unreliable. *Affect* as a word seemed more scientific, more rational.

Nevertheless, the influence of emotion on human thought and behaviour remained no matter how psychologists tried to dismiss or disguise it. Neither behavioural analysis nor cognitive theory could explain how and why we had feelings and new directions in the study of emotional influences had to be developed. Thus in recent years emotion as a topic of thought and investigation in psychology has gained ground and there is now a considerable interest in the subject (Mascolo and Griffin 1998; Eisenberg 2006). This growth in interest coincided with, and perhaps was driven by, the explosion in neuroscience research. Neuroscience helped focus attention back onto emotion as work in neurology made it clear that emotional states are central to the brain's functioning. The discounting of emotional factors in psychology research has reduced somewhat in the last two decades, though it has not been completely eliminated in certain quarters. However, in general psychologists are now more willing to countenance emotional elements as factors of importance in their research.

It may seem surprising that this turn of events has taken so long but at last many psychologists are recognising the importance of emotion in explaining human beings. Indeed it has come to be recognised that if emotion is not a major element in a person's life then that person is somewhat aberrant. No normal conscious human being lives without the subjective feeling that is the essence of emotion. We all feel something all of the time even if it is a bland emptiness. We have no experiences that do not involve feeling; that do not, in fact, involve some degree of emotion. Feeling and experience are part of every conscious second that we exist. Can we envisage a mental state where we have no feelings at all, no emotional context for our thoughts? We can use computing devices that think, that do not involve emotional states, but we cannot conceive of a human being operating in the same way without ceasing to be human. In the famous TV series *Star Trek* Mr Spock was recognised as an alien precisely because he had no emotion. Emotion in fact defines our very humanity.

Emotion, learning and decision making

Consider two important aspects of life, learning and decision making. In the past it was thought that these were, or should be, essentially independent of emotion.

Let us consider learning first. Though emotion is not the only factor in learning, have you ever tried to learn something when you were flustered and emotionally upset? Why do students and pupils fail at tasks and subjects that they do not like? Liking or disliking a subject are emotional reactions; reactions that often appear unavoidable but usually are misplaced. People who learn well are not flustered or annoyed or anxious they are generally calm and emotionally content. Children do well at subjects they have been encouraged to like or at least not encouraged to dislike. A person's emotional state is one of the key factors in learning (Pringle, 1958; Hascher, 2010). Rewards and praise increase learning because they induce a positive emotion that children want repeated. A class of children will learn best if the classroom atmosphere is happy and calm and disruption is not alarming or exciting the class emotionally. It is not that feeling needs to be removed from learning situations rather it is the development of the right feelings that secures learning objectives. A classroom should not try to eliminate emotion rather it should cultivate feelings of security, respect and mutual obligation. Yet, when we look to research to advance education, the majority focuses upon purely cognitive aspects of the process. It is only in relatively recent times that the study of motivation has flourished and more recent still that the role of emotion in motivation has been examined (Meyer and Turner, 2002; Linnenbrink, 2006).

Decision making, especially in regard to human relationships, is likewise enhanced, not by a lack of emotion, but by the development of the appropriate emotions. Damasio (1994) refers to a patient who, due to a tumour, had a large section of his brain removed the result of which was that he could no longer feel emotion. The problem faced by Damasio and his patient was that the patient could no longer make decisions. Though his intelligence was intact he could no longer decide on anything. He was free of emotion and had all his rational powers yet decisions were beyond him. This is in stark contrast to the view that the best decisions are made when emotions are eliminated and pure rationality is employed. For Damasio's patient, faced with a number of alternatives, decisions were impossible because none of the alternatives 'felt' right. Even decisions in financial matters will be advanced in the long term by emotions like respect, trust and empathy. This has been recognised by the Nobel Prize winner and economist Daniel Kahneman (2000) who has challenged the pure rationality assumption as the correct basis for business decisions. Business and financial dealings depend on the trust of strangers and this trust arises from one's emotional experience and one's respect and empathy for others. In general business cannot proceed unless the majority of business people expect others in their trade to treat them well, that is, with empathy and honesty. This is borne out at times of financial crisis when trust breaks down. Trust and its concomitant confidence are hard to re-establish as the 2008 financial crisis has shown. In normal times most business people expect the same positive feelings towards them as they have towards those they deal with. Of course there are exceptions, but, on the whole, business and financial affairs depend on the exercise of the appropriate positive emotions between people. Such affairs are not an emotional free zone (Gabriel and Griffiths, 2002). The right emotions are central for business to succeed. No wonder deals are confirmed with a smile and a handshake!

Emotion and personal success

The importance of emotion in dealings between people was emphasised by Goleman (1996). In his bestselling book *Emotional intelligence* he put forward the thesis (based on a survey of research) that a child's ability to control positive desires and delay gratification was twice as powerful a predictor of academic and worldly success for that child as the child's IQ score. Goleman's book followed closely the views of Howard Gardner (1984) who first developed the idea of multiple intelligences and emphasised the crucial importance of understanding ourselves and others for success in life. By developing the concept of emotional intelligence (EI), Goleman showed how, in many aspects of life, the exercise of appropriate emotional understanding was more important than the exercise of pure intellect. According to Goleman succeeding in this world and getting on in society are more determined by EI than by IQ. In this book we hope to provide clear explanations of different pathways in emotional development and how they impact upon later life.

Emotions, social relationships and development

Goleman's finding is hardly surprising because people are dependent on one another for success or failure in life. Relationships between people are the key factors and emotions are of central importance in these relationships. Emotions are the necessary mental elements to allow us to do things together (Oatley, 2000). A teacher cannot deal with students except on an emotional basis, nor can a boss deal with employees without using or evoking feelings. As Keith Oatley has concluded "emotions are the very heart of social cognition; without them we wouldn't be able to do anything at all" (Oatley, 2000, p. 291). Emotions are the enabling factors in human relationships.

The most important emotions that facilitate human relationships are those that develop in children under the influence of their social environment. Emotions are not only important givens in life (basic emotions) but many of them are a product of the very social interactions that they serve (secondary emotions). This increases the significance of emotion as far as development is concerned. From a neurological perspective, Lise Eliot neatly sums up this importance "Yet this aspect of development [emotional] is in many ways the most important one of all, because it establishes the critical foundation on which every other mental skill can flourish" (Eliot, 2001, p. 290).

The central importance of emotion in child development is increasingly being emphasised (Eisenberg, 2006). In the last two decades new neurological scanning methods have allowed the study of the developing infant brain. What has been learnt from these observations has revolutionised our knowledge of child development. We now know much more about the development of the physical structure of an infant's brain. The most dramatic findings from such studies indicate clearly that an infant's environment and his or her interaction within this environment actually change the physical structure of the infant's brain (National Scientific Council on the Developing Child (2007). The environmental influence establishes and confirms certain connections between neurons (brain cells). Alternatively if no environmental influence is present certain neural connections will wither and be discarded. After infancy these processes of establishment and elimination continue under environmental influences but the physical changes to brain structure will decrease as the child grows older. A very important part of a child's environment is his or her social environment. From an infant's earliest days social interactions are fuelled and developed in many ways by emotional exchanges. This means that as the infant interacts with other people his or her brain is actually changing physically according to the emotions that he or she is experiencing. The most important social interactions that a child has are between the child and those who care for him or her, normally the parents. A child's physical brain structure is therefore moulded or sculpted largely by the influence of his or her early social experiences process (Shonkoff and Levitt, 2010).

Because emotions are often the mediating factors of social interactions and are also the product of such interactions they are of central importance in the developmental process. In the 6th edition of *The Handbook of Child Psychology* (2006) Nancy Eisenberg and her colleagues recognise the central importance of emotion in child development. Eisenberg sees emotion as playing a central role in social interactions and in developing personality from inherited temperamental traits. She also postulates emotion as an integral aspect in a child's conception of self as well as linking emotion to the development of moral behaviour. This central role of emotion within child development processes is explored throughout this book.

Emotion and moral behaviour

Emotion is also the central most important element in moral action. In infancy the beginnings of intentionality are linked to emotionally loaded situations and this linkage develops throughout childhood. Thus according to Coady (1999) sympathy and compassion, resentment and indignation are moral emotions.

We feel a good case can be made that justice and mercy, as they are understood by ordinary people, are at their root founded in the emotional experiences of infancy and childhood. These concepts develop as much through emotional experience as they do through the development of cognitive capacities. If this was not the case, and moral action depended solely on intellectual ability, most of the intelligent people would be moral, and all those of lesser intellectual ability would be immoral.

A child's cognitive capacities allow for the level of his or her moral judgements, but give little indication of the child's moral actions. In contrast a child's emotional history may well give accurate pointers to his or her moral actions. As anyone who has worked with delinquent children knows, a child's moral actions are not always coincident with his or her moral judgements. Some children carry out moral actions that they cannot explain in moral judgement terms. Other children are good judges of moral action, as indicated by their interpretation of stories, yet in their own lives act quite immorally. Remarkably, as we will explain, it is the physical influence of the social environment on the developing brain that lays the basis for moral action. Factors can be found in the close mutually satisfying relationship between child and caregiver that will influence that child's moral or immoral behaviour. This link between emotion and moral action is explored further when the consequences of emotional development in various situations of rearing are considered.

Emotional development in adverse circumstances

Understanding emotional development and how it is affected by adverse situations is often the key to helping children who end up as delinquents, having transgressed the law in some respect. Children whose upbringing has been abusive or insensitive to their needs often develop unwelcome challenging behaviours. These are often based on a negative reaction by the child to his or her social environment; an environment which has lacked supportive nurturance and has forced the child, in the most extreme cases, to adopt basic primitive survival behaviours. These often anti-social acts are the result of poor, inconsistent, or absent nurturing where the child's essential dependency needs have not been met or have only been met on an inconsistent basis. The emotional development of children in such circumstances is often warped because of their need to resist and survive. Perhaps the most important aspect of emotional understanding is the realisation that not all people possess the emotions that develop as a result of good nurturance in infancy and childhood.

We tend to presume that everyone possesses the emotions that we ourselves have. Though this is true of basic instinctive emotions it is not always the case with those emotions developed in a social context. Depending on the degree of social deprivation and lack of nurturance, children in adverse situations may not develop certain emotions at all or else develop them in a much weakened form. Emotions are a spur to action, they move us, and they are motivating. Where socially developed emotions are absent or weakly developed they will not motivate socially responsible behaviours. Children and adolescents who come from backgrounds of insensitive or abusive rearing often have weakly developed or absent social emotions. These children must be understood on their own emotional terms, not on the expectations of society. Most societies develop their expectations of acceptable behaviour from the emotions and motivations developed by children in that society who are reared in conditions of optimal nurturance. Where children are not raised in such conditions we must not pathologise them or see them as suffering from inherent mental illness (Luvmour, 2011). Rather we should understand them and their emotions and actions as products of their upbringing. The adverse and insensitive nature of such upbringings moulded and physically changed the brains of these children and compelled them to behaviours that we often find socially unacceptable. Of all the reasons why emotions are important perhaps this realisation that emotional development is not fixed or invariant is the most salient.

This chapter has highlighted the importance of emotion with a particular emphasis on its importance to children. However, we cannot proceed to discuss emotional development without first attempting to define emotion and to understand its variations. This is by no means an easy task. All of us experience emotion but defining it is more difficult, even for psychologists. Where definition is difficult, understanding may be limited because different people may be talking about different things. Our next chapter defines emotion in a way that makes sense for most people and will allow a common understanding. Some authorities think that emotion does not develop very much at all whilst others believe that all emotions are the product of development. Our second chapter seeks to reconcile such differences in order that we can proceed to an accurate description of emotional development.

Questions to think about

1. Why did psychologists take so long to recognise and study the importance of emotions?
2. Make a list of the abilities and achievements discussed in this chapter that are influenced by emotions.
3. What are multiple intelligences and what is emotional.
4. What are challenging behaviours?

Suggested further reading

National Scientific Council on the Developing Child (2007). *The Science of Early Childhood Development* http://www.developingchild.net. Available at: http://developingchild.harvard.edu/resources/reports_and_working_papers/science_of_early_childhood_development/.

National Scientific Council on the Developing Child (2004). Children's Emotional Development Is Built into the Architecture of Their Brains: Working Paper No. 2. http://www.developingchild.net.

Luvmour, J. (2011). Nurturing children's wellbeing: A developmental response to trends of overdiagnosis and overmedication. *Journal of Humanistic Psychology.* 5(3), 350–368.

Goleman, D. (2006). *Emotional Intelligence: Why it can Matter more than IQ.* Random House Digital, Inc.

Or . . .

Goleman, D. (2006). *Emotional Intelligence.* New York: Random House LLC.

Eisenberg, N. (2006). Introduction. In W. Damon, R. M. Lerner, and N. Eisenberg (Eds.). (2006). *Handbook of Child Psychology, Social, Emotional, and Personality Development* (Vol. 3). Wiley. Com, pp. 1–23.

Chapter 2

What is emotion?

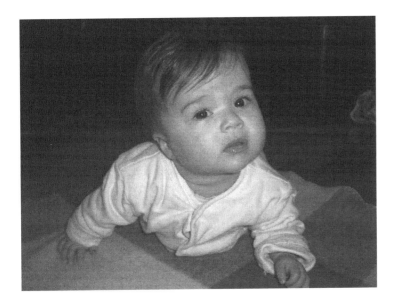

- There are multiple definitions and theories on emotion and a single unified approach is yet to be developed.
- In this book we define emotion as subjective feelings and differentiate between primary (basic, innate) emotions and secondary (social, developed) emotions.
- Primary or basic emotions are universal but secondary emotions are subject to culture and developed in diverse ways, with different strengths. The development of secondary emotions can go wrong when children are reared in adverse circumstances.
- Emotional development is complicated; there are multifarious interactions between social, cognitive and emotional development.
- The majority of researchers agree that each emotion has three components: physiological, subjective and expressive.

ANY ATTEMPT TO DEFINE emotion will lead to a picture of considerable complexity. It is only to be expected that complexity rules in human affairs and a wish to simplify may be against the reality of the situation. When he considered emotion from a philosophical standpoint Stocker (1996. p. xxi) stated, "Complexity is the rule not the exception".

The reason why emotion is complex and hard to define is because, on the one hand, emotion is closely bound up with other aspects of human functioning, but on the other, it is not reducible to these aspects. Emotion is closely related to cognition, but is not reducible to it. Emotion is often closely linked to action, to behaviour, but it is not just an impulse to act, it can be much more. Emotion is linked to physiological processes, but these cannot accurately define emotion. Emotion can usually be judged by emotional expression, but this is not always the case.

What do we mean by emotion? Emotion, mood, and affect? If we are to consider emotion we must, to some extent at least, define its meaning and distinguish it from similar but not identical terms. We need some shared understanding of the terms used in a discussion of emotion, but it is doubtful if we need a very precise and invariant definition of emotion. When Izard and others considered the problem of the definition of emotion in 1984, they asserted that where knowledge is lacking, formal definitions may sometimes do more harm than good (Izard *et al.*, 1984). In the same year Kagan suggested that emotion was a superordinate term, and as such did not require definition. What Kagan claimed was needed was clarity in the definition of the elements that made up the superordinate entity, and clarity also in the way these elements related to each other.

Nevertheless, if a coherent discussion is to occur concerning emotion, some shared ideas as to what is being referred to are necessary. Dictionary definitions are ultimately dependent on usage, and sometimes usage is imprecise. Emotion comes to English from the Latin emovere <ex-out + movere-to move> via the Old French emouvoir – to stir up. Emotion therefore as used historically refers to movement or to stirring up, in effect to strong feelings which move a person's awareness or consciousness. It is implied in modern psychological and psychiatric usage that this stirring may well be time limited, and probably occurs for only a relatively short period of time.

In contrast the term mood refers to a weaker less stirring but pervasive feeling which hangs about for longer periods of time. Mood, it seems, is a diluted drawn out emotion (DSM IV-TR, American Psychiatric Association, 2000). A mood is usually a feeling of low intensity that is, to some degree at least, involuntary. One mood changes to another. We always have a mood of some sort. Perhaps one way of considering mood is to think of it as the quality of consciousness that we experience at a particular time. Consciousness is always coloured, to some degree at least, with feeling, with mood.

The term affect is usually used in psychology to refer to a subjective feeling. This may well be the central and most important part of an emotion, but not all feelings stem from emotion. Feelings can arise from sensations such as heat or cold, or from events that cause pain, or from fatigue or energy (Mayer & Salovey, 1997). These feelings would never be sensibly described as emotions. Feelings can arise from sexual impulses, which may or may not be described as emotions depending on the context. Are these sensations and sexual impulses also affects? It would seem so. However, some psychological usage and most psychiatric usage (DSM IV-TR, American Psychiatric Association, 2000) defines affect, not as a subjective feeling component, but as an observable behavioural expression of that component. As pain, heat, cold, fatigue, energy, and sexual desire, can all have observable expressive elements this means that, even with this definition, affect includes more than is normally understood by the word emotion. For all that, emotion and affect have often been used interchangeably (Sroufe, 1995; Fox, 2008). Perhaps surprisingly the new psychological manual, DSM-V, does not provide a definition of emotion or affect and, despite the recent surge in neurological research in this area, it provides little mention of this core concept in psychology. When considering diagnostic criteria the DSM-V tends to rely on reports or accounts of "subjective distress", "subjective difficulty", "subjective experiences", to assess emotional aspects of psychological disorders (American Psychiatric Association: DSM-V, 2013).

The term affect confuses the issue of emotion and its definition. The term was coined in psychology and psychiatry at a time when emotion was not a popular topic amongst psychologists. Perhaps it was used to avoid confronting the more easily understood word emotion, and the obvious implications that such a word brings to either clinical or experimental work with people. Affect is a word not normally understood by those outside psychology or psychiatry. It has been used to mystify the practice of both psychology and psychiatry. It is confusing and tends to obscure rather than clarify. The use of the term affect will be limited in this book to those occasions where its use by other authorities requires that it must be mentioned.

What then is emotion?

We all know what emotion is but nevertheless, as is becoming apparent, it is difficult to define. Perhaps part of this difficulty is due to the fact that human beings function as wholes, and when we introspect about how we operate, we examine our whole functioning and do not break it down into isolated processes such as emotion, motivation, learning, and memory. Indeed we find such a breakdown difficult. We should not be embarrassed by our inability to dissect our performance; our mental and physical processes are intertwined in most that we do. Even when a task is mostly mental we use many systems coordinating with and feeding back to each other. Emotion is one such mental system. When we feel emotion it is usually linked, indeed intertwined, with other mental systems. We can experience emotion, because of what we perceive, because of what motivates us, because of what we think, because of what we learn, because of what we remember, or, in most cases, because of a combination of these processes. An emotional experience frequently involves cognition. Cognition, volition, and emotion are intertwined in most psychological events in very complex interactions. Edelman (1992) summarised the situation concisely when he stated "Emotions may be considered the most complex of mental states or processes in so far as they mix with all other processes" (p. 176).

Thus if we consider the development of secondary social emotion in children it becomes clear that these emotions do not develop in isolation. Their development is closely interwoven with what happens to a child, particularly in his or her social environment. Secondary emotions are also interwoven with a child's ability to understand. A child's cognitive development undoubtedly influences his or her emotional development, just as cognitive growth is influenced by emotional development. Social, cognitive and emotional development all proceed together in complicated interactions. Strongman (1987) makes much of developments where cognition, emotion, and social experience all interact. He suggests, following Arnold (1970) and Aronfreed (1968), that both cognition and memory processes influence a child's development of emotion. Thus a child appraises each emotional episode and, by an automatic process, thinks about the experience and links it to what has happened previously: memory and meaning allow the child to evaluate the emotional experience. We find it difficult to describe or define our emotions without reference to these other mental systems. Indeed science has made it clear that at neuronal level cognitive, emotional and social development are highly interactive (Shonkoff & Levatt, 2010) Thus if we consider emotion in a way that preserves its meaning, we must consider the various aspects that link it to other elements of our functioning.

Elements of emotion

Emotion interacts with other mental systems, but nevertheless, as a component of mental functioning has emotion any distinguishing features? Has it elements that either singly or in combination allow it to be distinguished from other mental systems? Can we, as Kagan (1984) suggests, clearly define these elements and the relationship between them?

Most emotional episodes have the following elements.

- *Physiological concomitants.* These can be divided into two main groups: (a) neurological aspects; and (b) visceral and dermal aspects. Of course these aspects are linked and some emotions involve the activation of many body systems.
- A *subjective feeling.* This is the experiential part of emotion and, for most people, is the essence of emotion.

- *The expression of emotion.* This is the communicative part of emotion and it is influenced by context, culture, age and gender.

People who interpret emotions must be aware of these three elements of emotion, of how they combine to form the emotion, and of the variations, combinations and possibilities involved. We shall now deal in some detail with each of these elements in turn

The physiological concomitants

(a) Neurological

All mental events have their origin in neurological activity. An emotional experience takes place in the brain. Though some basic emotions sweep over us without involving much thought many emotions involve cognition. Indeed, as we have already stated, in most of what we feel and do cognition, volition, and emotion are intertwined. This complexity means that many parts of the brain are involved in simple cognitive or emotional events. Nevertheless, certain areas of the brain seem central to some mental events much more than to others. We will explain brain systems in detail in the next chapter but for now a little explanation is required.

The human brain is an evolutionary development of earlier mammalian brains and has highly complex parts that are not well developed in other animals. However, the human brain has, in its central and lower parts, retained the same structures that occurred in our mammalian ancestors. Some of these mid-brain structures are closely involved with emotion and are part of the *limbic system* that is central to emotional reactions. The newer complex areas of the brain which are distinctly human are concerned with thinking and reasoning, that is, with cognition. They constitute what is called the *neocortex*. This new cortex, new because it is most highly developed in humans, is extensive and deeply convoluted. It forms the outside, top, front and sides of our brain. It is widely thought that this new cortex is generally the controller of thinking and consciousness. However, certain parts of this cortex are also essential for the subjective experience of emotion and these also form part of the *limbic* system. See Figure 2.1.

The limbic system has then two parts both often concerned with emotion. One part is in the older mid-brain while the other forms part of the new brain, the cortex. The word limbic means border and this is an apt name for a mental system that covers parts of both the old and the new brain.

(b) Visceral and dermal

We often describe emotions with reference to our internal bodily feelings. Thus we tremble with fear, flush with pride, have 'butterflies' in our tummies, etc. Emotions have bodily correlates that can involve every physical system, but seem particularly

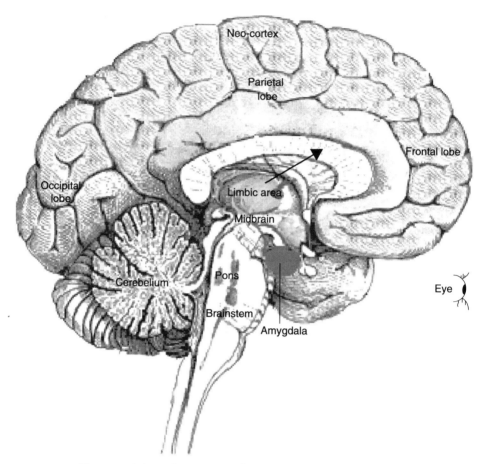

FIGURE 2.1 The amygdala and projection of the limbic systems to the frontal cortex.

associated with our visceral and dermal systems. Our autonomic nervous system orchestrates this arousal. This nervous system controls our vital organs, and is generally only under very limited conscious cortical influence. Thus our hearts can race, our breathing change, our skin sweat, or flush, our blood pressure increase or decrease, as a result of an emotional episode. These physiological correlates of emotion have been much investigated. For example, many studies have examined the flight or fight responses associated with fear. Many physiological responses are mediated by hormones. However, though much has been researched, it seems that emotions in most instances cannot be easily differentiated one from another on the basis of their physiological correlates. Bodily reactions to emotion seem fairly general rather than specific.

When we have an emotional episode we usually become more aroused both physically and mentally. However, some emotional episodes produce more physiological arousal than others. Emotions arising from memory, or from what Damasio (1994) calls "as if" perceptions (such as we may have if watching a film), often have very limited physiological correlates of the visceral or dermal type. It is also quite possible to be physiologically aroused without experiencing a particular emotion, for example after or during, vigorous exercise (Cannon, 1927). It also is possible that certain instances of autonomic arousal may not be perceived, initially at least, as a specific emotion (Zajonc, 1984). On the other hand one can, in certain instances, experience emotion without bodily arousal (Lazarus, 1991), and the degree of autonomic arousal may be very limited for developmentally advanced secondary emotions. Certain people suffer damage to the link between their autonomic nervous system and their cortical appraisal of that system and its associated physiological responses. This happens in cases of spinal injury. However, such people report emotional experiences, even though their cortical awareness of the physiological correlates of their emotions has been largely eliminated (Linton & Hirt, 1979; Bermond *et al.*, 1991). All these facts suggest that though physiological reactions especially of the visceral and dermal kind are, in most instances, an integral part of an emotion, they are not the central defining part.

A subjective feeling

For most people this is the essence of emotion. Izard (1977) states that we feel emotion all the time; we always have a mood or a feeling. What do we mean when we ask, 'How are you?' or, 'How are you going?' or 'How do you do?' We mean, 'How are you feeling?' We ask the question in recognition of the fact that we all feel something all of the time. Nevertheless, specific emotionally charged episodes occur as well as our general mood, and these are what most of us refer to as emotion. At these times we feel frightened, or angry, or anxious, or guilty, or joyful, or envious, or whatever.

Each subjective feeling is somewhat unstoppable. Few of us can talk ourselves out of our emotions, and though we can have them under some degree of control, we feel them because they have happened to us, and not because we planned their occurrence. This is not to say that our thought processes (cognitions) have little to do with our emotions. Recent work suggests that developed (secondary) emotions and cognitions are inseparable. Emotional labels are attached to various experiences, reflecting our cognitions of the external stimuli involved and the meanings they have for us. However, cognition and emotion are not identical, and whereas most of us can, to a considerable degree, program and control our thought processes, strong emotional feelings (and even moods) often just sweep over us, and our ability to control them is limited. They even sweep our thoughts along with them, and thus have considerable motivating force.

This unstoppable uncontrollable element in emotion is what differentiates it from most other mental processes. This lack of control is the factor that has given emotion a bad name in human affairs, even in the science that addresses the operations and nature of human beings, psychology. However, it is a central defining element in emotions. If, hypothetically, we were given another mental process that was somewhat unstoppable and uncontrollable, we would quickly subsume it under 'emotional reactions' no matter what its other characteristics might be. This is because, if we experienced the uncontrollability, we would immediately recognise the process as emotional. Other mental events do not stir us up, this only happens, by definition, with emotion. Some workers have defined emotion as occurring only when it causes disturbance to the person, that is, when it upsets or stirs up. Brown and Kozak (1998) define emotions as reactions to maladaptation, which consist of involuntary behaviour, feelings, and re-equilibration strategies. The key word here is involuntary. It indicates the unstoppable uncontrollable nature of emotion. However, Brown and Kozak also make the distinction between emotion and feeling. Following Janet (1928), they see feelings as everyday affective "secondary regulations" that are constantly present in ordinary life, whereas emotions, they postulate, are much stronger events intended to correct mental disturbance and restore mental harmony. This view of emotion, as separate from feelings, cannot be sustained, because if feelings do not have the uncontrollable element that is present in emotion, then feelings (secondary regulations) can easily be reduced to what Janet called "primary regulations", that is to cognitive processes. No, the unstoppable nature that is so defining of emotion is there precisely because it is a quality of feeling. This unstoppable uncontrollable quality is also true of other feelings that are not usually regarded as emotions such as fatigue, heat, cold, pain, and purely sexual desire. All conscious emotions and moods have this quality. If they did not we could simply think ourselves out of our emotional or moody state by an effort of will. Most of us have tried this and failed.

The surging quality of emotion comes from its unstoppable nature. Motivations that arise from emotions are often very strong and override those that come from other sources. This is because the unstoppable uncontrollable nature of emotions impels action. Frijda and Mesquita (1998) see emotion as having "control precedence", that is, as overriding and interfering with other mental processes. The overriding quality they recognise in emotion is there because, to some degree, emotion is unstoppable and uncontrollable. It overwhelms us and it often spurs us to action.

As Goleman (1996, p. xii) states *"impulse is the medium of emotion; the seed of all impulse is a feeling bursting to express itself in action"*. Yet Goleman goes on to discuss emotional control. How can something be unstoppable, overwhelming, and overriding, when it can also be controlled? We have little control over what emotion will affect us, or over when we are swept by that emotion, because, Goleman explains, the design of the brain dictates such a lack of control. However, Goleman states (1996; 2006) that we can have some say in how long an emotion will last. It is more likely that we can gain control over the length of time that we *express* an emotion, rather than how long we *feel* that emotion. This brings us to the control of the *expression of emotion* by cognitive forces and social experience.

As has already been frequently stated, emotion is often closely interwoven with cognition. Using our cognitive ability, and with considerable practice in social situations, we can learn to control our emotional expression. However, in controlling our emotional expression we are not necessarily controlling the emotion itself. We still can have the feeling. We can go a bit further. We can by means of emotional self-knowledge and the techniques laid out by Goleman influence our internal subjective feelings, but we can only influence them to a certain degree. *We cannot control them entirely*. The idea that emotion is not entirely controllable is not new; perhaps the first to mention it was Descartes (1649). If we could, emotion could easily be reduced to a sub-set of cognition, and people could easily think themselves out of their emotions. Some people perhaps, can think themselves out of some of their emotions, but, if a person is able to approach total control of their emotions we tend to regard them as psychopathological, rather than estimable. We feel that they have no emotions. We can use the term rationalisation to refer to a totally cognitive explanation of an event which we know, in fact, was in part emotional. If it were possible for emotional control to be total, then rationalisation would be considered a valid mode of thought, rather than a form of self-delusion and ego defence.

Can we have an emotional experience without this powerful subjective feeling? Certainly we can *express* emotion without feeling it; many children from adverse circumstances do so, as do actors, presumably; but one cannot experience an emotion without feeling it, the subjective feeling is essential. However, it may be possible that some emotional processes have an unconscious or preconscious origin. Many of us, especially children, are not conscious of the origins of our subjective feelings. We may even be unaware that we harbour certain emotions. In times of stress these emotions can break into consciousness, and in some instances when there is an emotional overload, the unstoppable nature of the emotions can cause a breakdown of normal functioning.

The expression of emotion

An expression of emotion usually accompanies the feeling. The expression of emotion is in behaviour which is subject to variation depending on age, gender, context and culture. Some specific physiological processes such as weeping, or laughing, or shaking, express particular emotions. Much emotion is expressed verbally by words, or vocally, by yells, sobs, or whatever. Non-vocal or non-verbal expression, particularly facial expression, is also ubiquitous. Emotional expression can thus be in words, or sounds, or looks, or movements, or postures, or gestures, or touch, or, as is usually the case, a mixture of these features.

Usually emotional expression links to underlying subjective feelings, and to physiological and/or neurological arousal, as is the case with tears or laughter. However, this need not always be the case. As we will explain later the emotional expressions of early infancy are not connected to more mature subjective feelings. Emotional expression can also be feigned by older children and people; it can be separated from the feeling that should accompany it. Actors do this regularly, as do teachers, and even parents. Contrariwise, some deep emotions, strongly felt, have limited expression in some people.

It is obvious that the expression that accompanies an emotion can vary considerably and may not even be genuine although in most communications the expression of emotion relates directly to the subjective feeling. This is particularly true of children who rarely try to deceive with their emotions and if they do try they do not often have the skills needed to succeed. Professionals working with children from adversity need to remember this.

Lang in 1988 classified responses to felt emotion into three categories. Some emotions are chiefly expressed in a cognitive/verbal fashion. Others have strong bodily expressions that are essentially physiological in nature. Still others have their chief expression in non-verbal behaviour. Though many emotions have expressions that include elements of all of these categories, on the whole Lang found a low correlation between these systems of expression. Lang's classification of emotional expression explains why, for example, emotions felt currently but aroused by memory do not, in general, have a strong physiological expression. When something emotional is brought to mind by imagery the expression of that emotion is often predominantly cognitive/verbal. In this instance there is no need for mobilisation of the body because the situation is imaginary. It is due to what Damasio (1994) calls "as if" perceptions. The picture with regard to emotional expression is indeed complex. Sometimes we can have strong emotions that occur with no physiological changes at all, whilst at other times the physiological reactions can occur in relation to several simultaneously felt emotions. Later when we discuss the development of emotional control in children, we will be discussing, for the most part, not the control of what a child may feel, but how he or she expresses that feeling.

In general many people confuse the expression of an emotion with the emotion itself. The key issue is whether an emotion is felt rather than whether or how it is expressed. Confidence tricksters and seducers know only too well that expressed emotion does not necessarily equate with the real thing, but many people fail to see the distinction, a fact attested to by the large numbers of people who are tricked or seduced. Many counsellors and therapists also appear to evaluate emotion by its expression, and some even consider the expression of an emotion as if it were truly the emotion itself.

The relationship between these elements of emotion

Whereas it is relatively easy to define each element of emotion it is more difficult to give a clear picture of how these elements relate to each other in every emotional experience. Most emotions have clear indications of all the elements we have mentioned but in some emotions one, or sometimes two, elements predominate. Emotion is very diverse. The emotions of early infancy may not have a strong subjective component. The second hand "as if" emotions that we experience when seeing a film or reading a book may not have strong physiological aspects. Some emotions may be deeply felt but may hardly be expressed at all. It appears that there is considerably variation in the combination of the elements of emotion. Is an emotion like instant fear essentially the same as an emotion such as shame in all of its components? What is obvious is that there are many emotions. What is less clear is whether these emotions or feelings are all essentially the same in terms of their constituent elements. The difficulty is that emotions vary in their neural mechanisms, their origins, their development and their functions.

Variation in emotion

Whether all emotions are in essence the same, or whether they are not, there is plainly a great deal of diversity in emotion. The English language has about 600 words that refer in some way to emotion or feeling (Oatley & Jenkins, 1996). This variation in emotion forms part of the definitional problem. Are there universal emotions shared by all humankind, or have some societies developed their own unique emotions? This question has created much heated debate since emotions were first studied scientifically by Charles Darwin in the nineteenth century (1872), and we will return to it when we consider theories of emotion in the next chapter. More immediately we need to consider the ways in which emotions vary.

Emotions vary in many ways, and we can infer some of the ways in which this variation takes place from what we have already discussed. Some of the variation is obvious and needs little explanation, whereas other variations needs considerable elaboration.

Relatively simple ways in which emotion can vary

(a) By interpretation

How do we interpret the emotions we feel? The most basic qualitative distinction that can be made between the perceptions that impinge on our consciousness is the distinction between perceptions that give pleasure and those that give pain or displeasure. Emotions are generally perceived with the same qualitative distinction. Thus there are pleasurable positive emotions, and negative emotions the experience of which is unpleasant, if not painful. There are, of course, mixed emotions where positive and negative feelings may both be present, but, in general, emotions divide into positive feelings like joy or love and negative feelings such as fear or anger.

We subjectively interpret many of our emotions as positive or negative. There is no completely agreed classification of emotions in this way. Anger, for example, may be a positive liberating experience for some people, on some occasions, but for the most part is experienced as a negative emotion. Likewise the fear generated on the roller coaster, accompanied by screams, may nevertheless be sought out and evaluated positively, whereas on most occasions fear is experienced as a negative emotion. Likewise, on certain occasions love can be painful.

(b) By intensity and duration

Emotions can vary in their intensity or strength and in their duration. Most emotions are strong episodes occurring over a short period of time that move or stir us up, whereas most moods are weaker feelings extending for longer periods. When we consider the progression from arousal to mood to emotional episode, we have a scale of variation in intensity and duration. In general, this is a progression from long-term feelings of limited intensity to shorter-term feelings of greater intensity. Intense emotions tend to be of shorter duration than vague moods, but again this is not invariably true. Certain strong feelings can persist in an intense form in certain people over long intervals of time. As any dramatist will tell, both intense love and revenge can be strong long term motivators of human action.

(c) By expression

Emotions vary in the degree to which they are expressed and this is particularly influenced by display rules of gender and culture. One might suppose that an intense emotion was one that was expressed forcefully and in varied ways. Generally this would be an accurate observation of most people in most circumstances. Yet the variation of emotion that can be seen in the expression of emotion cannot be completely correlated with the intensity of the emotion. What is expressed is not always that which is felt. Some intense strong emotions may not be frequently expressed, or may be expressed in feeble form.

Some emotions experienced only vaguely may be acted out in an intense way. Therefore we cannot be satisfied that variation in the strength of an emotion is directly related to the expression of that emotion. We must consider how emotions are variously expressed. In general terms people have considerable control over the expression of their emotions. A person can cognitively influence the emotion that they feel, and though they cannot totally control the emotion itself, they can with practice learn to completely control the expression of that emotion. The ability to control the expression of emotion is an important skill needed for harmonious social relationships, and may be acquired during childhood.

(d) By function

What are emotions for? This is a difficult question. In some ways it is like asking what life is for. Nevertheless many people have considered the evolutionary function of emotion. Essentially they feel that emotions, which are most highly developed in the social mammals, have survival value, and this has caused their selection and evolutionary development. This idea has been elaborated by Sroufe (1995) into a list of functions as follows:

i *A social/communicative function.* We communicate with others by way of our emotions and our emotional expressions. We usually communicate our inner state of feeling, though we can also deceive with this form of communication. Social communication by way of emotions is particularly important for infants and young children who are particularly dependent on others for their survival.

ii *An exploratory function.* Particularly with children but also with adults certain emotions promote a desire to explore and a desire to learn to control the environment. Emotions, it seems, are central to interaction or non-interaction with the environment.

iii *An instant response to emergency.* This is the function most often quoted as having survival value especially for instinctive quick emotions. (However, we must understand that survival, for a social animal, depends not only on instant responses to emergency, but also on the maintenance of the social group. This maintenance is usually advanced by emotions that are socially developed rather than instinctive. In social affairs the communicative function of emotion can also be crucial.) In response to emergencies the physiological changes that accompany instinctive emotion, such as those that prepare us for fight or flight are important elements in survival. By developing physiological readiness these emotions allows us to avoid or to cope with danger in an optimal instant way.

However the survival function of some emotions is not clear. This is particularly true for negative emotions such as despair and excessive anger; when expressed these emotions can lead to severe difficulties in life. (This can also happen sometimes when they are not expressed.) Far from being desirable adaptations such emotions speak against survival.

Emotions tend in many instances to be reactions. Most emotions start with a cause, proceed by means of a subjective feeling and an outward expression, and result in a consequence. The function they serve is often related to their cause. This cause is not always of the dangerous emergency type.

So again there is much variation if we consider the function of emotions. Emotions tend to be mental elements that motivate and guide a person's behaviour. Emotions often cause behaviour and they also regulate it. Thus the function of emotion is often idiosyncratic and related to the goals objectives and desires of the person concerned. Because people are vastly varied, and their desires and objectives likewise varied, so therefore will there be large variations in the function of emotion.

More complex variation in emotion

(a) By physiology

Physiological reactions are often concomitants of emotion. Emotions vary in their accompanying physiological reactions. However, this variation is complex and in our present state of knowledge is far from clear.

Emotional systems can, to some degree, be distinguished one from another by their physiological and anatomical attributes, including their neuroanatomy, their neural functioning and neurochemistry. For example, some neural elements concerned with the experience and expression of positive emotions are situated in the *left* frontal cortical lobes of the brain, whereas those for negative emotion are situated in the *right* (Fox & Davidson, 1988; Davidson, 1992). It is also known that different chemical neuro-transmitters in the brain are involved with different emotions (Oatley & Jenkins, 1996).

However, the accurate identification of a precise emotion solely by physiological or neurological indicators alone has proved to be extremely difficult. Whereas positive and negative emotions may be differentiated by physiological and neurological correlates, similar but different emotions cannot be separated by these means. For example, anger, fear, and sadness, cannot be distinguished one from another on the basis of their physiological correlates (Ekman *et al.*, 1983). This is not to say that closely related negative emotions do not vary in their physiology and neurology, only that we cannot, with our present knowledge, clearly distinguish between them on this basis. It is, however, very likely that the socially influenced emotions, such as guilt, have more neurological correlates in the frontal cerebral cortex than the faster, more reflexive, instinctive emotions, such as instant fear. The neurological correlates of certain types of fear may not involve higher brain centres.

Some emotions often felt with intensity do not have any obvious physiological concomitants outside the brain. Emotions that are, for example, evoked by memory alone often have few if any visceral and dermal concomitants (Cacioppo *et al.*, 1993). In emotions that arise from imagery there is no need for the body to have a flight or fight response. The situation is imaginary, yet the emotion felt may be quite real.

From this we can see that emotional variation may lead to, or reflect, physiological and neurological change, but the relationship between different emotions and these changes is very complex and not readily understood.

(b) Due to development

This is the most important and complex way in which personal secondary emotions may vary. Differences between people in terms of the socially generated emotions can be understood in developmental terms. By studying emotional development we can see how certain emotions change with circumstances, and how people come to possess different emotional repertoires. An understanding of this developmental variation in emotion is very important for those who work in professions that deal with people. Knowledge of this developmental variation is particularly important for understanding children from adversity, and the adolescents and adults that they become. All socially generated secondary emotions possess shared characteristics, but they may also have different developmental histories and ontogenetically can often be distinguished one from another. Are all emotions subject to developmental influences? Basic emotions are innate or 'hard wired' as we now say. These emotions are more governed by genetics than others, but we must realise, that the debate about the importance of rival genetic and environmental factors is futile. The simple fact is that even behaviours that are postulated to be innate develop (Sroufe, 1995) at least to a degree. Development influences everything. Everything exists in time; all living things have a developmental history. One could even argue that inanimate things also have a developmental history. Time changes everything to some degree. There is more on this in the next chapter.

We have outlined the complexity and diversity that constitutes human emotion by looking at the constituent parts of an emotion and considering ways in which emotion can vary. Are we any closer to defining emotion? Can we now say what it is? What aspects of emotion most clearly specify its nature? Two points stand out.

Defining aspects:

1. The most defining aspect of emotion is that it cannot be totally controlled. All emotions are, to a degree at least, unstoppable.
2. No matter what psychologists or physiologists may state, for most people the experience that they have when subject to emotion is the essence of emotion. For this reason we feel that this subjective experience is another defining aspect of emotion. We are, however, aware that the emotions of early infancy may not have a strong subjective element.

And what of the diversity of emotion, can this be more easily understood? How many types of emotion are there? What basis in defensible theory can we have to distinguish one type of emotion from another? In the next chapter we consider theories of emotion and select those with the most rigorous empirical basis. This will allow us to make clear distinctions between two main types of emotions (basic and secondary) and give us a better understanding of emotional development.

Understanding emotion

Would the difficulties in the definition and description of emotion mentioned in the last section be reduced if emotion itself was not one entity but had more than one form? Are all variations of emotion essentially the same, or are there distinct types of emotion, each of which can be more easily and accurately described and defined than the overarching term 'emotion'?

Multiple explanations

If we are to understand a phenomenon we usually turn to a theory that purports to explain it. In the case of emotion we have a plethora of explanatory theories. Things would be much simpler if every investigator of emotion had worked around a single theory. Unfortunately those who investigate emotion have found the complexity of the subject hard to explain from a single stance and have usually opted to explain an aspect of emotion rather than cover the whole field.

One would think that when a mental element was so important in very many aspects of human life it would be analysed with clarity by psychological investigators. Unfortunately this is not the case. There are nearly as many theories concerning the essence and origin of emotion as there are prominent psychological investigators. This diversity of explanation generally leads to confusion in the reader who rarely gets a complete picture of every aspect of emotion.

In 1998 Mascolo and Griffin summarized psychological perspectives on emotion in their book *What Develops in Emotional Development?* They outlined five major approaches in psychology to the study of emotion; Discrete Emotions Theory; Cognitive Perspectives; Structural Developmental Theory; Functionalist Approaches; and Sociocultural Perspectives. We need not discuss these at length now but each theory differed from the others in many ways. Theories differed in how they defined emotion. They also varied in what was included in or excluded from their concept of emotion. Each psychological perspective might include all or none of the following; moods, feelings, passions, sensibilities and attitudes. They also differed concerning the origin of emotion whether it was innate or learned or both. Each perspective had a different view of the function or purpose of emotion. Each theory outlined different components of emotion though some components were shared between theories and they also disagreed on which of the components initiated emotion. Each approach gave a different account of the development of emotion. Some approaches stated that emotions are largely innate and develop very little over the lifespan. Others took a completely developmental approach and yet others suggested that emotion was entirely dependent on context including cultural context. Finally there was no agreement as to the degree to which cognition influences emotion and the degree to which emotion can be controlled by other mental processes.

You will realise, reading these disagreements, that competing theories lead to a lot of confusion. This confusion in the reader is quite justified. It often seems as if different theorists are not talking about the same thing. Indeed this may be the case. Emotion may well be more easily and clearly explained if we realise that it is not a single mental entity. Emotion varies in many ways and this diversity has not been sufficiently recognised. Each psychological perspective may be correct concerning certain types or variations of emotion but not an accurate account of other aspects. Emotions can be very different one from another and the intensity of an emotion can also vary greatly. For this reason a number of approaches may be needed to adequately explain our emotions.

At this point it is instructive to consider some important questions. Are there universal emotions or are emotions developed solely by the environment, by context? If emotions are developed entirely by context we would expect different cultures to have developed different emotions. If, on the other hand, emotions are universal we would not expect them to be governed totally by context. Something in such universal emotions must be hard wired, (genetic), or else all human cultures must possess common contextual features. It is possible, of course that some emotions are universal and some are culturally specific.

Emotion is indeed not a single mental entity but consists of two distinct types each with its own variations. How do we know this? The justification and evidence for two distinct forms of emotion comes from studies of the brain particularly from advances in neurology and it is to this topic that we will now turn.

The neurology of emotion

As we stated earlier the human brain has evolved from less complicated animal brains. Generally vertebrate evolution has gone from fishes to amphibians, to reptiles, to mammals, to primates, to hominids, to humans. With each change the brain of the animal has become more complex. The reptilian brain, for example, had areas that detected smells and reacted to sight as well as an area that controlled movement, the cerebellum. As mammals evolved from reptile ancestors the basic brain was preserved but was added to by development above the reptilian brain. This development was the cortex, a bulge above the reptilian brain, and it allowed mammals many neural connections that reptiles did not possess. The mammals that developed the largest cortex were the primates, apes and monkeys, with the apes having the largest development of this part of the brain. However, the largest development of the cortex was in that branch of the ape-like primates known as hominids, our ancestors. Even this spectacular development of the upper brain was eclipsed by the explosive enlargement of the cortex that took place when one hominid group developed language and became human. Humans possess a huge cortex, sometimes called the neocortex, covering the whole outside of the brain with the exception of the underpart. This development amongst other things allows for thinking, planning, and the control of impulses as well as language. The most expansive development in this new brain was in the front part, that part above and behind your eyes. It was in this part that a unique function developed: consciousness. Some other mammals may have a degree of consciousness, we do not know to what degree, but the development and maturing of the frontal lobe of the human brain gives all of us that mysterious experience, that subjective feeling of being alive and aware of our life.

What has all of this to do with emotion? As the brain of animals evolved towards the human form the earlier structures were not discarded. With each change they remained in the lower parts of the expanding brain and these earlier structures are still active in all of us. Their action is still part of the human experience but in general it is not a conscious part. These older areas of the brain can and do generate emotions but this generation is often unconscious.

Underneath the cortex lie the structures that are older in an evolutionary sense. They include the amygdala, the hypothalamus, the thalamus and the hippocampus (in each hemisphere or half of the brain).

These mid-brain structures are referred to as the *lower limbic system* and lie deep towards the centre of our brains. In contrast the *upper limbic system* involves the frontal lobe of the cortex, that part of it closest to the mid-brain called the prefrontal cortex. Think of the area of your brain behind that part of your forehead just above your eyes. Now imagine that part of the cortex folded under itself and stretching back under the upper cortex towards the centre of your head, ending roughly where your temples are, just before your ears. You now know the part of the frontal cortex most concerned with emotion; it is the edge of this cortical fold (see Figure 2.2). These

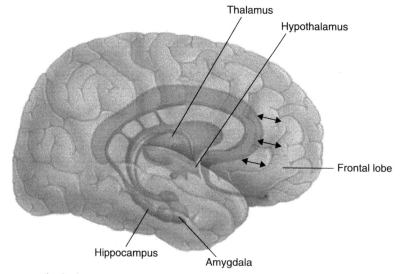

FIGURE 2.2 The limbic system.

upper and lower systems together form the *limbic system,* a system that spans the evolutionary older and newer parts of the brain and whose central concern is the generation of emotion (LeDoux, 1993; Eliot, 2001; LeDoux & Phelps, 2008).

We have defined emotions as being essentially uncontrollable subjective experiences. The word subjective means that they are, by definition, conscious experiences. How then can we talk of unconscious emotions? Although the human brain retained its more primitive underparts, as the cortex developed it grew from and above these primitive parts and developed many connections with them. The rear part of the frontal lobe of the cortex has many connections to the older mid-brain structures. This means that, although emotions may be generated in the mid-brain area, through these connections they soon become conscious subjective experiences. At least this is what usually happens.

The researcher who outlines this situation most clearly is Joseph LeDoux (LeDoux, 1996; LeDoux & Phelps, 2008). LeDoux states firmly that the brain structures that generate emotion are rooted deeply in our evolutionary past. He sees emotional generation as largely an unconscious process; and confirms the unstoppable nature of emotions, stating that we cannot completely control our emotions directly. This is because emotions emerge from the mid-brain, from the largely uncontrollable unconscious. LeDoux states that the wiring of the brain favours emotion in that the connections from the emotional centres of the mid-brain to the thinking cortex are stronger than those that run in the reverse direction. This means that in many situations when an external stimulus has provoked an emotion, a person's reaction is more governed by emotional imperatives than it is by considered thought. In an emotional situation, by definition, feelings dominate thinking.

LeDoux's most informative investigation was into fear. This basic emotion is almost universal in humans and also appears prominent in many other mammals. LeDoux showed that when confronted with a fearful stimulus a person may act in quite an unconscious fashion. So when suddenly confronted by a poisonous snake a person may leap backwards without thinking at all. What has happened is that the primitive mid-brain has reacted very quickly to the sight of the snake and has caused an automatic reaction. The feeling of fear comes later when the prefrontal cortex evaluates the situation and the person thinks about the danger that the snake signifies. LeDoux refers to such an emotion as a "quick" emotion. The reaction to such an emotion (leaping backwards) is caused directly by mid-brain structures and does not involve the thinking cortex. Thus some emotions can bypass the thinking brain. This is a useful function if danger threatens and reactions have to be fast. Nevertheless, though it is possible for some emotions to bypass the cortex, most emotions are quickly registered in the pre-frontal cortex and then, in the case of fear, the person will consciously feel fearful. LeDoux's work has been criticised (Rolls, 1999; Matthews *et al.*, 2004) but even his critics have to agree that on occasions, perhaps rare occasions, emotions can be hijacked and can bypass the cortical system of subjective awareness.

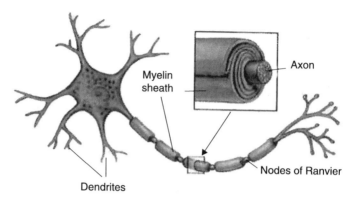

FIGURE 2.3 Myelination.

> **Myelinated** means insulated. A myelin sheath is a cell which forms on the axon or dendrite extension of a neuron and insulates the passage of electricity along the neurone. Myelination is essential for efficient communication between brain cells.

In mature people, on most occasions, the upper limbic cortical system allows them a subjective experience of emotion and indeed some measure of control over that feeling, though the control is not total. However, in early infancy there is no involvement of the upper limbic cortical structures in the production of emotion. These structures are still immature, only starting myelination at around six months, thus emotional events for a very young infant are not influenced by either subjective consciousness or thought. For young infants emotion is quite spontaneous and is concentrated on emotional expression. All their emotions are quick and bypass the immature cortex. There is little point in shouting at a very young infant who is crying bitterly; he or she has no control over emotional expression. The emotional expressions that young infants show are not regulated by their thoughts or their motivations (but by their needs). These mental connections have yet to develop (Gibson, 1991; National Scientific Council on the Developing Child, 2007). We do not know what young infants feel when they express emotion, they may be responding instinctively to some general sensor, but we now realise that they do not experience the subjective feeling which older people call emotion. Perhaps this is just as well because the depth of passion expressed in early infant emotion, if experienced subjectively, would be more than most of us could cope with!

As the frontal lobe begins to be myelinated (see Figure 2.3), after six months of age, infants begin to have a subjective view of the world and the emotions they are experiencing. Brain scans show that, as a child develops, there is increasing involvement of the upper limbic system (pre-frontal lobes) accompanying the experience of emotion. Increasingly in toddlerhood and early childhood emotional events may involve many other parts of the frontal lobes as well as the pre-frontal cortex. In later years scans show that in addition to frontal lobe activity several other areas of the cortex and mid brain may be involved in emotional experiences. This is because in advanced developed emotions cognition and memory are often an integral part of the subjective emotional experience (Carter 2000; Eliot, 2001).

Theories of emotion

We will now return to the many theories of emotion in the light of our knowledge of the limbic system and see if we can reduce the postulates of the main theories to some common ground that will help us when we consider the development of emotion in children. Theories of emotion tend to emphasise one of the three elements (1. physiological, 2. subjective feeling, 3. expression) of emotion we mentioned earlier over the other two, though most theories recognise the three parts.

If we consider theories that emphasise the expression of emotion one of the earliest investigators was the famous naturalist Charles Darwin. In 1872 Darwin published *The Expression of Emotion in Man and Animals*. In his earlier travels on the ship *HMS Beagle* Darwin had noticed and recorded the emotional expressions of the peoples that he met. He paid particular attention to the facial expressions of young infants. Later Darwin corresponded with people who had contact with other cultures and asked them to observe infant expressions and report the results to him. From this information Darwin deduced that there were *basic emotions* that were universal. These could be seen in the facial expressions of young infants in every society that he had observed or had been reported to him. Darwin felt that such expressions were instinctive and indicated innate emotions that everyone inherited. Darwin's theory of emotions depended on interpretations of emotional expressions particularly those on the face. It was from these expressions that he developed his conclusions about emotion. Other theorists have also concentrated on facial expression particularly the discrete emotion theorists (Ekman, 1984; Ackerman *et al.* 1998). Facial expression of emotion has even been suggested as the causal element in emotion. Izard (1981) and Tomkins (1981) have both suggested that, in certain circumstances, feelings may arise due to feedback from facial muscles to the brain. There has been no evidence to confirm that this is so, but some studies suggest that facial feedback may enhance or intensify an already existing emotion that has a facial expression (Adelmann & Zajonc, 1989).

Just as some psychologists and other scientists investigating emotion concentrated unduly on the expression of emotion, so others have laid their primary emphasis on the bodily concomitants of emotion. These physiological correlates of

31

emotion have often been seen as the central originating element of emotion. The origins of emotion in purely bodily processes dominated the discussion of the nature of emotion for many decades of the last century. Even before the beginning of that century, the James-Lange theory was developed, and it dominated the psychology of emotion for many years (James, 1884; Lange, 1885). This held that bodily processes caused the subjective experiences associated with emotion. In the 1920s and 1930s this approach was modified in the Cannon-Bard theory (Bard, 1934). This approach considered emotional feeling to be part of a general reaction that was essentially concurrent with bodily changes.

The Cannon-Bard theory emphasised the central importance of brain processes in emotion, and confounded the idea that emotion was simply the brain's explanation for bodily arousal. For all that, the idea that bodily processes initiate emotion surfaced again in the 1960s as the Schachter-Singer two factor theory. This held that, though physiological arousal does not cause a particular emotion, it is still the origin of emotion. Physiological arousal is the first factor in emotion, and this arousal is subsequently labelled by cognitive processes that take into account the context of the emotional occurrence. An emotion is a person's explanation of an aroused feeling (Schachter & Singer, 1962).

One must ask why theories, which place cardinal importance on the physiological processes of the body, as being the origin of emotion, have been so dominant in the investigation of emotion by psychologists in the best part of the last century. Psychologists have always aspired to be seen as scientific researchers, and approaches to emotion that have measurable variables, such as physiological reactions, at their core are judged to be harder science than those that do not include measurement. However, simply because something can be measured and varied in a controlled way does not mean that it will lead to better, more applicable, more accurate, scientific hypotheses. Psychology has been diverted by physiology in its study of emotion.

Le Doux's work illuminates several theories of emotion: the Schachter-Singer two factor theory of emotion, where the emotion is experienced first as a bodily reaction, and only later labelled by cognition as a specific emotion, fits with LeDoux's description of fast emotions. However, the theory that links most with LeDoux's work is the differential emotions theory sometimes called the *discrete emotions theory*.

Discrete emotions theory

Discrete, or differential, emotions theory has been put forward by Izard (1977; 1993) Tomkins (1982) Ekman (1984) and others. These theorists resisted the 'cognitive revolution' of the 1960s and 1970s, and proclaimed that emotions were discrete entities, separate from though interacting with other psychological systems including cognition. These theorists postulated that emotion had three components. Of most importance were the physiological component, which was largely neural, and the expressive behavioural component. Their third component, the subjective experience of emotion, was of lesser importance, and arose as a consequence of the interaction of the other two components. These theorists were particularly interested in facial expression, especially infant facial expression.

The lists of *basic* in-built *emotions* that each theorist of this school offered differed slightly, but they all held that fear, anger, joy, sadness, disgust, interest, and surprise, were basic discrete emotions present from birth (Ackerman *et al.*, 1998). The evidence for this they proclaimed was found in the facial expressions of infants. They held, with Darwin (1872), that these expressions were invariant across cultures, and must reflect in-built genetically determined neural features. According to this theory as time passes these basic primary emotions interact with cognition to form "cognitive-affective structures", but the basic emotions do not change their structure in these processes. What others might call the *secondary* emotions; these theorists refer to either as "cognitive-affective structures" or "dependent emotions" (Ackerman *et al.*, 1998). Although they mention dependent emotions they concentrate on the *basic primary emotions*. These they see chiefly as motivators, and emphasise their importance in initiating cognitive processes.

This theory was useful in emphasising that emotions are not simply part of cognition. It also has considerable support from recent neurological observations made in early infancy. These observations suggest that the amygdala, the hypothalamus and other neural connections are fully formed at birth. This lower limbic system operates to give the six or seven emotions that are clearly observable as emotional expressions in early infancy and it appears that these expressions are universal. However, these same neurological studies also clearly show that the upper limbic system particularly the frontal lobes of the cortex are not operable in early infancy and only become significantly myelinated, and thus operable, from the age of six months onwards (Deoni *et al.*, 2011). When we consider that these upper limbic cortical areas are essential to give the subjective feeling that we have defined as central to emotion, we come to the conclusion that early infant emotional expression, though genuine and clearly observable, is different in kind from later emotional developments. These later emotional developments are subjective experiences mediated through the limbic cortex, whereas the lower limbic system gives emotional expressions in early infancy that are probably genetically determined patterns of response to external, particularly parental, stimuli. These responses though emotional in expression may not be emotional in feeling. We do not know what a young infant feels but the neurological evidence suggests it is different from the clearly subjective feeling of emotion that arises later (Eliot, 2001).

LeDoux's (1993) finding that the amygdala can, if necessary, bypass the cortex and deliver instant initially unconscious emotion to older children and adults also gives some support to discrete emotions theory. LeDoux's work, however, does not imply that in the majority of occurrences basic emotions are unconscious. He recognises that most emotions generated by the mid-brain are experienced subjectively. Nevertheless, it is easy to envisage these basic emotions as quick emotions even if the conscious upper limbic system gives them a subjective feeling. These emotions are innate or hard-wired and though felt subjectively on most occasions are not much influenced by thought processes.

All in all, the discrete emotions theory continues the mind set of many psychologists in that it emphasises physiology and expression over subjective feeling. Its refusal to contemplate real changes to the basic emotions (that are seen in early infant expression) puts it at odds with any truly developmental approach. However, the theory has considerable strengths. Perhaps some emotions are more discrete and less open to change and development than others. This must be borne in mind as we go on to discuss emotional development.

Discrete emotions theory does not emphasise the effects of social interaction on emotion, and its reduction of secondary emotions to 'cognitive-affective structures' is unconvincing to those who observe unstoppable feelings of guilt, pride, and shame, in their clients, or themselves! This theory has been criticised by Russell (1994), particularly in respect of the interpretation of expressions in cross cultural settings, and by Sroufe (1995) in respect of the interpretation of facial expressions in childhood. It is always a temptation to equate emotional expression with emotion, and whereas in most circumstances this equation is true, it is not invariably so. Sroufe (1995) explains early infant facial expression in terms of reflexes and other factors.

Discrete emotions theory	Structural development theory
Principal proponents: Tomkins, Izard, Ekman.	Principal proponents: Sroufe, Lewis, Case.
Emotions are discrete from other mental elements.	Emotions are part of holistic development.
Emotions not changed by the environment though interaction occurs. Emotions generally unchanged throughout life but 'cognitive-affective' structures can form.	Emotions changed and formed by interaction with the environment. Emotions also influenced and changed by cognitive and other development.
Concentrates on basic (primary) emotions. Listed as fear, anger, joy, sadness, disgust, interest and surprise. These are invariant across cultures and identified from early infant expressions.	Suggests emotions develop in year 1 from non-emotional antecedents. Later these emotions, anger from frustration, anxious fear, and love can be transformed by environmental/social/cultural influences into further 'secondary' emotions.

Basic emotions present from birth. Hard wired into brain. Invariant.	Emotions change and develop new forms under environmental influences, though earlier forms can also be retained.
Concentrates on early infant expression.	Concentrates on later infant social interaction. Sees earlier infant expression as reflexive.

A structural developmental approach

We will now consider those cognitive affective structures (or dependent emotions) that have been mentioned but not emphasised by the discrete emotion theorists.

Are all our emotions innate and only slightly modifiable, usually in expression, during our lifetime? Does the context of our lives merely influence our emotion or do new emotions grow from our experiences particularly our early social experiences? Do emotions develop and do new emotions form?

Everything that is inherited can be altered by development and basic emotions are no different in this respect from other features. The basic emotions, referred to by LeDoux and the discrete emotions theorists, that are expressed and presumably present in early infancy may well be modified later by experience. This modification is usually in the expression and control of the emotion. The expression of basic emotions alters as we grow older, become more socialised, and more practised in emotional self-regulation. These quick innate emotions are with us throughout life and their modification is development of a sort. However, the development of emotions is much more than modifications to these innate emotions. As brain scans of older infants, toddlers and children show new emotions can form during development. These emotions are seen to involve many parts of the brain not just the mid-brain and the pre-frontal cortex. Such emotions are complex mental events often involving cognition, particularly appraisal, and other mental processes. These developed emotions have a place in the discrete emotions theory though proponents of this approach are reluctant to regard such developments as true emotions and they give them other names. Nevertheless, brain scans on children and infants of different ages show clearly that there is such a thing as emotional development both in regard to basic emotions and the other emotions that arise from our experiences, particularly our early social experiences. In later infancy and then, as toddlerhood progresses, more and more areas of the brain light up as emotional development involves other mental systems, usually located in the cortex. There is neurological evidence for a developmental approach to emotion (Carter, 2000).

This emotional development like all development occurs in a context. In the case of emotional development the environmental context is largely social. We develop our emotions for the most part in association with other people. We become emotional beings at the same time as we grow into social beings. Social and emotional developments are very closely linked. For this reason we call these emotions which arise in development secondary social emotions. A human being has certain innate emotions, fear for example, even if their interactions with other people are very limited, but other emotions (secondary emotions) may not develop at all in these circumstances. By and large social interaction is essential for emotional development (Lewis & Michalson, 1982; Grusec, 2011).

Theorists who believe that emotions are the result of development can be grouped under the structural developmental title. The developmental explanation of emotion was first put forward by Kathleen Bridges in 1932. The best known current proponents of this approach are Lewis (1990; 1995; 2005), Case (Case, Hayward *et al.*, 1988) and Sroufe (1995; 2009). Sroufe, for example, sees every aspect of a child as developmental. This development is holistic; it is all of a piece. As far as emotions are concerned, all systems, whether physiological or psychological, interact with each other and with the environment, particularly the social environment, in the developmental process. The environment is always a partner in the developmental process, but genetic unfolding also has its place.

In Sroufe's (1995; 2009) approach all emotions have antecedents. The precursor to an emotion in later development can be an earlier secondary emotion, but in the first half year of life precursors can also be physiological states not usually referred to as emotions. Sroufe considers that the more advanced later emotions are structural transformations of earlier secondary emotions, and have developed under environmental, especially social, influences, but also in concert with the child's cognitive growth. Generally in this theory, emotions develop from the simple to the complex, and they can do this either by differentiating, or by integrating, or by a combination of both processes. Sroufe outlines three early emotions which develop at some time during the second half of the first year from physiological precursors. These emotions are anger, fear and joy. Each of these emotions is by this time a separate entity and can continue to differentiate. However, it is also possible for these emotions to blend, to integrate, and be transformed into qualitatively new emotions. These theorists emphasise interactions between systems. For later emotions they emphasise the continual interaction between emotion and cognition, though they hold to the point that emotion never loses its distinct character. Emotion can feed back to cognition, and Case (Case *et al.*, 1988) sees cognition as always coloured by emotion. Emotion can so affect cognition that it can be motivating. For these theorists, therefore, cognition is important, but so is context.

Other theories of emotion

There are other theories of emotion besides the two we have outlined. One of these centres on the mental mechanism of cognitive appraisal following the recognition of a stimulus in the environment (Arnold, 1970). Sroufe does not deny the importance of appraisal and in the two factor theory of emotion it is one of the two factors (Schachter & Singer, 1962). Indeed Sroufe defines emotion as follows "a subjective reaction to a salient event characterised by physiological experiential and behavioural change" (Sroufe *et al.*, 1996, p. 200). The use of the word reaction infers an appraisal of the salient (or meaningful) stimulus.

Other approaches emphasise socio-cultural factors and some refer to attribution which is really an appraisal of social interactions (Weiner 1986). Yet other theories emphasise the functional nature of emotions. All of these theories see context as a key element in emotion and as context varies so will emotion whether this variation refers to a change in a stimulus or a change in social or cultural environments. It is this proliferation of theory that can cause confusion when we read about emotion; however, when we realise that brain studies point to two types of emotional reaction things become clearer. These neurological investigations can be seen to separate the quick instinctive innate emotions from the more complex, usually slower, emotions that involve other mental systems. The discrete (or differential) emotions theory deals centrally with the quick emotions and the structural development approach deals with the development of the more complex considered emotions. These later emotions, developing in the second half of infancy, are closely involved with the child's environment (context) particularly his or her social environment and the child's appraisal of events in this environment and how these events serve the child's needs. We are convinced that these two main theoretical approaches cover many of the basic elements of the other theories and are therefore the most important paradigms on which to base a study of emotional development.

Basic and secondary emotions

From what we have explained above it is plain that to fully understand emotional development we must consider two forms of emotion that have different theoretical explanations. On the one hand we have *basic emotions* which are innate, quick and genetically determined. These were first postulated by Darwin and are elaborated by the discrete (or differential) emotions theory. At times these emotions have been called primary emotions but the name we will use for these emotions is *basic*. On the other hand we have emotions that arise in development. These we will call *secondary* emotions; because they arise from social interactions these emotions can also be referred to as *secondary social* emotions. They and cognition develop together and are strongly linked. A child's emotional capacity is based, at least in part, on that child's ability to think and reason.

37

BASIC EMOTIONS

Fear, Anger, Joy, Sadness, Disgust, Interest and Surprise. Shown by infant expression consistent over cultures. Under discrete emotions theory.

SECONDARY SOCIAL EMOTIONS

Love, Anxious fear, Anger/Frustration, Jealousy, Bitterness, Disdain, Envy, Sorrow, Guily, Shame, Pride (last three self-conscious), Sympathy, Empathy. Plus others influenced by culture. Varied expression, sometimes very little. Under Structural developmental theory.

As we describe emotional development we must keep the differences between these emotional types in mind. For example we must realise that cognitive influence on some emotions is much more powerful than on others. Basic emotions are instantaneous, like the anger we may feel when someone strikes us unexpectedly or the fear we will feel if the earth shakes under our feet. We don't need to think to produce these emotions. Secondary emotions are much more incubated and develop over time (though even these emotions can have components or episodes that contribute instantaneously to their development). Thus guilt, resentment, and jealousy, belong to this slower category (though surprising your lover in bed with another adult can, depending on the adult, add *instantaneously* to your feelings of jealousy that may or may not be already present).

On the whole, the basic quick emotions have less cognitive control than secondary incubated ones. This is because cognition has less influence on intense emotions and these quick emotions are instinctive in-built features. Quick emotions tend to be those first expressed in infancy, when cognitive capacity is limited in any case. Over the life span their expression can develop but generally they remain unchanged otherwise and are not a significant part of the developmental process.

The secondary emotions of later infancy are not instinctive but have developed from earlier features (but not from the basic emotions). They develop under the influence of the environment, and in concert with developing cognitive processes. These emotions start as reactions to the social environment and the type of care that the dependent infant is experiencing. In the early stages they are based on associations related to a general sensor (Bridges, 1932) but later secondary emotions often involve an awareness of the self and an awareness of one's social relationships (self-conscious emotions). If the development of initial infant associations is warped, as can happen with infants in adverse circumstances, then the secondary emotions may develop in ways different to that which we would normally expect.

This in turn will affect the development of later secondary emotions. Where cognitive processes have also been damaged the situation becomes even more complex, because, where cognition has no control at all over emotion, a child or young person can develop self-justifying perceptions that are not rational.

The approach that we will now take to the development of emotions is influenced by both these theories. As far as discrete emotions are concerned, we are convinced that emotions are distinct entities, and we are also open to the possibility that certain emotions are more instant, and thus appear to be more hard wired, than others. Nevertheless, our stance is essentially a developmental approach. This approach emphasises not only the importance of holistic development, and the interaction of psychological systems, but also the crucial importance of environmental factors. In this it is very similar to the structural developmental approach, but in what follows the effect of environment is emphasised even more than in Sroufe's account. This is in accordance with the latest findings of environmental neurology (Schore, 1994; National Scientific Council on the Developing Child, 2004).

However, before we describe in detail the development of secondary emotions in infancy and toddlerhood we must once more consider the organ that is the driving force in development. We look at brain development in the next chapter.

Questions to think about

1. Review this chapter and list the number of ways in which emotion can vary.
2. Consider your male and female friends, how do their emotional expressions vary given the following:

    (a) Failure in an exam
    (b) Success in a job interview
    (c) Attending a football grand final
    (d) Guest at a wedding.

    Is the variation due to gender or other factors?

3. Over a few days make a record of your emotional episodes. Can you identify the physiological response, the unstoppable subjective feeling, and the emotional expression? Are they quick basic or slow thoughtful secondary emotions. Some people may need more than a few days to record different emotions.
4. In your own words describe both basic and secondary emotions.
5. In your own words describe the difference between primary and secondary emotions.

Suggested further reading

Izard, C. E. (2009). Emotion theory and research: Highlights, unanswered questions, and emerging issues. *Annual Review of Psychology, 60*, 1–25.

LeDoux, J. E. & Phelps, E.A. (2008). Emotional networks in the brain. In M.Lewis, J. M.Haviland-Jones & L. Feldman Barrett (Eds), *Handbook of Emotions* (3rd ed.). New York: The Guilford Press, pp. 159–179.

The basis of development

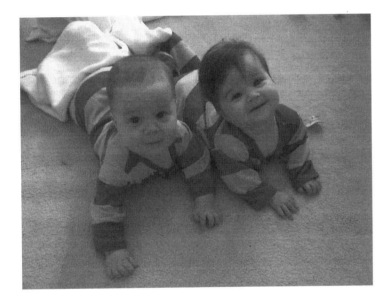

- Recent insights have changed how we view brain development. It is not simply a case of developing from simple to complicated systems.
- In some ways the infant brain is more complex than the adult brain. There are processes of proliferation in brain architecture before processes of reduction.
- General development can be understood from a normative perspective, however wide variation within normative processes means we also need to consider individual development.
- Understanding of genetic influences has advanced greatly but fails to fully explain diversity in development. We now believe it is a case of

'nature via nurture' and studies show how environment impacts upon genetics and developmental outcomes.

• Environment is important to all aspects of development even those with a genetic base. In emotional development the environment and social interaction is strongly influential in the creation of secondary, social emotions.

HOW DOES ONE LIVING form become another? This question is central to the study of evolution. It is also central to the study of development. Unlike manufactured goods living forms are not assembled from components. All apparently new forms have precursors in either evolution or development. In both evolution (phylogeny) and development (ontogeny), new forms seem to grow out of existing forms.

It used to be thought that in both phylogeny and ontogeny systems develop from simple to complex. However recent insights have shifted this view and we now know that in both cases development is highly complex and often is often goes in fits and starts.

In ontological development, the infant becomes the toddler, who in turn becomes the child, and then the adolescent and so on. Most of the body you have now is different cell by cell to the body you had seven years ago!

In evolution, life has, we assume, developed from the single cell to the multicelled, to many invertebrate forms, to vertebrate forms, to mammalian species, and so to primates. In each case, succeeding forms are often, but not always, more complex than those from which they arose. Is there a plan in all this, an inbuilt ascension from the lower to the higher?

In the nineteenth century, and most of the twentieth, it was thought by many that the evolutionary story was a 'right royal progress' from the simple and primitive to the advanced and complex. Indeed Bronowski (1973) spoke at length of the *ascent of man*, and made a popular television series on the subject. In evolutionary terms at least, it seemed that the ascent to forms of higher complexity was pre-ordained, perhaps divinely pre-ordained (though divine control was not Bronowski's view). Though chance had been a factor, things had come right at the end, (which is where we are now). This type of thinking was very human centred. It was wise after the event, and we all realise how easy it is to be wise in retrospect. This type of approach tended to justify the dignity and complexity of human beings by alluding to some type of evolutionary hierarchy, some type of progress towards forms that are better and more in tune with a plan for creation. In ontogenetic terms this upward progress signified development from the immature child to the mature adult. It was also felt that this progression was in some way guided by forces unseen, be they divine or natural.

In 1989 Stephen J. Gould published some seminal thoughts in *Wonderful Life: The Burgess Shale and the Nature of History*. In this book he challenged the "right royal road" approach to evolution and suggested that evolution was a matter not of progress but of chance. Yet the chance that Gould spoke about was dictated chance. As far as the development of life was concerned, this chance was dictated by environmental change, and was random only in so far as environmental change is random. Gould connected the development of life with the development of the earth, indeed with the development of the universe. If earth had been different the right royal road to higher forms would have been different. Gould explained that, in the far distant past, certain complex developed Precambrian life forms could have led to quite different complexity than we have now. That they did not is because, in some way, they were ruled out by changes in the earth's environment, or even by intervention from beyond the earth. Gould restated the importance of environment in the evolutionary process, and pointed out that some simple forms have survived for eons, and in a sense are just as evolved as we are. Evolution is adjustment to environmental requirements not a royal progress to "higher forms". In 1997 Diamond considered socio-cultural evolution and made much the same point as Gould.

As far as development (ontogeny) is concerned the same general idea applies. There is no predestination. What happens is that the organism adapts to its environment. It may of course do this according to some DNA blueprint, but we do not develop in a vacuum, the environment is an ever present factor and cannot be ignored. Plomin (1983) has written that the expression of hereditary influences, especially during sensitive periods such as infancy, requires transactions with the environment. If we ignore environmental issues they do not go away. Development takes place in accordance with the environmental influences whether we recognise them or not. In the development of emotions there is no inevitable progress, no rule to say that a child must develop guilt feelings at a certain age, or feelings of empathy, or feelings of affection or love. Yet our social policies in general, and our policies for children in particular, often assume an ascent from childhood to mature responsible adulthood, just as evolutionary theorists assumed an ascent from the 'lower species' to humankind. We assume, for example, that all people will have feelings of guilt just because the majority of us do. We erect systems of dispensing justice based on the idea that all young people can experience shame. We return children to their families, where we expect them to grow in an atmosphere of love and affection, because the human family is a higher form of experience and will produce higher beneficial emotional development. At the same time we often ignore the general environments in which families must survive, and the specific environmental influences that influence the growth of emotions in family members. It seems then that there are no absolute certainties in development, any more than there are in evolution. We are all subject to our genetic blueprints, but only as they interact with our environments. There is no certain course spelt out for us.

When it comes to children this orientation that nothing is certain and everything is environmentally dependent is very important. If we ignore the environmental influences on our children, and do not adapt these influences to cater for what we esteem as desired characteristics, we will get children and adolescents who display something else. A gardener may hope that the bulbs she planted will inevitably produce beautiful flowers, but in her heart she knows that the result is dependent on frost, and rain, and sun, and shade, and soil, and a host of environmental features that cannot be ignored. Neglected children will respond to environmental forces and many will survive, but perhaps not in the way we would wish. In terms of emotions, a harmonious society thrives on positive emotions, but these only grow from positive environments for children, not from situations where emotional development is left to environmental chance.

Many of the processes that occur in phylogeny are present in ontogeny. In particular we cannot study development without bearing in mind the importance of variation. Humans are immensely complex organisms largely on account of their brains, but they are also very varied. Any experienced psychological practitioner knows that no two cases are the same. Yet development is often explained by ages and stages, as if there was truly a "royal road", and variation did not count. Variation arises from genetics and environmental selection, and it is environmental selection, particularly in the development of the brain, that is vitally important in producing an individual in tune with his or her surroundings. Where adverse environmental selections occur, what will develop is an individual suited to adverse conditions, but perhaps not suited to the expectations of society. Almost all babies are cute but how do they grow, in many instances, into such coarse and unmanageable people? The answer lies in the environmental history of the child and in particular in his or her emotional history. A child's environmental history is the unfolding of environmental influences on the template of the child's genetic inheritance. The organ that is most subject to these environmental influences, and is central to the development of any human being, is the brain.

Early neurological development

The basis of development in a human being lies in the head, in the brain. Foetuses without brains do not survive. Genetic influence sets the general structural framework of the brain and turns genes on and off at certain points in development (that are determined in many cases by environmental influences). In the very early growth of the brain growth cone cells lead the migration of neurons to the head end of the embryo. The progress of these cones and their following neurons is genetically controlled and thus determine the general structure of the brain. The rate at which the brain matures dictates the general pace of development in children. The brain is the organ of the body that balances and controls development. More than that, the brain and its associated master gland, the pituitary, are often the driving forces behind development.

44

The human brain is perhaps the most complex entity in existence. It contains 100 billion nerve cells called neurons. These cells develop when we are still in the first trimester of our embryonic life. In the first trimester of our gestation neurons are produced at the incredible rate of 500,000 per minute (Eliot, 2001). We are born with almost our full complement of neurons or nerve cells (Kolb & Fantie, 1989). Strictly speaking we cannot get a brain cell cancer or tumour; most neurons don't multiply. Brain tumours are cancers of other cells in the brain, glial cells that service the brain cells. The division of neurons is largely completed in the foetus at 18 weeks but a few new neurons are produced later in pregnancy and even in the early weeks after birth (Eliot, 2001). Recent work with stem cells has also indicated the possibility of neuronal division at a later stage and it is now accepted that some new neurons can form over the lifespan. However, it seems we are born with *nearly* our full complement of grey matter! Is intelligence then fully determined at birth? By no means! Though neurons, for the most part, do not form or divide after birth, they do grow, and most importantly connections form between them. Tree like branches grow out of our nerve cells and these join with protuberances from other cells called axons, what we think of as nerves. Where axons and dendrites almost meet we get a joining of nerve cells, called a synapse which paradoxically is a tiny gap (see Figure 3.1). Axons and dendrites grow and synapses proliferate in the foetus and later in the young baby at an astonishing rate. Trillions of connections are formed. It is this multitude of connections that gives the brain its vast complexity. The connections are of course not total, a tiny gap is left between dendrite and axon, the nerve cell extensions, and that final gap can be bridged biochemically by neurotransmitters (see Figure 3.1).

However, simply having connected or synapsed neurons is *not* the key to development. The brain is a living developing organ. It changes radically during childhood but it also continues to change throughout life. In a sense the brain is never finished, never completed, even in old age. It is always adapting to environmental demands, and compensating, where it can, for injuries that it may have incurred. Thus a woman who has had a stroke in her 80s can still recover, at least to some degree, some of the functions taken away by the stroke. Though many neurons die or become unused during childhood the brain continues to have a large spare capacity in terms of neurons into the adult years, though it loses neurons increasingly after 25 years of age, (and more so if you drink alcohol). Despite increasing cell death after 25 the brain can still maintain its working competence in dealing with the environment for many years. It is only in extreme old age that this spare capacity may be used up. This excess capacity, in terms of numbers of neurons, is also useful if working combinations in the brain are damaged. The brain can readapt to the environment following brain damage by selecting other neural combinations to carry out its tasks. This is known as transfer of function.

Though the brain is capable of some recovery and a flexible redeployment of function at the end of life, its degree of flexibility at this stage is very limited. It is

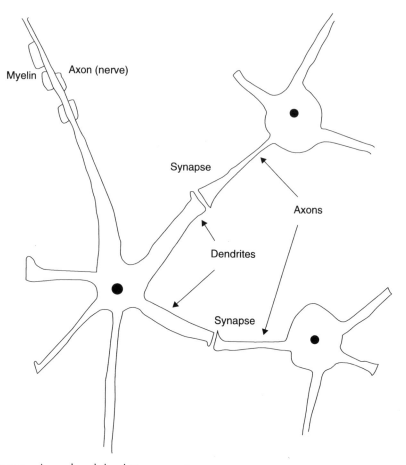

FIGURE 3.1 Axonal and dendritic connections.

at the other end of the life span, during infancy and childhood, that the brain has the greatest degree of flexibility and adaptability (Rakic, 1991). The brain of a newborn child, though it has almost all its neurons, is not finished. This does not matter because the brain begins working well long before it is finished.

We must be critical and wary of the analogies that are used to describe the brain. Currently the analogy that is most frequently used is that of the computer. However, the brain is living and developing and a computer is not. A computer is manufactured to a plan, components are assembled, and when finished the computer is turned on for use. The brain is not manufactured and turned on. Unlike any computer, it works well even before it is finished. For this reason a computer is not a suitable analogy for the brain. A systems model for the brain is a more appropriate analogy than that of a computer (Edelman, 1992).

Even before birth connections form between brain cells. After birth the brain develops by becoming more and more complex. The number of connections proliferates at an astonishing rate. A child's brain, at two years of age, contains twice as many connections between the nerve cells, and uses twice as much energy, as the brain of an adult (Shore, 1997). Complexity builds steadily on complexity, although new neurons do not form to any great extent. Rather what neurons there are, and there are billions, are integrated and rearranged again and again into forms of increasing complexity. How does this integration and rearrangement proceed? It proceeds by the development and use of trillions of connections between the nerve cells, and just as importantly, by the elimination of other previously formed connections. Connections that are not used, or do not relate efficiently to the environmental needs of the child, are eliminated (Huttenlocher, 1994). They are pruned. This process of connecting and pruning is referred to as "sculpting" by Tucker (1992). A sculptor does not add to his stone, merely works it into a new form.

With virtually all our neurons present at birth, after birth, for the most part, we cannot grow new brain cells, nor can we repair those whose nuclei become damaged. In fact the opposite occurs and during the first year of life considerable brain cell death occurs. More brain cells die during this first year of life than at any other time in the life history of most individuals. So it is not only connections that are pruned, it is sometimes the cells themselves see Figure 3.2. Unused neurons (as opposed to the connections between neurons) are eliminated (Hamburger & Oppenheim, 1982; Janowsky and Finlay, 1986).

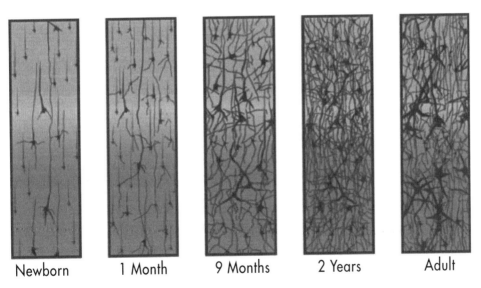

Newborn   1 Month   9 Months   2 Years   Adult

FIGURE 3.2 Neuronal density and connectivity in development.

Source: Corel, JL. *The postnatal development of the human cerebral cortex.* Cambridge MA: Harvard University Press, 1975.

Apoptosis is the medical word that applies to this process (Carter, 2000). It means programmed cell death and is a natural and essential process in any part of the body. When it does not occur cells do not die but proliferate and cancers may form. In infancy and toddlerhood many unused neurons die and are generally not replaced. The brain is consolidated to fit the developing child's environment.

Some neurons do not die but their processes are suppressed (Cowan *et al.*, 1979). Presumably these suppressed neurons remain dormant, having fulfilled their function during infancy. They form part of the flexible spare capacity available to the brain if anything should go wrong or brain injury occur.

In infancy and childhood therefore masses of connections are formed. (See Figure 3.2) Yet it seems that only those connections survive that relate to a child's experience of the environment, or that have the potential to relate to that environment. From what we now know about brain development it seems that unused connections have little chance of survival and indeed must be eliminated if effective future functioning is to take place.

From all of this we can see that what is happening *cannot* be described as an inevitable progress from a simple 'primitive' to a complex 'higher' form. The toddler brain is, in a certain sense, more complex than that of an adult, in that it has more neurons and more connections. What in fact we see is a process of fine tuning to the requirements of the environment. The infant brain is *not* the unfolding of a genetic blueprint. Rather it is the result of a biological potential influenced by early experience (Johnson, 1997).

What is happening is selection (Edelman, 1992), selection of those cells and circuits that relate to the child's environment. These selected cells are elaborated and preserved. At the same time the elimination takes place of many of those circuits and cells that are never used by the environment. These processes of selection, elaboration, preservation, and elimination, are the bases of brain development. The most exciting finding from developmental brain research in recent years has been that the electrical activity induced in the young brain by the action of the environment on the brain, *actually changes the physical structure of the brain* (Shore, 1997). The selection of new connections, and the concurrent pruning of unused elements, continues for the first decade of life (and even at a reduced pace in adolescence) and is guided by the experience to which a child is subjected.

In the early months of life, the development of brain operations is thus almost entirely dependent, initially at least, on *stimulation* from outside, from the environment. Stimulation from the environment via the sense organs activates certain circuits, or combinations of neurons, or neural maps, (or whatever we call them), in the brain. The neural connections involved in these systems will be confirmed and established as working elements in the brain. *This cannot take place without stimulation from the environment.* Connections and circuits in the brain that are not stimulated in infancy may fall into disuse, and in some instances, the neurons involved will die. Development, even at very young ages, involves not only the establishment of working neural patterns in the brain, but also the decay of others, and even the death of neurons. *Thus we can say that the environment selects the neural circuits required for development from a vast array of connections.* This process is not unidirectional. As the child develops the brain in turn can act on the environment, and by doing so develop and confirm certain neural combinations (Edelman, 1992). The selection of neural circuits, either by the effect of a stimulating environment on the brain, or by the effect of the brain on the environment, is only possible as each selected circuit becomes insulated by myelin, a lipid/protein produced by specialised glial cells. This process is called myelination.

Myelination is a very important aspect of brain development. Brain connections will not work consistently until they are insulated, that is, until they are covered by myelin cells forming a myelin sheath. Even when this process occurs in the young developing brain, selection may occur, and many already myelinated connections will be rejected and pruned. In general, during development, the lower mid-brain structures are myelinated before upper cortical brain structures. This is of crucial importance in the development of emotions, as we shall see.

Thus when it comes to emotional development, early emotional experiences will affect physical brain development. Likewise brain development will affect the type of emotional experience that it is possible for a child to feel. For example, those emotional experiences based on cognitive appraisal, if they are to be accurately felt, require a brain development, including myelination, that allows for such appraisal (Schore, 1994).

The overall process of selection of certain neural structures, and the competitive elimination of others, which occurs in infancy, has been called "parcellation" (Rakic *et al.*, 1986). This process is essential in infancy because development in this period often requires the creation of structures and functions necessary only for a distinct, time limited, period of growth. These structures and functions may be eliminated when not required for the next stage (Oppenheim, 1980). Parcellation allows structures and circuits used earlier to be eliminated, suppressed, or reorganised.

The selection of new connections and the concurrent pruning of unused elements continue for the first decade of life, guided by the experiences that a child is subjected to. At about ten years or so, a draconian pruning of connections takes place, and from this time on, though some adaptability and flexibility continues in the brain, the general sculpting process is complete. The environment will no longer have the distinct effect on brain development that it had in the first ten years. After ten years things are more set than they were. Nevertheless, during adolescence the final changes to the frontal lobe of the cortex are taking place and this involves some selection and elimination as before (Giedd *et al.*, 1999; Spear, 2000; Lerner, 2002). In adult life the brain retains flexibility and if injured it still carries sufficient spare capacity, in the form of unused circuits and neurons, to be adaptable. New skills can develop at any age, and functions can be transferred following injury, but the ease and alacrity of the process is much reduced in adulthood when compared with earlier periods.

What emerges from the study of a child's growing brain is that brain activity affects brain structure, and brain activity is closely linked with what happens in a child's environment. Thus environment can cause physical changes in brain structure and brain physiology. But must it be the environment that is the essential factor? Could genetics alone not account for all this establishment of inter-neuron connections and also their pruning? Is it not possible that what happens is dictated, not by the child's environment, but by an inbuilt program?

Genetics cannot account for the establishment of all the connections and eliminations that take place in a child's brain. The reason for this is that there are far too few genes in the human genome, 30,000, and far too many connections in a child's brain. Many of the 30,000 genes are shared with creatures with little or no brain. However, even if each gene accounted for one connection (to say nothing of prunings) the child's brain would indeed be very small. It would be under-developed. The child's brain is far too complex to be accounted for by genes alone. There must be other factors involved. It seems that genetics can determine the general structure and perhaps the potential of the brain. However, what is selected for use by the environment, and what is further integrated and diversified, is a function of the experiences that a child has. There is even evidence that the environment has an impact upon genetic makeup and genetic expression; this new science is called epigenetics (Roth & Sweatt, 2011). There is no escaping the fact that experience in childhood affects the actual physical structure of the brain.

Implications for child development?

The recent work on the developing infant brain emphasises some themes that are central to an accurate study of child and adolescent development. These themes are also of significance as far as emotional development is concerned and we will now elaborate them.

The essential nature of children

When a child is awake his or her brain is constantly interacting with the environment. What does this tell us about the essential nature of children? Children interact with their environment if allowed to do so, unless they are ill or asleep. Children are therefore *active*. In a sense we do not need to explain why children are active because they always are. It is in their nature. This could be seen as a circular explanation, but observations of children show it to be true, just as observations show the earth to be round. A child psychologist may be asked to explain why an atypical child is rather passive or inactive, a condition that should elicit great concern, but the normal activity of normal children begs no explanation. We cannot explain such activity, except that it is intrinsic to life itself, and is a product of the interaction between an active brain and a stimulating environment. This stance is an *organismic* one. It supposes that children are active intrinsically motivated beings, who will interact naturally with the world and try to make sense of it.

An opposite viewpoint is that children are reactive when impinged upon, and passive otherwise. According to this position, the environment is the important agent making the child react. The child is like a machine, and this stance is said to be *mechanistic*. Needs and drives theories often infer a mechanistic child. Children react because they have needs, and when these are satisfied, so are they. If we satisfied all their needs they would be content and passive. This does not gel either with our experience of children, or with research observations. When a child (and especially an adolescent) has all immediate needs satisfied, he or she looks for others (higher needs). If these can't be found, the adolescent becomes bored! Boredom is natural activity that has nowhere to go. If mechanistic theories of children were correct the satisfied child would be passive, rather than bored and very restless.

This is an important point, because later we will develop the idea that children are motivated and directed in their activity very largely by their needs, particularly their emotional needs. However, one need leads to another, and thus true satisfaction cannot be obtained. A resort to needs as an explanation for children's behaviour does not have to deny the essentially active nature of the child.

The importance of environmental stimulation

The natural growing state of the brain is a constant dynamic interchange with the environment. Stimulation from the environment is crucial and formative in a physical sense. Without such stimulation neural circuit selection could not take place. Such stimulation can be pleasant or noxious. Generally children will seek out pleasant stimuli and avoid noxious ones.

Children may have inherited genetic potential by way of brainpower, but it is the environment that makes use of this potential. Brain development and growth are determined by an *interaction* with a stimulating environment. Infants must be allowed to interact with their environment in some way if their brains are to develop. The mode of interaction may not always be by 'moving and shaking'. Infants can also listen, or even just observe a stimulating scene with which they interact by means of their sense organs. Toddlers can speak. What is true of infants and toddlers is also true for children and adolescents though the rate of brain development and change slows down considerably after infancy.

The importance of variation: normative and individual development

The third thing we learn from studying the ontogeny of the brain is that *each brain is unique.* Each person is unique; variation rules in development as it does in evolution.

Not only do we all inherit different numbers of neurons and connections between them, but also much more importantly, we all experience somewhat different environments. It is the effect that the environment has in selecting neural combinations that ultimately multiplies human variability. No two human brains are alike, essentially because their histories are different, in terms of the establishment of certain neural combinations, and the death of others.

Identical twins have different brains, yet they have the same genetic inheritance. Even when such twins are raised in the same household, selective factors, that operate from the environment and impinge on the neural structures of the child, will be somewhat different for each twin. Thus the patterns of neural connections that are established and consolidated in each twin's brain will be different, at least in part, because of the somewhat different interactions of each child with the environment. They will have similar, but not identical, histories and this will be reflected in different neural circuitry, certain circuits being established in one twin but not the other. Post-mortem examination of the brains of identical twins shows this to be the case (Edelman, 1992). If it is possible to show that identical twins can vary, then one can conceive of the importance of variation in people who do not share an identical genetic inheritance or similar environments.

It has been shown that certain behavioural functions in people can be related to fairly specific areas of the brain. This is known as localisation of function. However, the most recent brain research shows that the location of these areas in the brain cannot be established in an absolute sense because it varies somewhat from person to person. Localisation of function is a fact but exactly where each function is localised in the brain varies considerably in each person. Our cerebral layout may be as distinctive as our fingerprints!

It is the brain that lies at the heart of the developmental process. In the end, all developments in human beings are ruled by the interaction of brain with environment. Every brain is different, so development must be immensely varied, and be very different for different people. This variation in developmental pattern is an important reality, and is not always emphasised in developmental psychology. When we consider children their development and their psychology, and their growth into adolescence, we are considering a very complex field. The human brain, as we have said, is one of the most complex entities in existence, even when we consider it at a specific point in time. How much more complex then is its development over many years? This complexity is further multiplied when we realise that developmental psychology is a consideration of many, many brains, each with its own genetic endowment, and its own environmental history. We are obviously looking at a topic that is very elaborate and complicated.

One of the key issues in developmental psychology is how to account for variation. No two children are identical. Variation is not an exceptional thing between people, it is the rule; it is a fundamental fact of life. Without variation life could not have evolved. Developmental psychology is about variation as much as it is about commonalities. When we consider the commonalities and features in development that many of us share, we must also allow for variations on the general theme. We must not be lulled into thinking that everyone obeys the rule, or conforms to the stage and its standards. In fact most people vary from the rule, or the stage of development that is being discussed. Most people only obey a rule or a stage in development if it is expressed as a range, rather than a mean, or a definite point. And of course a range allows for considerable variation. Even with this, there still will be a considerable number of people who lie outside the conventional range of a development, and who must also be considered.

When we study children and adolescents we need to comprehend the changes we see in our subjects. Children and adolescents change and often change quickly over time. We call this development, and of course it continues through life. It is, however, most dramatic in childhood and adolescence.

An infant of three weeks is quite different to an infant of three months, who in turn is different to a child of three years. These changes from one age level to the next are qualitative changes, and development unfolds in a series of qualitative changes until the young child is transformed into the adult. "Development during childhood and adolescence refers to certain age related changes that are orderly (sequential), cumulative, and directional (towards complexity)" (Waters & Sroufe, 1983, p. 79). How do we comprehend and describe the many qualitative changes in childhood and adolescence?

We can do so by referring the changes to ages and stages. We decide what stage the child is at, and whether this stage matches his or her age. Stages are set down by considering the orderly sequence of qualitative changes seen in development. We measure the average age at which children reach and accomplish each change. Children develop at different rates so a change is accomplished over a range of time. This range will have a point within it that can be considered as the average age for the accomplishment of this task. One change leads to another. A constellation of changes can be described as a stage and stages can be demarcated by age. So, knowing a child's age, one is able to predict what stage he/she is at, and what tasks he or she can accomplish, if the child is within the normal range of development.

This approach is *normative*. The general changes undergone by most children are measured in relation to age, and norms are set up for the achievement of these tasks. Using norms we can determine the developmental position of a child with respect to his or her peers. Norms are usually given as ranges of time within which a developmental change can be achieved by *normal* children; hence the word. Children who lie outside the range could be considered as *abnormal* in respect of the change under consideration.

However, development need not be viewed from a normative perspective. Let me give an example. Children with an intellectual disability, by definition, lie below the norms for intelligence at each age level. Thus the IQ (developed from norms and therefore a relative measurement), for a person with a disability can go down from say 70 at 3 years of age to 50 at 10 years old. This normative approach paints a gloomy picture. It seems the child with a disability is getting worse. Even professionals can interpret the norms in this way! In fact all that is happening is that by growing older the child falls increasingly behind his or her age peers as far as intellect is concerned. We are not getting any real details about development other than this.

From an *individual development perspective*, the child with a disability may be making good progress, and growing mentally from year to year. If we measure what this child can do, (rather than measure him or her against age peers), we find that the child can do a great deal more at ten years than at three. Development has taken place, progress has been made, effort has been expended, and achievements have been gained. It is only by comparison with others that this development is seen in a negative light. As far as individual development is concerned, the child is making good progress. See Figure 3.2 for an illustration of this. Similar issues may arise when a child does not follow the normative pathway in emotional development. In such a situation a child may still make substantial progress in emotional development.

As we investigate emotional development, we will not only study ages and stages, but we will consider individual development and progress, where a child is measured only against him or herself. Many of the children seen in welfare, or other social science practice, are the very children who lie outside the norms that have been established. Their development and behaviour is often best understood by an *individual* rather than a *normative* approach.

Development in context

The brain does not grow in isolation. Development never takes place except in an environment. Development is therefore always in a context. Our world throws up many different contexts; during development the context of the child changes. To begin with there is the context of the caregiver, usually mother; then there is the family context, the social and community contexts, and the cultural context. One context can affect another. The cultural context is particularly powerful. It has a very strong influence on the family, and on social and community contexts, and even on the caregiver context.

Culture has many aspects that influence development, but perhaps the most important is language. Language is always linked to society and develops only in

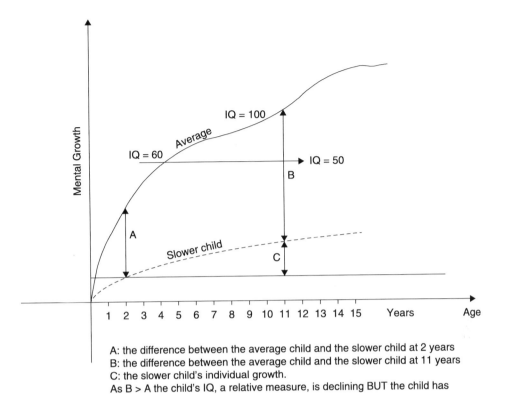

A: the difference between the average child and the slower child at 2 years
B: the difference between the average child and the slower child at 11 years
C: the slower child's individual growth.
As B > A the child's IQ, a relative measure, is declining BUT the child has mental growth, see C.

FIGURE 3.3   Normative versus individual growth.

association with social life. It is of considerable importance because it can greatly influence many other areas of development. Language (and thus culture) may well influence the development of thought (cognition). One can easily see how a context such as culture is a pervasive and powerful influence in many aspects of development.

All development occurs in context, in fact in many contexts. We cannot, and should not, compare developments if their contexts are different. Yet in practice we frequently do! For example, children from different cultures, or different social groups, are compared in a normative way. As far as development is concerned this is neither scientific nor is it fair or reasonable.

One could consider the family context, and wonder if it is reasonable to compare the development of children from different families. As you realise, this type of comparison is very common. Comparisons are odious, especially if they are based on a fundamental misunderstanding of the nature of development. We should compare less but understand more. What is important to understand is the influence of context on development. It is by the detailed understanding of development in different contexts that we will make progress in resolving children's difficulties, and tolerating diversity, rather than trying to change it.

Nature versus nurture

This phrase was introduced by Francis Galton in the Victorian era, and at the time seemed to usher in a debate of some importance (Kimble *et al.*, 1991). Even today it is used as a heading in almost every developmental psychology textbook. Are we a product of our genetic inheritance or our environment? Which means most in our development? The debate is old and sterile. As Donald Hebb (1980) pointed out, our behaviour is determined 100 per cent by genetics and 100 per cent by environment! We can see from a study of infant neurology that genetic endowment and environment influences are linked, indeed intertwined, in a complex pattern. Both are important. Nature always acts through nurture. Genetics sets potential but only an optimal environment can fulfil this promise. We will debate this no further at this point. Both influences are intrinsic to human development. We will now proceed to investigate how these play out in emotional development in infancy.

Questions to think about

1. Write a paragraph of 100 words in favour of the statement 'nothing is certain and everything is environmentally dependent'.
2. Explain to yourself why the human brain is the basis of human development.
3. Can you answer the following?

   (a) In what ways is the brain pre-determined at birth?
   (b) Is this an important issue for child development?
   (c) Why?

4. Debate with yourself the importance of the statement 'each brain is unique' in terms of understanding child development.
5. Explain how a normative developmental approach can distort the interpretation of an individual's development.
6. Why are children active?
7. What is meant by

   (a) an organismic stance?
   (b) a mechanistic stance?

Suggested further reading

Eliot, L. (2001). *Early Intelligence: How the Brain and Mind Develop in the First Five Years of Life*. Harmonsworth: Penguin Books.
Or, her latest . . .
Eliot, L. (2010). *What's Going on in There?: How the Brain and Mind Develop in the First Five Years of Life*. Random House Digital, Inc.
Perlman, S. B. & Pelphrey, K. A. (2011). Developing connections for affective regulation: age-related changes in emotional brain connectivity. *Journal of Experimental Child Psychology*, 108(3), 607–620.
Panksepp, J. & Smith-Pasqualini, M. (2005). The search for the fundamental brain/mind sources of affective experience. *Emotional Development: Recent Research Advances*, 5–27.

Chapter 4

Emotional development in infancy

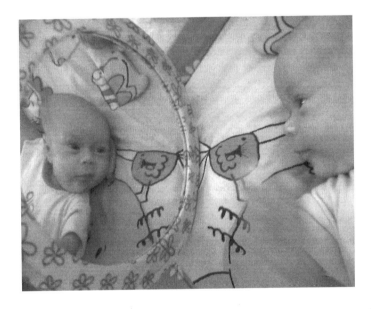

- Infancy is defined by dependency. The dependency evokes relationships with carers and it is through these relationships that development, including emotional development, occurs.
- Children are born with basic primary emotions but development of the social, secondary emotions is founded in infancy from non-emotional antecedents called proto-emotions.
- Carers' effectiveness in meeting infants' dependency needs through attachment influences the development of the first secondary emotions.

> - The proto-emotions of satisfaction and frustration and the infants' perception of change are precursors to the development of secondary emotions.
> - In this first year, through increasing awareness and cognition, infants develop, to varying degrees, their first secondary emotions: anger from frustration; anxious fear; and love of their caregivers.

THE NECESSARY ELEMENT THAT defines childhood and particularly infancy is dependency. When we think of an infant we immediately think of a helpless babe. It is the dependent state that is the core of childhood, and it is the gradual progress from this state to independence that constitutes the developmental pathway for most individuals.

Immediately after our birth we are totally unable to look after ourselves. If we cannot gain help from our caregiver we will die. In this we are unlike some other animals who are able to assume an independent existence (be it hazardous) as soon as they are born or shortly afterwards. We are dependent, totally dependent for a long period. In most cases we are dependent for our survival on our caregiver, usually mother. In this respect we are not unique as a species.

Some other animals are born helpless and some are born blind as well. Consider the contrast between the newborn rats and newborn guinea pigs. The little rats remain blind and helpless for some considerable time and if their mother does not attend to their needs they will die. The new born guinea pig is a fully functioning replica of the adult animal and in a short time after birth is able to graze on grass and run away from predators. What does such a distinct difference between these neonates suggest? Is this difference reflected in the adult animal?

Rats are one of the most adaptable animals. They have followed humans across the globe and have adapted in a very short time to every environment that humankind has created. They can even live in refrigerated cold stores. Their numbers are increasing in spite of many campaigns for their elimination. Their adaptability often puts them one step ahead of those who would destroy them. In animal terms the rat is intelligent and learns quickly. The guinea pig by contrast is largely a domestic animal (originally domesticated in Peru by the Incas as a source of meat). It lacks adaptability and will not survive in most instances if released into the wild. It could readily be considered a stupid animal, guided for the most part by a few genetically programmed routines of behaviour. Are these differences between rats and guinea pigs in the adult animal related to the distinct differences between their neonates? The answer is that they probably are. It is hypothesised that the rat's relatively long period of dependency in infancy, and its early need for maternal care is positively correlated with its ability to learn and adapt to new circumstances. A major element in this period of early dependency and learning is the mother rat.

This relationship between early dependency and learning has often been commented on. Many biologists believe that those animals which must possess flexible learning patterns in order to survive need a period of extreme dependency in infancy. It seems such dependency is needed for important survival learning to take place. In human beings the dependency period is proportionally the longest of all species, and presumably the opportunity for learning is therefore the greatest. One can also extrapolate and suggest that the role of the caregiver, usually the mother, is of central importance. How our mother treats our dependent state will greatly influence our initial feelings about our existence.

From the child's viewpoint the caregiver–child relationship is crucial and very intense. Through it the child survives. Through the mother child interaction the child learns if he or she is valued or not. In the relationship he or she begins to trust or mistrust the world and those in it. So mother (or principal caregiver) appears essential to appropriate growth and development. Is she the key factor, the central element leading to developmental success? It often appears that she is. *However, there is nothing essential or magical about mothering except that it satisfies the child's dependency needs.*

Dependency needs

What do infants need from their caregivers? Human needs have often been counted and classified. Abraham Maslow in 1954 arranged human needs into a pyramidal hierarchy see Figure 4.1. He suggested that some needs were more important than others. Maslow said those needs at the bottom of his pyramid were the most important and he felt that the fulfilment of these basic needs was essential for survival. As illustrated in Figure 4.1, at the very bottom forming the base of his pyramid were *physiological needs*. For example, the infant needed food and drink, usually combined in milk. Above these physiological needs were *safety and security needs*. For example, the child needed a safe place to sleep. Next highest up the pyramid was *the need to have love and to belong*. Above the need to belong Maslow placed *esteem needs*, the need to achieve and gain recognition. Beyond this moving towards the apex were *cognitive needs* (knowledge and understanding), *aesthetic needs*, and the highest need, *the need for self actualisation*.

Maslow's pyramid of needs is useful in that it lists the dependency needs of infants and children. It is much less useful as a way of ranking the importance of each need. For example, children probably have as great and as essential a need for love and comfort as they do for food or security. In places like Bosnia, or other war torn regions, children often had great difficulty gaining enough food, and often lacked a safe place to live, yet they still formed ties of love, still knew where they belonged, and even in famine and insecure conditions, went on to develop self-esteem (Neher, 1991).

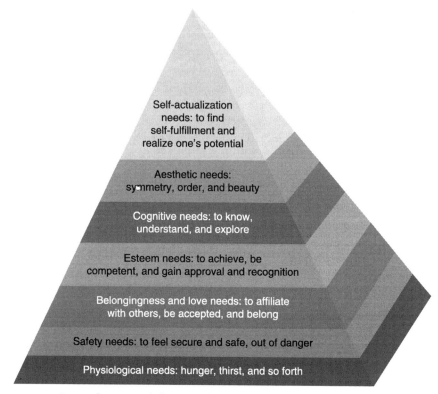

FIGURE 4.1   Dependency needs from Maslow.

It is inadvisable to rank physiological needs as more important than security needs, and security needs as more important than the need for emotional warmth and belonging. There is no need for a hierarchy of needs. To the infant, and later to the child, they are all of crucial importance though the satisfaction of different needs is related to different aspects of survival and development. For appropriate emotional development the child needs to be cuddled and comforted with emotional warmth and physical cosiness. Indeed, if human infants are like Harlow's young rhesus monkeys (Harlow & Harlow, 1962), then the need for warmth and belonging may outrank the need for food. However, ranking a child's needs in importance is rather futile and it is best to think of all the dependency needs of an infant as extremely important without giving them a rank.

For an infant to survive and develop optimally the caregiver (or caregivers) must initially supply all physiological, safety, and security needs, and equally importantly satisfy the child's need for touch, warmth, and human contact. Only when these things are given to the child does he or she have an environment that allows him or her to develop full potential.

Thus if a mother leaves her baby hungry and wet, allows the child to fall, and does not cuddle the infant, the child's view of subsequent interchanges with the environment will be quite different to that of a child who is satisfied, dry, secure, and cuddled. The neglected child may not trust those who surround him in future years because early dependency needs have not been properly met. He or she may not respond to the emotional demands of socialisation because personal relations hold little reward. Thus when basic dependency needs have not been met, or have not been met in an appropriate way, the child cannot proceed, or finds it very difficult to proceed, to the higher levels of social interaction and therefore emotional development.

In most circumstances the degree to which the infant-caregiver relationship satisfies the dependency needs of the child is the key factor in setting the tone for future developments. This factor provides the base on which the process of socialisation is carried out and this process is in turn central for the development of the secondary emotions. If a mother cares for her child, she will allow him or her to develop trust. In time this trust will not simply relate to the child's comfort but become a sentiment attached to mother. The child's survival and development including emotional development depends in part therefore on mother and the quality of her care. Mother in this context means the child's principal caregiver. It usually is the child's biological mother but need not be so. Mothers or carers must be attracted to infants in order to adequately service their needs. Many factors contribute to such attraction but there is no doubt that early infant expressions of emotion reinforce this attraction and it is these expressions that we will now consider.

Dependency, care and the earliest emotional expressions

Infant development covers the first year of life and is the basis on which a child's future emotional, social and intellectual progress is founded. As we have explained the neonate is completely dependent and must be fed and cared for if he or she is to survive. Has this newborn baby any emotion? Most certainly the newborn has emotional expressions. In the first few weeks of life infants exhibit emotional expressions that correspond to all six or seven basic emotions mentioned in the last chapter. These expressions have been selected throughout human history because it is through emotional expression that the young infant attracts the adults who attend to his or her dependency needs. If babies do not attract adult care they die. Young babies may also instinctively sense the reactions of others to their needs. This may be part of a subconscious general sensor that tells young infants if their situation is good or not good. If it is not good a baby may start to cry. Babies are, in fact, instinctive communicators of their needs even in the first days and weeks of life. They are successful in that they usually get the adult attention they require.

It would seem therefore that if you define emotion by expression young infants are highly emotional. However, signs of emotional expression are not a sufficient basis on which to infer subjective emotional experience in very young infants and this component of emotion is central to our definition of emotion. The emotional expressions that a baby can generate in the very early weeks of life are seen by many theorists including structural developmentalists as instinctive in-built features (Sroufe, 1995). Thus surprise, indicated by a startle, is a reflex action, to which the very young infant cannot attach meaning, because awareness is lacking (Ekman *et al.*, 1985). Disgust, indicated by a curl of the lip, or a wrinkled nose when something with an unpleasant odour is presented, is likewise a reflex response in the early weeks of life, and not an emotion, according to Sroufe (1995). A smile, in the very early weeks of life, can also be like a reflex action, and can occur without awareness, for example, in sleep in response to a stimulus (Emde *et al.*, 1976; Eliot, 2001). Of course smiling can occur when the very young infant is awake. In this case it may be less of a reflex but remains essentially an in-built instinctive reaction. An infant of five weeks, or even younger, will smile quite readily, when certain stimuli are presented. Children of this age will smile particularly at a human face (Johnson *et al.*, 1991). It need not be a face that they know, any active human face will do. This action, like many others, is intended to ensure the survival of the infant. Smiling is very attractive to adults, who coo, gurgle, and smile back (Keller & Scholmerich, 1987). In smiling the infant has a device to make him or herself attractive to adults, thus increasing the chances that he or she will be given attention and care (Johnson *et al.*, 1991). The smile at this age is more a survival function than a truly social communication, and many authorities see it as resembling a reflex action (Shaffer, 1999). Fear, expressed as a cry, or a fearful face, can also be a like a reflex reaction in the early weeks in response to pain, or an intense noxious stimulus. As the infant grows beyond the early weeks, increasing neurological development in the cortex modifies and transforms the operation of these in-built emotional expressions. What then is happening in the first few months of life? What are the processes that lead to awareness, and thus to subjective emotion?

The growth and importance of awareness

Internal and external stimulation impinging on the very young infant are the precursors of awareness. In the early weeks of life infant arousal can be seen by the increasing strength and/or frequency of response by the baby to various stimuli. This arousal can be due to internal physiological processes such as those which give rise to hunger. (This hunger may not be truly consciously felt by the infant in the way that hunger is felt later in childhood.) Arousal can also be achieved in the neonate by external stimulation. The infant is, at this stage, refining his or her perceptual systems, and is beginning to perceive more accurately. If a child at this stage is subject to prolonged stimulation, he or she will become distressed. This distress, or arousal, is general, and usually involves the whole body of the neonate. However, as this distress is not subjectively experienced by the child, it cannot be defined by us as an emotion. Rather it is a physiological reaction to a stimulus.

From birth to say eight weeks infants sleep a lot and cry a lot. They have facial expressions that indicate emotions, but we do not know what they feel in association with these expressions. As the first weeks progress, arousal (including distress) slowly becomes less general and takes on more focus. When this happens we get the first glimmers of conscious awareness. It is this early awareness that leads to social life and thus to emotional life. After 8 to 12 weeks the infant increasingly sleeps less and seems more aware in his or her waking periods. The child appears at this stage to have more time to look around, to consider things, and to be less ruled by instinctive reactions though these still predominate. The emotional expressions the baby produces at this age seem more focused than before, slightly more responsive to social situations, and not quite as instinctive. Indeed this change has been noticeable in some infants as far back as six weeks and in most from eight weeks onwards. At 12 weeks this change is clearly recognisable. The change in infants over this period can be explained by a growth in awareness. We can trace arousal back to earlier weeks, perhaps even to before birth; before 12 weeks we have processes that give general arousal, and, as arousal is focused, the child becomes aware. At 12 weeks though arousal is more focused the child's upper limbic system is only just getting started and is little involved in emotional reactions. Thus, though baby has an emotional life, full of expression and recognition, it is still not felt in a distinctly subjective way. Yet the emotional life of infants in their early months is of great importance to future development and emotional stability. If an infant is mistreated his or her feelings will not be recorded in conscious cortical memory, but they will be recorded nevertheless at a subconscious level where memory and learning operate very effectively. Where mistreatment is predominant subsequent subjective emotional growth may well be influenced in a negative direction. Likewise consistent warm nurturance in response to an infant's needs lays a good base for future positive emotional developments.

We have emphasised the importance of a subjective experience in defining an emotion. A subjective experience requires a person to be conscious of their feelings. For the first few weeks of life an infant does not possess this type of awareness. However, the brain grows very quickly in the first few months and precursors of subjective awareness also develop quickly. The neurological evidence suggests that true subjective awareness is noticeable in most infants at six months (and in some babies earlier) and becomes increasing important from this time onwards (Eliot, 2001).

What this means is that in the earlier months of life there can be no true emotional experiences as adults experience them, because there is no conscious subjective awareness. Subjective emotion can only occur when awareness is developed to the degree that allows for a conscious experience. This type of awareness becomes possible when the upper limbic system becomes increasingly myelinated from six months onward (Eliot, 2001; Deoni *et al.*, 2011). What then does an infant feel before this neurological change happens? Certainly young infants react emotionally, we can see this clearly from their emotional expressions but they do so generally without reference to the social context that they are in. Before six months infants are very spontaneous in their emotional reactions, for example, they seem to react instinctively with natural involuntary smiles when stimuli, particularly faces, are pleasant. After six months things change, increasingly children give emotional reactions specific to social situations and in accordance with their place in such situations. Growing awareness is the process that mediates emotional expression from now on, and, as the frontal cortex of the brain matures increasingly after six months, it further develops emotional life as a subjective remembered experience (Eliot, 2001).

Emotions in the first year of life

We should now consider what emotions can be present in infancy. On the one hand there are the basic emotions that are probably present at birth and are universal. These are instant fear, sudden anger, instant joy, sadness, disgust, interest, surprise. Infants can express all of these emotions on their faces early in life. After six months of age infants will also increasingly feel the subjective feeling that accompanies each of these emotions. Though these emotions will be modified to a degree by the environment that the child grows up in they are inherited genetic features not products of the environment and in general they do not develop or change greatly throughout life though their expression can change quite distinctly as the years progress.

On the other hand the growth of awareness in the early months of life allows the child to experience and interact with his or her environment. This interaction is usually with people and it allows emotions to develop from non-emotional precursors. These emotions are the secondary emotions the only true developmental emotions and it is to their development that we now turn.

However, we must not forget the basic emotions as we consider others that arise from environmental, especially social, experience. Developed secondary emotions (Plutchik, 1980), do not replace the basic emotions; rather additional emotions arising from social experience are added to a child's emotional repertoire.

Dual coding of mental events: positive and negative emotions

Writing in 2000 Scherer stated (p. 146) "Many early psychologists stated that the pleasantness-unpleasantness dimension was the most important determinant of emotional feeling". This dimension of experience fits with the behaviouristic classification of reactions as either approach or avoidance; a division that has a long history in psychology (Schneiria, 1959) and which has more recently been applied by Greenspan (1997) to sensations and emotions.

Initially awareness may be merely focused arousal, but slowly in the early weeks of infant life it becomes a factor in its own right. When this happens a child's interaction with the world changes dramatically. From this point on children become active players in their own development. Children are naturally active, and from this age a child can actively seek stimulating contact with the environment. What age are we talking about? Birth is an exciting moment for most parents, but much less commented on is the wonderful experience that many parents have when their child is between 8 and 12 weeks old. It is then that parents have the full realisation that they have been joined by a new conscious social being, by a new member of the family.

From the time of this early awareness, which is still not yet truly subjective, each sensation that is registered by a child will nevertheless be coded, not only as sensory information, but also as a pleasant or an unpleasant or a neutral mental experience. Thus most sensations from this time on will be registered with a dual emotional coding, that is as positive or negative (Greenspan, 1997). Sensations will have a dimension, be it loud, or bright, or heavy, or soft, or whatever, but they will also have an emotional feel. This is sometimes referred to as the valence of the experience. All experience is essentially mental experience, and as soon as focused awareness is gained, all mental events are coded according to their properties. They are coded as pleasant, neutral, or unpleasant. This is why, in one sense, we have emotion all of the time (Izard, 1977). This colouring of experience is the essence of emotion when some months later subjective feeling begins to develop. This is, in a way, so obvious to all of us that it is almost tautological to point it out. However, the fact that emotional tone, however slight, pervades all that we do, has not, up until now, been widely accepted as a basis for child developmental psychology.

The coding of mental experience as pleasurable, or neutral, or unpleasant, which occurs when awareness has reached a critical level, sets the scene for future emotional development. Secondary emotions are usually classified as positive, and related to pleasurable pleasant feelings, or as negative, and related to unpleasant, sometimes noxious, feelings. This division appears early in development but as development proceeds through childhood and complex secondary emotions emerge the division into pleasant and unpleasant becomes more difficult to apply and therefore less useful. Nevertheless, it is a useful starting point for the consideration of emotional development in the first year of life.

Early bases for emotional development

After three months of age, all experiences to which the infant is subjected are coded, both cognitively and as a quality of feeling, pleasant or otherwise. This is possible because of the development of awareness. Awareness is a form of focused arousal that has, by means of the dendritic elaboration of cortical networks, developed a neurological existence of its own. This early awareness, with its relationship to pleasant or unpleasant stimuli, leads quite quickly to the first truly developed emotions. It is from these early emotions that all the other developed or secondary emotions will eventually spring. Some authorities (Sroufe, 1995; Elster, 1999) call these first feelings of awareness proto-emotions. They are proto-emotions because when they begin they are not subjectively experienced.

The earliest proto-emotions are not imbued with a great deal of meaning. In the earliest stage of infant awareness, from say three to six months, proto-emotions remain responses either to external stimuli or internal physiological states, though by six months they can be subjectively felt. At the earlier stage the stimulus is the meaning but as cognition advances, slowly before six months and increasingly after this time, an infant's secondary emotions become infused with meaning. If we consider, therefore, the period between three and six months, we can see three bases, or proto-emotions, from which subsequent secondary emotions grow. These bases for future emotional development are:

(a)   satisfaction;
(b)   frustration; and
(c)   an infant's perception of change.

The first two bases for secondary emotional development, frustration and satisfaction, are both physiological and perceptual states, as far as the baby is concerned. However, physical and perceptual states usually involve caregivers and their ability to deal with the infant's dependencies. For baby this involves being touched and cuddled, or not being touched and cuddled, as well as attention or non-attention to more specified physical needs. Our selection of these three bases for emotional development has been influenced by the earliest account of the ontogeny of emotions, given by Bridges in 1932. It has also been guided by more recent work by Sroufe (1995). We will now consider each of these bases in more detail.

Satisfaction

The development of satisfaction, (and frustration), is linked to the ability of a normal infant, after three months, to discriminate between the pleasant and the unpleasant. Satisfaction is often the absence of discomfort, a neutral state where an infant's dependency needs are met at least for the moment. In this state stimuli can bring a delight which is expressed in the form of smiles and coos. The baby is showing his or her pleasure. He or she is pleased, we might even say happy. Certainly the infant is satisfied and prepared to show this with pleasant expressions. Satisfaction is a word that subsumes, to some degree, feelings of joy and happiness, indeed this proto-emotion can exist in both intense and attenuated forms that go by different names. According to Stern (1990), joy first appears around six weeks, and is in essence a response to people. Satisfaction, which Stern considers as centrally important, has appeared earlier.

In the early period, around three months, satisfaction is related to an internal feeling of bodily equilibrium and contentment and is often expressed in response to a stimulus of a particular quality or intensity. Emotional expression at this stage is closely related to perceptions and indeed, in certain instances, this relationship does not disappear as we grow older. The physiological and perceptual origins of emotions cannot be denied. However, over time, as cognitive capacity increases, satisfaction becomes a secondary emotion related to a child's meaningful interpretation of the situation he or she is in. This is certainly the case increasingly after the age of six months.

Meaning comes to feature more prominently in the development and interpretation of emotions as an infant grows older and develops a memory for experiences. These experiences arise increasingly because the child has interacted with the environment. The most important parts of the environment for the child are those aspects which nurture and sustain him or her. Central to this sustenance is the social environment, and at the centre of this, the child's caregiver, usually mother.

The active and increasingly reciprocal inter-change between caregiver and infant changes the nature of satisfaction. As satisfaction develops we tend to use new words for the usually positive secondary emotions that evolve, though most of us can still, at any age, experience primitive satisfaction.

Frustration

The inability of an infant to change his or her environment and especially the inability to influence carers to provide relief is experienced emotionally after six months and this is the essence of frustration.

The development of the proto-emotion of frustration is, like that of satisfaction, linked to the ability of a normal infant after three months to discriminate with some awareness between the pleasant and the unpleasant. In the early weeks of life arousal due to internal physiological factors, or intense or prolonged external stimuli, can produce a distress reaction in the infant. However, because awareness has not yet developed, this reaction has no meaning attached to it, and cannot be considered as a subjective experience. When the child becomes aware, unpleasant stimuli related to internal physiological processes or external stimuli continue to evoke distress and when this is not relieved frustration arises. After three months of age distress, and thus frustration, can also be caused by the cessation of a pleasant stimulus. The infant reacts to restore the pleasant stimulus, but if this does not happen quickly, protest and crying will ensue. After six months feelings of continuing unrelieved displeasure can be experienced subjectively, and true frustration has arrived. The infant, now aware, increasingly tries to make sense of his or her distress, and focuses on certain stressful aspects of the environment that are linked to his or her feelings of discomfort. These may include not only external unpleasant stimuli but also carers who do not relieve the internal discomfort that the child is suffering. In addition at this age distress can develop from an infant's own action on the environment, or an infant's thwarted desire to act on the environment. So though frustration has its origins in the early months of life it changes. It is increasing awareness that brings it to full bloom.

Later still, in the second half of the first year, frustration with the environment is often focused on the key elements of the environment that having meaning for the child, usually because they cause pleasant or unpleasant feelings, and relate to the child's nurturance. In other words, frustration becomes related to meaningful objects and situations (Bronson, 1972; Tennes *et al.*, 1972). Among the most frustrating 'objects' may be the child's caregivers. At first frustration is a time limited proto-emotion. It occurs in the infant in response to certain environmental situations. However, as these frustrating situations become frequent and more prolonged a new emotion slowly evolves. It is a response to frustrations that cannot be resolved, an internal subjectively felt reaction, anger, slow anger from frustration.

An infant's perception of change

All of us exist in time. It is a fundamental dimension. Perceptions of time, and its passage, are closely linked to our emotional lives. Goleman (1995; 2006) comments that the ability to postpone satisfaction is a high predictor of success in life, and may be more important than traditional measured intelligence. This ability, to postpone satisfaction, is a higher order ability, which occurs late in the development of emotions. Infants have little or no ability to postpone satisfaction, as any parent knows, or should know. Does this mean that infants have no conception of the passage of time?

In the earliest weeks of life it appears that infants are purely present centred. Children of this age simply need care from day to day. They need consistent care, and it does not concern them as to who supplies this care. Memory is not yet properly developed, and the passage of time thus has no meaning. However, as soon as awareness develops, not only are pleasant and unpleasant situations registered in consciousness, but, by degrees, the passage of time becomes noticeable.

Infants become able to detect changes in their surroundings. Out of this they develop their experience of the passage of time (indeed all of us, at any age, notice time more when changes are obvious). At first infants give few signs that they are aware of time passing but by six months of age there are indications that children remember things, and that they are now aware of the passage of time. By six months of age most children can detect changes in their day-to-day environment. They have by this time sufficient memory capacity to notice that things are not as they were before. This realisation introduces into their awareness, into their consciousness, a new factor. It is a factor that can affect the child's contentment.

Like all perceptions that a child may have, those concerning changes in the environment are coded (Greenspan, 1997). Perceptions of change are related by thought in a child's mind to spatial and other elements in the environment, and they are also coded emotionally as unpleasant, neutral, or pleasant experiences. The perception of change therefore, and the passage of time, have an emotional tone that most children can feel subjectively after six months of age.

Children may be aware after six months that time passes, but if their needs are adequately met, and their environment remains stable, there will be little effect. However, in certain instances changes may have been coded with a negative aspect in a child's experience, and even children in the most stable of circumstances, at six months of age, may show a distinct wariness on certain occasions (Sroufe, 1995). This wariness is dependent on comparisons that are made in a child's mind from memories and may not be a very obvious feature for many secure children. Nevertheless, wariness is present in most children at this age, and from it can grow a much more widespread and intense emotion. For example, as any parent knows, a drastic change in environment, such as a change of house, is a very unsettling experience for an infant over six months. After the change of abode such an infant may become much more irritable and insecure, though many children settle relatively quickly. Generally for older infants new contexts are not easily comprehended, because infants lack cognitive experience, and for this reason new contexts are not welcomed emotionally by the child. They are too much to deal with. Such drastic change becomes aversive for the infant, and it is only a short step from a dislike, or an aversion, to an anxious fear.

A drastic change in environment has a very noticeable effect on most infants of over six months, but it is when a child's dependency needs are threatened by change, especially a change in caregivers, that a child becomes most acutely aware of the passage of time. Indeed so acute is this awareness that a new emotion is evolved, anxiety. This anxiety is based on a child's felt inability to predict what will happen, particularly in respect of his or her essential needs and supports. These infants come to fear change, and with this process anything that is unfamiliar may induce a negative emotional reaction. Unfamiliar objects, and especially people, indicate to a child that things have changed, and because change has produced wariness in recent experiences, this can easily generalise into a fearful anxiety of anything unfamiliar. The unfamiliar is a symbol to the infant of change and unpredictability.

The development of anxious fear in infants is very varied. Many, but not all infants, from situations where their essential needs have not been met consistently, may come to feel very insecure, and thus anxious and fearful of anything that is unfamiliar. Such children are very difficult and unsettled. Indeed their underlying physiological reflexes in response to distress may be reactivated, and they can be inconsolable for considerable periods. However, infants from what should be considered as situations of adequate nurturance can also develop anxious fears. This process is so pervasive that some children, who have not experienced much change at all, develop, as the second half of their first year proceeds, anxious fears of things that are unfamiliar. On the other hand, many children do not develop marked anxious fears in their first year, and even the widely reported fear of strangers (in the second half of the first year) is not shown by some children.

Our selection of an infant's perception of change, as the third base for emotional development, comes in part from a consideration of attachment theory, as postulated by Bowlby (1982). We will discuss attachment in infants in more detail later; however, whether we call it attachment or not, an infant's desire for security (in the second half of the first year) is a potent factor in the further differentiation of emotions. Infants need security if they are to have their dependency needs met, and as soon as they are able to foresee events, even to a very limited degree, this power of prediction will influence the growth and differentiation of their emotions.

The usual course of emotional development in the first year

Having considered the nature of the bases of emotional development we can now chart the development of emotions in the average infant in the first year of life. Children of three months can see and hear but not perfectly. They are still learning how to interpret sound and vision. Their awareness is already gaining in complexity, due to social and environmental associations, some of which are remembered unconsciously. However, this awareness is not well differentiated as far as specific stimuli are concerned and is more of a 'general sensor', a general feeling of well-being, or not well-being, of knowing if you are comfortable or uncomfortable.

Now look at Figure 4.2. This diagrammatic schema is a general guideline, not an absolute and invariant statement about emotional growth in the first year. Many children can defy any general outline. A few children reared in the most restrictive and disadvantageous of emotional circumstances develop quite normally in emotional terms. This is not usually true, but it can happen. What usually happens can be deduced from our schema, but the schema is not invariably accurate. Neither is it a product of a definite piece or pieces of research. It is a synthesis of a number of ideas. We feel it is useful to have such an overview of the infant, coping with his or her environment, because it allows one to infer what may have happened to a

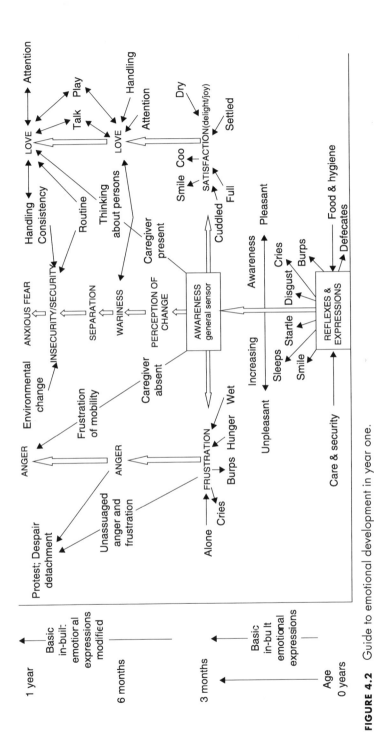

FIGURE 4.2 Guide to emotional development in year one.

particular child. This diagram is therefore an aid to understanding early infant emotional development, not a chart of the process. You can see the 'fixed response patterns' stage illustrated. This stage includes the reflexes present at birth and the instinctive genetically determined responses which include the expression of each basic emotion. The next thing to notice is an arrow showing increasing awareness, which is quite well developed at three months. At this point some of the reflexes come to develop inner meanings for the child. For example crying comes to mean frustration, is less of a reflex, and more under the child's control.

What develops out of awareness is *frustration* or *satisfaction* or for most children elements of both these proto-emotions. As the diagram indicates satisfaction is being dry, and fed, and cuddled, with no wind. It will be quite a frequent proto-emotion in any child whose dependency needs are adequately met. The generally satisfied child learns to enjoy his or her satisfactions, and the attention he or she is given. He or she comes to associate the pleasant feeling of satisfaction with the person who gives the pleasant feeling. Thus, as time passes, the generally satisfied child develops positive feelings of love towards his or her caregiver usually mother.

Difficulties arise when the child is often or always frustrated and never, or rarely, satisfied. Frustration is being wet, hungry, flatulent, and alone (not cuddled). Frustration on a continual basis can become anger, especially when it is augmented later by further restrictions on freedom of action. This is particularly so as the child grows older. A frustration, like being hungry, is added to by parental restrictions on freedom of action and freedom to move.

Paradoxically we all need a little frustration. Amsel (1962) refers to the "frustration effect". This is where an animal responds with momentarily increased vigour when extinction conditions (no reward) are first instituted. Thus it appears frustration, in limited amounts, can motivate us to action. After reward has been experienced on a number of occasions, non-reward, on a particular occasion, will elicit a primary aversive emotional reaction (frustration), which is related to the magnitude of the anticipated reward. For example, an infant crying before a feed is such an event. Components of this frustration can become conditioned to ante-dating stimuli (seeing Mum prepare for breast feeding, or mixing food, or whatever) and these can give anticipatory frustration (not being rewarded quickly enough). All infants experience such frustration. If they do not, the experience of reward will lose its power. This is why Spitz (1965) feels that it is probably as harmful to deprive a child of all short-term discomforts, as it is to deprive him or her of pleasure. Without discomfort and displeasure there can be no satisfaction when a need is met.

We are sure that this paradoxical situation, where some discomfort or frustration is needed to energise an infant and give them intense pleasure when satisfaction occurs, is an essential part of balanced development. However, we may well be concerned not with short-term or momentary frustration, but with long-term distress when children's needs are not met. In this situation long-term frustration, rather than stimulating children, uses up their resources of energy. We are inclined to caution in the view that children need discomfort and frustration. They do so only in very limited short-term amounts that lead ultimately, and fairly quickly, to satisfaction. For many children, where long-term frustration has no outcome in satisfaction, emotional growth will be adversely affected.

Our third base for emotional development is the child's *perception of change*. Starting about 6–7 months of age children become increasing aware of change, particularly in the people who care for them. By, say, 9–10 months, the average child becomes particularly aware of separation from mother (caregiver) and feelings of insecurity may arise. In the second half of the first year such feelings grow and can give rise to more specific emotions, especially anxious fear. This usually develops if the child cannot predict what is going to happen in the environment, and what will happen to him or her in terms of pleasant, or unpleasant consequences. It is the undetermined possibility of unpleasant consequences that induces this anxious fear. The child needs to be capable of understanding the passage of time, and of cognitively recognising the changes it brings. A child who cannot do this will not develop this early emotion. Thus towards the end of the first year and the beginning of the second excess environmental change produces insecurity, while a consistent environment gives feelings of security. In the first year of life the child becomes increasingly aware of emotion. By six months, when their upper limbic system begins to operate to a noticeable degree, children are able to have their first subjective emotional feelings and between seven and nine months children increasingly think about their feelings (Sroufe, 1995). Thus cognition increasingly evaluates and colours the subjective feelings that constitute emotion. The child puts meaning on his or her emotional expressions, including the basic in-built expressions, and recent experiences involving the basic emotions can now be remembered with feeling, and usually with meaning. Increasing thought and memory are applied to emotional experiences.

Looking still at Figure 4.2 you can appreciate that by one year a number of developed emotions exist in a child. He or she still possesses the basic in-built emotional expressions that were present from birth and which in instant situations are evoked. However, these quick emotions may now, at one year, be experienced subjectively. In addition most children of this age have had some frustration, some experience of change, and a deal of satisfaction. They may feel and show the developed secondary emotions of anger from frustration, love from satisfaction and anxious fear if change is threatening. These first secondary emotions can in turn develop into a very wide range of further secondary emotions.

Surveying Figure 4.2, it can be seen that the proto-emotions, satisfaction, frustration, and the perception of change, fan out into other sentiments, depending on a child's individual experience. Let us now consider some individual routes through this schema.

When things go right

Consider the child who develops from a base of satisfaction with not too much frustration. From the child's earliest days attention to the child's overall needs by the caregiver produces secure attachment in the child towards this person. This developing attachment is particularly evident from about seven months of age. It is important to remember that secure attachment is based on care and attention that includes warm physical and affectionate verbal contact, as well as actions that cater for the child's need to feel comfortable. It is the child's feeling of comfort and satisfaction that is associated by the child with the caregiver.

Gradually this care and attention produces a feeling in the child that we can call love. This love can be quite demanding on the child's part, because it is built on the caregiver's ability to satisfy the child's dependency needs. It is not a detached disinterested form of love, it is very much cupboard love, but it is love for all that. Even from the early weeks the child attracts the caregiver, and when the caregiver satisfies the child, the attraction begins to develop a mutual element. The child begins to know that he or she is loved because his or her dependency needs have been met promptly in full by warm affectionate care, and in secure and predictable circumstances. The child in return feels affection for this person who gives this loving care. This experience of mutual regard in the relationship leads the child on to a positive view of himself or herself.

The mutual aspect of this relationship between care and child in later infancy can be seen in the development of joint attention. This is where both parties to the social interaction attend to the same issue or occurrence. This usually revolves around the child's body or behavior. This is an important development in that it is the foundation from which a sense of self will grow in the next developmental period, toddlerhood (Akhtar & Martinez-Sussmann, 2007; Moore, 2007).

When things go wrong

In contrast, those infants who have been frustrated for most of the time, and subject to frequent, prolonged, and unpredictable separation, develop strong emotions of anger, and are fearful of change. These children are constantly frustrated. Anger from this frustration may become predominant in their emotional make up. Such children may not feel affection for others. At one year of age these restless angry infants are forced to develop every possible strategy to survive. A considerable number of these children do not survive, but most do. However, they do so at a cost, as we shall see.

Consider the child who is constantly subject to change in infancy, especially after seven months of age. In this case, if the changes are frequent or prolonged, feelings of insecurity will arise, leading to a child who is generally anxious and insecure. A significant number of children of this age develop separation anxiety, when they become aware of change, and realise that it can break even the weak affectionate bonds that they have formed. If a child has no ties of affection then, paradoxically, change is less of a threat, as he or she has nothing to lose. Children come to fear mother's (or caregiver's) absence because they depend on her and are therefore attached to her. This anxiety is easily assuaged if the degree of mother's absence is moderate and predictable. However, if mother (or caregiver) is absent unpredictably for frequent or prolonged periods this can give rise to adverse emotional development in the infant, *unless the child's dependency needs are met in some other way.*

Thus for many children a lot of change between 6 and 12 months and longer can be very damaging emotionally. Welfare departments provide extensive evidence of children reared in constantly changing conditions. Nevertheless, some children take more readily to change than others. Changes of home or family can be very disturbing; some type of constancy is needed. Children who can't predict what will happen to them, and who therefore lack a sense of security, become particularly anxious, and later, out of this base may grow the emotion of despair.

Change as a factor in emotional development is an important consideration if older infants need residence in hospital or anywhere away from home and family. Children who experience prolonged absence from their caregiver when they enter hospital can suffer distinct adverse emotional reactions. Modern hospital admissions for children tend to involve mother/caregivers as well in order to avoid these reactions. Children taken into 'care' in the second half of their first year may also suffer feelings of insecurity and anxiety.

Infants whose early upbringing has been adequate and secure can, if sudden change occurs, suffer more than those who have had to endure inconsistent nurturance. Such children can suffer instant misfortune with a withdrawal of the good care they are used to and their reactions to such an event can be viewed as a series of stages. To begin with children in such circumstances *protest*. They cry and become distressed. Then there follows a period of *despair*, when apathy and misery take over, and the child gives up the hope of returning to stable known conditions. This is followed by a *detachment* phase, where protests cease and the child apparently recovers composure. Such a child loses interest in parents (or caregivers), and is often said by welfare or nursing staff to have 'settled down'. In reality the child has suppressed the hurt, but is still inwardly very unhappy. A child who is not loved at all and who has had few satisfactions is less influenced by constant change and separation. Such children do not despair, because they have had nothing to lose, and therefore nothing to become desperate about.

Children from situations of deprivation may suffer cognitive deprivation as well as emotional insult. As we have said, cognition and emotion interact in complex ways. This interaction is important because, unlike the average infant, these deprived children with cognitive deficits will not think increasingly about their feelings as their first year progresses. The result is that they experience emotional intensity, but are unable to understand their feelings. When questioned, at later ages, they often find it difficult to distinguish between feelings.

The first year summarised

The position we have outlined in this chapter is one where certain secondary emotions are differentiated from more generalised states in the first year of life. This is in agreement with the research conducted by Sroufe (1995), and others.

Those who support the discrete emotions theory have argued that emotions are inherent features, and that during the earliest weeks of life an infant can show clear expressions of six to seven basic emotions (Izard & Malatesta, 1987). These are usually listed as joy, interest, sadness, anger, fear, surprise, and disgust, (Ackerman et al., 1998).

Earlier we explained at length that the expression of an emotion is not the same as an emotion, though expression is obviously a part of emotional behaviour. When we view early infant expression we must be careful not to project our own understanding of the expression onto the infant. Very young infants may show the expression, but we do not really know how they experience the emotion. We have outlined the neurological objections to inferring subjective emotional experience from early infant expression. Nevertheless, these early emotional expressions persist and we know that by six months they can be experienced in a subjective way. However, other things are happening. The child's environment is selecting neural networks that will develop other emotions, secondary emotions, and in the later part of the first year these are also subjectively felt.

By three months the proto-emotions of satisfaction and frustration are firmly established, and the development of more complex secondary emotions has begun. Wariness develops a little later from a child's perception of change. The first complex secondary emotion to emerge is formed by the association of satisfaction with care, and can go under the general title of love. It is the first emotion dependent on adequate social relations for its development and for this reason is called a secondary emotion. Anger is more complex and more focused than frustration. It also forms under the influence of the environment, particularly inadequacies in the social environment. This type of anger from frustration is slow in forming and thus different from the basic quick emotion of the same name. Anxious fear is also different from instant fear, a basic emotion, and relates to the stability and predictability of the child's environment, particularly as far as unpleasant experiences are concerned.

So by one year we can in many children identify satisfaction, frustration and its product anger, wariness, anxious fear of change and strangeness, and love of that which brings satisfaction and security. Love, anger from frustration, and anxious fear have all developed and are not built-in reactions giving instinctive emotional expressions. They are the first secondary emotions and they lead on to further secondary emotions in the second year of life some of which depend on a distinct sense of self and an appreciation of other people for their development.

Questions to think about

1. What are the proto-emotions of early infancy that influence the development of emotion?
2. Why is a little frustration helpful in emotional development?
3. What are the first formed secondary social emotions?
4. What happens to basic emotions during infancy?
5. Discuss major change in an infant's environment such as shifting house or town?
6. Describe the emotional/behavioural cycle which takes place when a young child is left away from carers on a permanent basis.

Suggested further reading

Bridges, K. B. (1932) Emotional Development in Early Infancy *Child Development*, 3 (4), 324–341

Walker-Andrews, A. (2008). Intermodal Emotional Processes in Infancy. In M. Lewis, J. M. Haviland-Jones & L. Feldman Barrett (Eds), *Handbook of Emotions* (3rd edn). New York: The Guilford Press, pp. 364–375.

Izard, C. E., Woodburn, E. M., Finlon, K. J., Krauthamer-Ewing, E. S., Grossman, S. R. & Seidenfeld, A. (2011). Emotion knowledge, emotion utilization, and emotion regulation. *Emotion Review*, 3(1), 44–52.

Chapter 5

Emotional development in toddlerhood

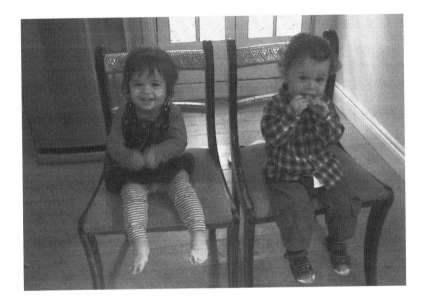

- In the second and third year much development takes place neurologically, emotionally and cognitively. All three of these aspects are interwoven.
- Social interaction is necessary for secondary emotions but a sense of self which develops in toddlerhood is also required for the self-conscious secondary emotions.
- The reciprocal relationship(s) is the arena for most of these developments to take place. There should be shared and rewarding experiences

> with a high level of mutual emotional warmth and a spirit of playful interaction between the child and the carer.
> - In toddlerhood love is the most important source of new self-conscious secondary emotions.
> - By the end of this period well cared for children have developed their full repertoire of secondary emotions. Children who have been emotionally deprived may not have developed positive secondary emotions to their full degree.

WHEN A CHILD REACHES one year of age the development of the early secondary social emotions, is well underway. The infant has experienced satisfaction and frustration. He or she may also have experienced wariness as he or she experiences change. The satisfactions that a child of this age can experience relate to a developing love of those who bring the satisfaction. The frustrations can give rise to anger, while experiences of insecurity give rise to anxious fear especially when confronted with strange situations and people.

The child of one year also has basic quick emotions. During this year the child had modified the innate emotional expressions that filled his or her early weeks because these expressions can now, with myelination of the appropriate sections of the cortex, be felt subjectively. However, lip curls of disgust and startles that indicate surprise can still emerge as quick emotional reactions as they can for adults. For the most part, however, in-built responses have been made conscious and the basic emotions that are shown by a one year old are truly felt subjectively.

We will now look at the second and third years of life and at the secondary emotions that develop in this period. This second year is when most children learn to both walk and talk, and, with the third year, we have called this period toddlerhood.

Of course development cannot easily be separated into phases demarcated by years, and many of the factors that greatly influence emotional development in the second year have their origins in the first. For some children developments that usually take place in the second year do not occur until the third. We will concentrate on what usually starts in the second year and extends into the third.

The second year of life is a period of great neurological and emotional change, and shows quite dramatically the link between development and environment. If children are deprived at this age they will be marginally more able to survive than if they were deprived in the first months of life. This is because they are a little less dependent and can do a little more for themselves in an instrumental sense. Nevertheless, in this second year they remain thoroughly dependent on adults for their well-being. If deprivation occurs at this stage it is likely to severely affect the development of the secondary emotions with all the implications that holds for future responsible and equitable adult life. However, deprivation tends not to start in the second year. Most deprivation circumstances are from birth, and there is evidence that early deprivation in institutions lasting longer than the first six months of life has a detrimental effect on all aspects of development (Rutter, 1981; Kreppner *et al.*, 2007). It is also apparent that such deprivation is reflected in neurological deficits and the architecture of the brain (National Scientific Council on the Developing Child, 2004; Pollak *et al.*, 2010)

The emergence of further emotions from the early secondary emotions is the central aspect of emotional development in the second year, though the roots of this process have been developed earlier. Secondary (Plutchik, 1980), self-conscious (Lewis, 1992), or social emotions, are emotions whose ontogeny is linked to a child's social relationships and the child's understanding of those relationships. There are differences in nomenclature for these later emotions but all researchers recognise the importance of social processes in the generation of these emotions and their development is referred to as socioemotional development (Brownell & Kopp 2007). We regard all the emotions arising from social processes as secondary emotions and those which require a sense of self as self-conscious secondary emotions.

Cognitive growth is intertwined with emotional development; therefore the development of these secondary emotions is linked to a toddler's growing cognitive capacity (Shonkoff & Levitt, 2010). The child is by this stage an active agent in his or her own development. Both cognitive growth and emotional development, if they are to proceed, require that the child actively gains a sense of separateness from his or her surroundings, including the humans who deliver essential care. The development of a sense of active agency is central to all future emotional and cognitive progress. The child has to be able to actively consider himself or herself with respect to other people and things. The development of this sense of agency is, by another name, the emergence of a sense of self and we must now consider it in detail. What are the foundations of a sense of self? How and when does an infant develop the ability to think for, and about, himself or herself?

The sense of self

Though a sense of self develops throughout life, and can be discussed in terms of identity or self-concept, its origins lie in infancy in processes like joint attention that involve both infant and carer (Moore, 2007). By 18 to 20 months most children can recognise themselves in a mirror (Lewis & Brooks-Gunn, 1979). Thus we can confidently say that at this age they have some idea of their separateness from others. This sense of separateness has probably been growing and developing in children for many months prior to their successful identification of themselves in a mirror.

What is certain is that a sense of self only grows in close conjunction with a sense of the separate existence of other people, especially the child's caregiver, usually mother. In other words, a sense of self is only developed along with a sense of the existence of other people as independent entities, and not just as caregivers. From our beginnings there is a self-other equivalence (Moore, 2007). A child's feelings about others are therefore of central importance. These feelings, if positive, lead to positive secondary emotions but they also, as Greenspan (1997) has pointed out, are the starting point of many cognitive developments. Many good educators over the years have guessed that positive and secure emotional development is a central plank on the road to cognitive growth and maturity. Now neuropsychology is gaining evidence for this guess to be confirmed. Schore's work in 1994, which outlines the development of cortical structures in the second year, supports the proposition that emotional developments hold the key to the development of an awareness of self, and that this, in turn, is central to the growth of cognitive ability.

It seems therefore that both emotional and cognitive developments, and their neurological correlates, evolve at least in large measure under the influence of other people. Of these influences the relationship with the caregiver is the most crucial as it is usually the first relationship and sets the pattern for others. Every experience that a child has with his or her caregiver will be coded emotionally by the child as positive or negative, (or sometimes neutral), and, if negative experiences predominate, the caregiver will be associated with feelings of frustration. These may develop into feelings of anger. It would appear that feelings of anger do not give as direct a route to self-awareness as do feelings of contentment and satisfaction. In many ways self-awareness is the key to the future, first emotionally, and then in a cognitive sense. Thus if adverse conditions lead to frustration and anger they hold up the interwoven factors of emotional and cognitive development. In fact is has been shown that children who experience early neglect have measureable differences in the connections in their pre-frontal cortex which is associated with reduced cognitive function (Hanson *et al.*, 2013) and emotional development.

Because it is central to the development of a child's feelings about himself or herself, the relationship with the caregiver must now be examined in detail. It is called the *reciprocal relationship* and is the final stage of attachment as outlined by Bowlby (1982), though it originates in much earlier stages of attachment, a fact that Bowlby recognised. An understanding of this relationship, and how it relates to the development in the child of a *sense of self and others*, is a crucial step in understanding the development of later secondary emotions, and the emotional and cognitive development of toddlers.

The reciprocal relationship

The developing sense of self and agency, that grows from the latter half of the first year into the second year of life, is very largely the mechanism that transforms the early associative secondary emotions of infancy into higher forms. This mechanism centres on a child's first enduring social relationship, and the way this relationship changes a child's reaction to his or her environment. The chief characteristic of this relationship is one of reciprocity. The relationship may begin in a one sided way but it becomes reciprocal, in that it works both ways, from adult to child, and from child to adult. It is possible that a child may develop several close reciprocal relationships simultaneously. Indeed this may be quite common. However, for the sake of clarity and simplicity we will concentrate on a single relationship.

The beginnings

The origin of a sense of others, and thus a sense of self, is in the positive interactions between infant and caregiver in the early months of life. We have pointed out already that a child comes to associate feeling satisfied with the warm presence of a caregiver. The word warm is very significant in this context. Harlow and Harlow's work (1962) with infant rhesus monkeys showed that infant primates need cuddlesome warmth as well as food, and, when pressed, will prefer the warmth to the food. This associative learning produces feelings of satisfaction in the child whenever the caregiver is present, even though at certain times, the caregiver may not actually be delivering care to the infant, either in terms of cuddles or food. This positive feeling on the child's part will grow into affection for the caregiver, and if the caregiver maintains a warm relationship with the child, a mutual love develops.

Although we are discussing toddlers in this chapter the reciprocal relationship starts in infancy but growths to full bloom in toddlerhood. There is evidence that caregivers and other adults have an in-built tendency to find infants "cute", and to play with them (Keller & Scholmerich, 1987; Johnson *et al.*, 1991). This playful interaction becomes much easier when, about three months of age, the infant is capable of staying alert for increasingly longer periods. It becomes further developed when the infant develops a social smile (6/7 weeks) (Eliot, 2001), and even further develops when the child is able to reach for, and touch or hold the adult. Skilled caregivers can develop this interaction by appearing responsive, or by stimulating the infant at the appropriate time. Though reactions are seen on the child's part much earlier, by three to four months this interaction is distinctly *mutual*, in that the baby now knows how to respond to mother. More importantly at this age we can observe the beginnings of the baby's ability to get mother to respond by stimulating her with a coo or a gurgle or a smile. Eye contact between the parties is very important (McDowell, 2002).

At four months the interaction is largely influenced by the caregiver. Nevertheless, it is out of this type of interaction that the infant has the first experience of self, and several months later the child will be able to interact with the adult in a more deliberate way, seeking responses from the adult, and even anticipating the adult's actions. Anyone who has played peek-a-boo with an infant will know the delight that anticipation gives. A sense of self develops further as an infant learns to take turns. By seven to eight months the reciprocal interaction may be equally weighted between the parties. As language develops the sense of self is greatly strengthened.

Fogel (1993) states that this reciprocal relationship allows the infant to develop a sense of give and take, a sense of social participation, and a concept of his or her own efficacy. Thus infants learn that they can affect the environment as well as it affecting them. Fogel sees the caregiver as the dominant partner in the first six months, but between six months and one year the infant becomes much more active in the interchanges. Greenspan (1997) says that feelings of self grow at this stage as the sense of purpose in reciprocity increases and the infant distinguishes more and more between the initiator and the receiver. By nine months the infant is initiating many interchanges, and when mobility is gained, about one year, the infant takes over the initiation of the majority of interchanges between the parties. As the infant enters the exploration phase, the caregiver goes into the background, but is, very importantly, still available.

Thus from the beginning there is a *reciprocal* relationship between the caregiver and the child. Though initially this is, in the early weeks, a relationship which is one sided and based on an adult's care for the infant, it increasingly becomes based, as the weeks progress, on playful interaction between the parties and on shared joyful experiences (Grusec, 2011). The relationship is most easily strengthened when the caregiver plays with the infant; that is interacts just to amuse and engage the infant. Playing with the infant, and generating positive mutually enjoyable emotions, is central to further emotional development, and we will now consider these aspects in more detail.

The importance of positive shared emotion

The relationship between the infant and the caregiver that develops in the first year of life, and is continued into the second, can to some extent at least, be explained on the basis of associative learning. However, such reasoning is more explanatory for the initial formation of the relationship than it is when it comes to how the relationship develops. The reciprocal relationship between caregiver and infant becomes a complex interaction, and it depends, as it develops, on personal interchanges that are themselves complex and subtle, and not easily analysed in terms of association, reinforcement, and other behaviouristic concepts.

Perhaps the most striking aspect of the relationship between caregiver and child is that it becomes a relationship full of fun and delight for both parties. Indeed without this element the relationship would become a chore and its psychological quality would alter. If the relationship does not involve fun and satisfaction it may not achieve its psychological and neurophysiological purposes. A funless and tedious interaction between the parent and child may keep the child alive, but without the elements that energise the relationship, and vitalise the infant and parent alike, the psychological and neurological outcome may be very limited indeed.

So fun, even mutual hilarity, is central to this developmental process. For Stern (1990), who uses the term "mutual hilarity", the intense pleasure and shared joy of the interaction are essential for it to achieve its psychological purpose. The relationship between the infant and caregiver should relieve distress, but it must also provide shared positive emotion. Where distress is not relieved the relationship will fail. Where there is no positive emotion in the interaction it will also fail, emotional growth will be limited, and in consequence cognitive growth will also be limited. We can easily see the effect of a cheerless adult disposition on the interaction.

Children from backgrounds of adversity often have to suffer care and relationships which are cheerless and without 'warmth'. The British Department of Health suggested in 1995 that lack of warmth on the part of parents was the largest problem in their child welfare system. As we examine the developmental benefits that arise from a fun filled positive relationship between caregiver and child we can easily agree that this may be so. We should not, however, conclude that poverty is the factor causing lack of warmth. Many poor people have very warm relationships with their children. We should also treat with sympathy and insight parenting situations where it is hard for the parent, for reasons of time and other pressures, to deliver a warm relationship. Some of these parenting conditions arise due to governmental policies or the lack of them.

In many ways the enjoyable and pleasurable interaction between caregiver and child in the first two years centres not on care but on play. Much has been written concerning the functions of play, but this interactive play with the caregiver in infancy and toddlerhood has a clear developmental function. Children who cannot interact with their caregiver in a playful way at this stage can be seen later to have psychological deficits. Play is an essential component of any growth promoting environment, and generates positive feelings that facilitate further structural growth (Greenspan, 1981; McEntire, 2009). Chisholm (1990) puts it quite simply by stating that play enriches the environment, while Tucker (1992) sees the ability to play with emotion as the key to the brain arousal which stimulates the development of neural networks.

What is being evoked here is the Freudian pleasure principle. A modern reading of the facts suggests that without pleasure, without the heightened energy that arises from it in the infant, certain neurological changes will not take place (Schore, 1994). Satisfaction, joy, pleasure, whatever we call it, has both psychological and physiological consequences. Positive emotion is an essential element of the interaction between caregiver(s) and child over the first two years of life.

Imitation, pretence and trickery

The reciprocal interaction between caregiver and infant not only contributes to an infant's sense of self but also allows the infant to learn to imitate the caregiver.

Neonates have some capacity to imitate adults and perhaps this early in-built imitation serves as a base for the more subjectively conscious imitation of older infants and toddlers. The older infant knows how the caregiver will respond in certain situations because the interaction in question has been repeated many times. It is a short step from such knowledge to an imitation of the caregiver's part in the exchange. Imitation is both a sign that the child understands that the caregiver is a separate person, and a mechanism whereby this distinction between people can be expanded and more fully understood.

When children imitate their caregiver they are in a sense pretending to be the caregiver. Imitation arises essentially out of the synchronised and frequently repeated routines that are seen in the reciprocal relationship between child and adult. In the first year, if the reciprocal relationship between child and caregiver is strong, infants can often look to their caregivers for emotional guidance when, in a novel or insecure situation, they are unsure about their emotional response. This is called social referencing (Boccia & Campos, 1989) and continues into later stages of development. The infant seeks to confirm his or her own emotional response by reference to the caregiver. In this process we can see the beginnings of conscious imitation. However, in the intimate environment of the reciprocal relationship threatening situations are not needed for the infant to directly imitate the caregiver. Infants will imitate caregivers if the relationship is pleasurable and secure. Novelty may, among other things, promote imitation, but it is not essential, and the infant seeks, not guidance, but participation and control.

When a child becomes a good imitator of his or her caregiver the skill generalises, and the child becomes able to copy other people and eventually other things. This ability to 'let's pretend' arises in the close caregiver/child relationship, and it is vitally important for future emotional and cognitive growth. Once the ability to pretend is developed it becomes of central importance for future play. When used in play pretence becomes the psychological driving force behind the development of symbolic thought. In symbolic thought there must be a symbolic function, that is a situation where something stands for something else. When a child pretends, something always stands for something else. Once this mental ability has been developed it becomes embodied as the central element in all imaginative play. Imaginative play always involves pretence to some degree, and prompts the child to think about mental states (Shaffer, 1999). Thus children in such play practise their relationships with others, albeit in a symbolic form (Harris, 1990). Practising imaginative relationships is essential if a child is to fully understand that other people are separate beings who have minds of their own. This realisation usually prompts the child to consider what other people may feel and to adjust his or her own behaviour accordingly. What we are now talking about is the development in the young child of a 'theory of mind'.

When, in the reciprocal relationship with the caregiver, a child realises that the other person has feelings of which the child must take account, the seeds of sympathy are sown. However pretence can go in a different direction. A toddler is often amused by trickery. At story-time before bed a toddler may be asked by a caregiver to point to the picture of the horse in his storybook. The child points deliberately to a duck and then waits for the caregiver's response. When she (the caregiver) pretends to be upset by the toddler's silly mistake the little boy laughs uproariously. He is tricking her by false replies and enjoying her emotional reaction. He knows a duck is not a horse but he is imaginatively testing the system, and, with the hilarity so common in interchanges at this age, is enjoying a new game of mistakes, which he can only truly play now that he has mastered the symbolic function. Later he will be able to consider 'what if' situations. What would the world be like if horses were ducks and ducks were horses? Out of beginnings such as these can grow creative thought, which in the course of development, is a long way from simple imitation. A child's use of deception and trickery indicates that he or she has developed a 'theory of mind', and the use of deception and trickery in play is a sharpening of this understanding.

Control and regulation in the reciprocal relationship

A great deal has been written about how children in the course of their development gain control over their emotions and emotional expression. In order to become properly socialised a child, it is said, must gain control over his or her emotions. The origins of this control process are postulated to be in the early reciprocal relationship between caregiver and child. The impression is given that control is imposed by the caregiver and somehow the child is brought to acceptable social behaviour. As we have stated already emotions, though modifiable to a considerable degree, cannot be entirely controlled. What is subject to control is emotional expression.

There is no doubt that emotional expressions change over the course of the reciprocal relationship between child and caregiver. However, our view of these changes is that they involve emotional development, not increasing emotional control. Nothing need be imposed by the caregiver, and if it is, it may be resisted by the child. Yet somehow the relationship, if warm and secure, does produce a child who will obey social rules and who can, as they grow older, adapt to new social conventions, or contrariwise object constructively, and in a civilised manner, to such conventions.

The key words are moderate and mediate rather than control. The child's emotions evolve into forms where the emotional expression appears to be moderate. These moderate emotional expressions mediate further friendly social interaction. The caregiver should not regulate the relationship otherwise the child will not grow in autonomy, rather the adult should regulate his or her own emotional input into the relationship in order to demonstrate appropriate responses to the child. This regulation is best achieved by an adult who loves the child, and reacts with appropriate natural emotions rather than behaving to a formula. After all, the relationship is natural and should flow easily from one emotional reaction to the next. The key elements remain security and positive pleasurable emotion. Where these are lacking it is probably impossible for the adult to influence the relationship much less control it. In fact the relationship will break down.

The reciprocal relationship is important particularly at play-time, but also at bath-time, feeding-time, and bed-time. Let us consider bath-time with a vigorous toddler. Such a child may splash a lot in the bath and then he or she splashes Mummy quite violently in the face so that soap gets in her eyes. Mum should not ignore and suffer such an incident, but should react with her natural emotional reaction and be offended by such splashing. Mother should withdraw temporarily from the positive fun and enjoyment of the bath-play and be offended. This should be drawn to the toddler's attention with the appropriate verbal disapproval. When the toddler desists, after a very brief time of emotional withdrawal, the adult should again join the toddler in the fun of bath-time. In this situation the adult has given a natural emotional response, but has also regulated the interaction between her and the child. The toddler will have perceived a change in their positive emotional relationship.

The message to the toddler is that fun has limits and respect should be shown. What is happening at a deeper neurological level is that the influence of adult regulation is creating new neural pathways, that will, when this type of event is frequently repeated, give the child the possibility of self-regulation of his (or her) emotional expression. The child will develop this self-regulation in order to remain within the limits of civilised bath-time that allow for the continuation of mutually pleasurable experiences. If we give the impression that such self-regulation is instantly and easily achieved let us correct it. Such self-regulation only comes with repeated experiences, each perhaps slightly different from the previous one.

However, the patient consistent adult, who preserves the fun of bath-time and the child's respect for their caregiver, will eventually see that the child has responded with a degree of self-regulation. What makes the difference is the positive emotion of fun that is energised at bath-time by a water loving child. It is positive emotion and a desire to keep it going that, in the end, makes the child respond to what happens to the adult, and eventually establishes within the child limits to the expression of his or her joy and excitement. If bath-time was not enjoyable self-regulation and respect could not evolve. In fact the child wishes to retain the mutual pleasure of the emotion and slowly realises that without mother's involvement such mutual pleasure is destroyed. Rather than deflate and control the positive emotion involved in the joy of bath-time the child wishes to continue it. What changes over time in the child is not the emotion but the control of the expression of that emotion.

Emotional expression is initially moderated by others but, as development proceeds, becomes increasingly regulated by the child (Thompson, 1990; 2011). A secure reciprocal relationship facilitates the transfer of regulatory capacities from caregiver to infant (Wilson *et al.*, 1990). The child, in time, is able to self-regulate, because neurological connections have become established due to repeated episodes of positive emotion, each of which has been subject to outside moderation. Schore in 1994 emphasised the caregiver's role in moderating and mediating environmental inputs to the reciprocal relationship. He suggested that a caregiver's influence in regulating these processes may represent the essential factor for experience-dependent neurophysiological maturation, the outcome of which is a higher level of neurological control of emotional expression. This development, Schore stated, takes place as a maturation of the frontal lobes of the cerebral cortex, particularly the orbitofrontal areas.

Let us consider the issue of respect in more detail and return to our bath-time example. It is most important for the continuation of a harmonious balanced reciprocal relationship that respect should also be shown to the toddler, with an apology, if the adult makes a mistake and splashes the child in the face, or rubs too hard on sensitive skin while trying to remove paint marks. Both parties should learn to moderate the relationship so that, not only does fun and joy proliferate, but in time its limits are also understood, and with them the first glimmerings in the toddler of the sentiment we call respect. Respect is the emotion that prevents the development of a hedonistic self-love that can easily arise from pleasurable situations. Instead respect allows for the development of mutual love.

Respect is considering the other, and is a very important element in the reciprocal relationship and the psychological developments that flow from it. Notice that it arises in an environment of security, positive emotion, and warm feelings shared by child and caregiver. Experience with children from adverse situations indicates that respect tends not to be shown by those children who are insecure and have limited experience of warm positive emotions.

The relation of reciprocity to other concepts

The processes of the reciprocal relationship between child and caregiver strengthen many of the essential mechanisms of what child psychologists label as *attachment*. Secure attachment is the condition that allows the secondary emotions of mutual love and respect to develop; indeed it is possible to equate secure attachment with the emotion that arises from it, namely mutual love. It is based on the satisfaction of dependency needs and warm human interactions. We will describe attachment in more detail later. These same processes lay the basis for a child's '*theory of mind*' (Baron-Cohen, 1991). In this theory children understand that other people have minds and use this understanding while developing their own thoughts and behaviours. In short, a theory of mind is the ability to infer what others are thinking and feeling, and to act on the basis of this inference. The reciprocal relationship is also the venue where most of the *negativism of the 'terrible twos'* is worked out. We will examine this in more detail later, but the later reciprocal relationship is the arena where eventually the child pushes for control and, by experiencing resistance to that control, comes to a fuller understanding than before of his or her psychological separateness from others. He/she learns that the caregiver cannot be pushed around, and this gives an increased understanding of the position of others, and through this understanding, a greater conception of self.

The reciprocal relationship that is so important to appropriate emotional development must, if emotional growth and cognitive growth are intertwined, also be of great importance to *cognitive development*. According to Greenspan (1997) this is undoubtedly the case. For example, a child's concept of the meaning of 'a lot', or 'many', arises because he or she got, as part of a request or otherwise, more than they wanted or expected. In the same way the meaning of 'too little', or 'a few', grows from the emotional experience of not getting what you wanted or expected.

Thus concepts like 'too much', or 'too many', may well develop in situations that have a strong emotional component within the reciprocal relationship. At breakfast a child may take too much but eat too little. Emotional comments may well be made by the caregiver on these situations. Likewise bath water may well be too hot, or too cold, or, for the properly nurtured child, 'just right'. We are reminded in this context of *Goldilocks and the Three Bears*, a story well understood by older toddlers, where the concepts of too much, too little, too big, too small, too hot, too cold, etc., and just right, are given much repetition, usually to the intellectual delight of the listening toddler. Such a toddler can follow the story because of his or her own experience in an essentially emotional reciprocal relationship. The story forms an imaginative setting where the toddler can rework and examine these cognitive concepts.

However, perhaps the most important area of development that starts in the reciprocal relationship relates to a child's conception of *appropriate social behaviour*, and the concepts that arise from this. Essentially the moderating and mediating experiences of the relationship allow the child to understand 'give and take'. In a good reciprocal relationship the child will learn the basis of taking turns. Not only will children learn this but they will practise what they have learnt over and over again. Long before they can articulate the cognitive concepts of moral judgement they will have a strong and impelling emotional feel for what is fair equitable and right.

Children will know, if they have been through a warm nurturing and secure relationship, what they ought to do, and indeed they may do it long before they can explain their actions. Morality and justice grow from actions and experience rather than detached thought, and such experience is infused with the emotions that arise first in the close but equitable relationship with the caregiver. Justice is at its root emotional. So are many moral concepts that relate to pleasurable and equitable human interactions. These had their origins in the first important interaction of a child's life, and the moderation and mediation that took place in that interaction.

Ask any toddler and he/she will tell you, 'I am a good boy (or girl)'. Goleman (1995; 2006) was so convinced of the importance of the first emotional experiences that he listed the following features as having an origin in those experiences, *confidence, curiosity, intentionality, self-control, relatedness, capacity to communicate,* and *cooperativeness.*

We have talked for simplicity's sake about a single reciprocal relationship, that of an infant/toddler with a caregiver. However, as we shall see, when we discuss attachment, many children rely not on one but on a number of reciprocal relationships. There are many arrangements whereby emotional warmth and the joy of play can become available to a child. What is important is that the arrangement, whatever it may be, satisfies the functions that we have outlined above. Different cultures and contexts may have different arrangements. We must now, having set the scene with a long discussion of the central relationship of the early years, return to the development of emotion, specifically in the second and third years of life.

The secondary self-conscious emotions

Once a child has a notion of his or her separate existence and the existence of others, the secondary emotions of the first year, mutual love, anxious fear, and anger from frustration can be moulded into new forms. These first developed secondary emotions were largely generated from early associations of the proto-emotions satisfaction, frustration and the perception of change. The moulding of these early emotions into new forms takes place in toddlerhood under the influence of the child's interactions with people and his or her growing cognitive capacity. It is important to remember that there is a feedback mechanism involved here. Cognitive ability is itself changed by emotional events and the interactions that a child has with people. So cognition can cause changes in emotion, but likewise emotion can cause cognition to change.

Earlier we stated that many secondary emotions were incubated emotions; that is 'slow' emotions that needed some time to form. This is because they arise out of human interactions and often involve the processes of rumination and memory. Some secondary self-conscious emotions are not slow but sweep over the child quickly. We can become jealous or indignant very quickly indeed. Whether quick or slow, these later secondary emotions possess the defining characteristic of emotion; they are to some degree uncontrollable and are not totally reducible to cognitive thought processes.

The early secondary emotions in the second year come under the influence of the developing self. Lewis (1992) states that emotions which develop due to a sense of self, what he calls self-conscious emotions, are quite different from the basic in-built emotional expressions of early infancy and the early secondary emotions of the first year. He sees shame, guilt, and pride, as being present in the second year in some children and in many by three years. Sroufe (1995), on the other hand, believes that many of these emotions are not fully formed in the second or even third years and he suggests true secondary self-conscious emotions only come to full development in the later pre-school years.

Whether self-conscious emotions in the second year are fully formed or not is not important. There is clear evidence that secondary emotions, involving a sense of self, start in the second year in many children and are present in most by their third birthday. The presence of self-conscious secondary emotions in toddlers is inferred not only from what they might say, but also from their facial expressions and other actions, and, in particular, from their bodily posture. Thus Lewis (1992) has inferred shame from a 'collapsed' body position, and pride from a cocky strut with shoulders and head held high.

These secondary emotions are developed with reference to the self and others and toddlers clearly show, during the second year when they exhibit certain behaviours, that they have such points of reference. Zahn-Waxler and others (Zahn-Waxler *et al.*, 1992) have shown that toddlers respond to distress in other people; Kochanska (1993) that they understand what is forbidden, and that they act in an anxious (guilty?) manner when they transgress; Dunn and Munn (1985) that they recognise wrongdoing by others; Cole (Cole *et al.*, 1992) that they know they have done wrong things, and wish to make amends. Therefore by 18 months of age children know things. Not only that, but they know that they know things. It goes even further; children at this age know that other people know things. They are aware that other people have thoughts, and they may even be concerned, to a degree, as to what these thoughts are. Children at this age have an unarticulated theory of how other people think, a 'theory of mind'. This awareness of others and their thoughts shapes emotional development from this point onwards.

The ontogeny of emotion in toddlerhood

Look at Figure 5.1. At the base of this figure is the situation as we left it after Figure 4.2; that is after the first year of emotional development. As you can see, (although satisfaction and frustration are still very operative), three early secondary emotions predominate *anger from frustration, anxious fear,* and *love*. These three emotions act as bases for further development. The child's growing cognitive capacity, and particularly the growing sense of self and of others, adds to and reworks these emotions into further secondary effects.

Secondary emotions arising from anger

Though some children are never very angry, a child's anger from frustration in the second year can become intense and be exhibited as rage or fury. This anger can be

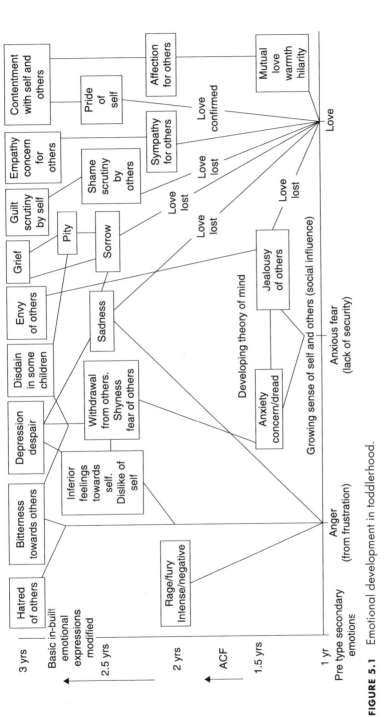

FIGURE 5.1 Emotional development in toddlerhood.

quite a normal development; part of the negative stage sometimes called the terrible twos. In infants the expression of anger is associated with being effective (Lemerise & Dodge, 2008). However, where such anger is the predominant emotion that a toddler shows to the exclusion of other feelings, which frequently occurs in situations of poor nurturance, it can lead to further negative secondary emotions. The secondary emotions that arise from this type of anger in the toddler period are feelings of inferiority, resentment, hatred, and later, in association with pride, itself a secondary emotion, indignation. Thus the child who predominantly feels such anger may divert this anger towards him or herself giving *feelings of inferiority* and dislike of self.

If the anger is directed at others it becomes *hatred* or *bitterness*. In every case the anger is transformed either in relation to the self or to others. Emotions such as bitterness are festering. The child who experiences them has thought about them, and they have grown and developed with such thought. Nevertheless, thought does not control such feelings. Like all true emotions these negative secondary emotions have an uncontrollable quality. We cannot talk or reason ourselves out of such emotions. No matter how much we know that it is wrong to hate, many of us cannot stop hateful feelings breaking over us when circumstances are ripe for the expression of this secondary emotion. In many cases children may direct anger at themselves *and* at others. In this way they can have considerable feelings of inferiority but also harbour anger and bitterness towards others.

Secondary emotions arising from anxious fear

The basic emotion of fear is present in the first year as a reflex response to pain, or as a reflex response to an intense noxious stimulus. Later in the first year anxious fear is related to an infant's perception of change, and arises from wariness when a child cannot predict what is going to happen. This other fear is a secondary emotion and is related to anxiety.

Children predominantly feel anxious fear because they cannot predict what will happen to them. This lack of predictability can develop further in the second year and third years as children develop cognitively. Anxious children are those who think about their fears in relation to themselves, and, in some instances, in relation to other people who are of importance in their lives. Anxiety is, to some degree at least, cognitive fear, in that it is produced when a child thinks about fearful things. This ability to think about fear is undoubtedly present in many children by three years of age. However, anxiety is a true emotion, it has an unstoppable quality, and, though produced by thought and lack of predictability, it cannot be totally controlled by thought. If such total thought control was possible in relation to fear, both instinctive basic fear and the secondary emotion we can call anxiety would disappear as emotions.

Anxiety can range from concern to dread, and it is often related to a child's feeling of security. Children from a secure background of loving nurturance may well be frequently concerned by what is happening, but they are unlikely to feel the intense dread that sweeps over children in adverse circumstances when they believe that their very survival is at risk. When we consider anxiety that arises from a fear of other people, one of the solutions for a child with a high level of anxiety is to withdraw from social situations. Such children can become very shy and uninvolved in wider social experiences. This withdrawal can, in some cases, negatively affect the self-concept and lead the child to the view that they are unworthy and unpopular.

Secondary emotions arising from love

The mutual love that arises from the affection that the infant feels for a nurturing caregiver is itself a complex emotion. It evolves first by simple association, but is developed further in the reciprocal relationship over the first years of life. It evolves from an infant's experience of satisfaction and what is associated with that satisfaction, but becomes a very strong force in its own right. From the earliest months satisfaction can vary from contentment to pure joy. Love in turn varies in intensity.

However, when it is associated with a strong secure and playful reciprocal relationship between child and caregiver, love can become the strongest of the positive emotions. Love is often expressed by acts of kindness. These have considerable social implications which eventually feedback to the emotional development of the child. In the year second and third years of life, love is under much cognitive consideration in the toddler's mind, and under the influence of the toddler's growing sense of self and of others, this consideration gives rise to further strong secondary emotions.

Jealousy

Where love has to be shared, as when a sibling arrives in the family, jealousy can arise. Jealousy is an emotion that is both quick and slow but it is a secondary emotion for all that. It can arise in certain situations without the involvement of much thought, but usually it festers with time and is developed through thought and memory processes. Essentially jealousy stems paradoxically from love, but it also arises in part from anxious fear, and it always involves a third party. Thus the child fears losing the love of the caregiver to another (Dunn & Kendrick, 1980). A child fears the loss of the close reciprocal relationship that serves his or her dependency needs. This is a fear of change and this relationship with anxious fear is illustrated in Figure 5.1. Anxiety fuels jealous feelings. Jealousy is extremely common (Buhrmester & Furman, 1990), and a moderate amount is normal in development. Where jealousy is left unassuaged and love is not reinforced, a further secondary emotion, *envy*, can grow. Envy can be directed towards a class of people or to people in general.

Jealousy is an important factor when another baby arrives in the family. Quite normal children can have ambivalent and jealous feelings when a sibling arrives, but in the case of a child who has had inconsistent care and has often been frustrated, and subject to unpredictable change, such feelings may not easily subside. These children have had a minimum of affection directed to them but sufficient to let them know what love is. Children in this situation are insecure but they know what benefits love brings. This causes them to consistently seek affection and attention even when these feelings are not regularly reciprocated by those who care for them. If another child arrives in the family they dread the loss of even the small amount of comfort, satisfaction and affection that they had gained at certain unpredictable times before the new baby's arrival. To have to share a meagre, randomly given, amount of parental love with another child is quite devastating for these children. Thus jealousy adds to their anger and anxiety. For a child who has a lot of loving care in life, jealous feelings are more easily reduced when parental love and concern is reasserted, and when the child begins to realise that there is enough love to go around and a newly arrived sibling does not matter. Jealousy is thus a complex emotion. It cannot be felt by those who have not loved or been loved at all. Sociopathic (psychopathic) people do not feel jealousy, nor do they understand jealousy. These persons have managed to survive without love, and where love does not exist jealousy cannot develop.

Shame

Shame is a secondary emotion that, like jealousy, arises largely from the base of love and positive feelings. To feel shame a child has to be self-conscious and to be aware of the thoughts of others. Sometimes this awareness of the thoughts of others occurs unexpectedly and suddenly when the toddler does something to please, and finds instead a distinct disapproval. A toddler has, in the reciprocal relationship, learnt to expect a positive reaction from the caregiver on most occasions. Emde (1992) has shown that in such a relationship toddlers develop a sensitivity to adult reactions but particularly to negative reactions. When a toddler experiences not the positive response that he or she expected, but instead a quite unexpected disapproval, this has a very deflating effect on the toddler. This is often the beginning of the secondary emotion that we call shame.

Shame arises in the second half of the second year and is definitely present in many children at two years (Malatesta et al., 1989). By this time the child has a knowledge that others think about him or her. He or she may be concerned about such thoughts. So when he or she is discovered doing something wrong or distasteful, the child's own thoughts, when cast upon what others might think, produce the emotion of shame. Malatesta et al. (1989) makes the telling point that both shame and pride arise in conditions of loving attachment that is in the positive emotional experiences of the reciprocal relationship. Secure attachment, which we will discuss at length later, is based on positive interactions that serve the child's dependency needs. Positive interaction experiences can occur consistently for the child (secure attachment) or inconsistently (insecure attachment). Malatesta states that when attachment is secure, experiences of pride will outweigh those of shame, whereas when it is insecure, experiences of shame will outweigh those of pride. Nevertheless, both of these secondary emotions depend on positive interactions with the caregiver and thus can be seen to arise from love.

Context is also very important in the expression of shame. The cultural context largely dictates what actions are shameful. A child has learnt to feel worthy because they have been loved and nurtured (even if, in some cases, this has been inconsistent). Shame arises essentially from a temporary loss of this worthiness, and therefore of love and respect. The child who commits a shameful act realises that in the caregiver's thoughts he or she is less worthy, at least at that instant. This induces shame.

When children, including toddlers, experience the emotion of shame their reactions can vary considerably. Some, mostly from backgrounds of a secure recip-rocal relationship, may attempt reparative behaviour or say that they are sorry (Cole *et al.*, 1992). Others, often from more insecure backgrounds (though some secure children can also act in this way), respond to shame by a resort to anger. Shame has frustrated them and they cannot tolerate the feelings it brings (Tangney, 1995).

Guilt

Guilt occurs somewhat later in the toddler period than shame (Sroufe, 1995). According to Hoffman (1984) it begins in the second year of life. Guilt evolves when the expectations of adults with regard to the child are internalised in the child's mind. We can think of guilt as internalised shame. It is a secondary self-conscious social emotion, but one where others are not *directly* involved, instead their representations have been internalised. Freud explains guilt as the strictures of the super-ego on the ego when it surveys the actions and desires of the id.

Whether we take a psychoanalytic approach or not, guilt is a self-critical emotion that does not, unlike shame, require public exposure in order to be gener-ated. It is a product of internal rather than external scrutiny, and like shame, arises essentially from the experience of love, and the possibility and actuality of love being withheld and lost. This is an important point because those who survive without much love, (or maybe none at all), have not got well developed emotions of shame or guilt. Attempts to control or influence these individuals by resorting to their expected feelings of shame or guilt often prove ineffective.

Pity

Pity occurs when we see others who are not loved as we are. We feel on their behalf. We may not do much about the plight of others yet we do not want to be in their position. We pity them. A child of three years can understand that others may not be loved. Essentially the child can comprehend this because he or she knows what it is like to be loved and what it is like to be temporarily unloved. The child knows which state is preferred and thus can pity those who are unloved. Though pity as a secondary emotion arises from experiences of love, a conscious consideration of love, or the lack of it, is not always prominent in pity. We can pity those who are simply less fortunate than we are. Unfortunately we can also despise them for this reason. Pity, when weakly developed (because its base in love has not been secure), can easily slip towards a lack of respect and a despising attitude to certain unfortunate people.

Pity arises essentially from an experience of love and the understanding that others also can love and be loved, or be deprived of these experiences. Where children have been little loved, pity on their part is usually a scarce emotion. Where a child is emotionally deprived the little pity he or she may initially show for others who are weak and unfortunate can easily degenerate into rejection and contempt. For people who are somewhat insecure in their own affections pity is a difficult emotion to sustain.

Sympathy/empathy

Sympathy is more than pity, and is one of the manifestations of empathy. Sympathy and empathy have very similar meanings and are often used interchangeably. There has been considerable debate as to the difference between these words especially as applied to young children (Lennon & Eisenberg, 1987). Both words imply an ability to put oneself in the position of another person, and to vicariously feel what they are feeling. Perhaps the best distinction between the words is given by Denham (1998). She insists that empathy is an overarching social emotion, which is in essence the ability to feel the emotions of another. Although it is obviously developed after the sense of self and the sense of others have matured, according to Denham, empathy is not just a self-conscious emotion. Rather it is a motivational emotion that spurs us to action on behalf of others in need. Denham sees two types of empathic response. On one hand a child can react to another's difficulties with distress. On the other hand a child can react to the misfortune of another child with sympathy. This analysis places sympathy as a sub-set of empathy. All of this is quite academic; what matters is that sympathy is an emotion that requires children to understand how other people feel. The emotion can only be felt with reference to others. Essentially when we are sympathetic we are sorry for others, who have had misfortune, because we can put ourselves in their position.

Sympathy arises from love because, for the young child, love heals misfortune. A child knows this is so from his or her experience of loving nurturance, gained in a positive reciprocal relationship. When the child sees another person in difficulties, the child wishes to overcome the other's difficulties by offering understanding and help, just as these elements were offered to her when she was in trouble. To develop sympathy a child needs 'a theory of mind' to apply to other people. Sympathy is the emotion that most clearly illustrates that a child has developed a 'theory of mind'. It is hard to imagine how a child would have sympathy if he or she had not developed ideas of the separateness of others and a 'theory' of how others felt.

Children as young as 18 months can express sympathy, or carry out actions from which we can infer that they feel sympathy. For many years, under the influence of Jean Piaget, it was thought that infants and toddlers were extremely egocentric. That is, they were dominated by their own perceptions, and could not conceive of a viewpoint that was not their own. More recent work has suggested that this is not the case, and children as young as two years are aware, not only of their own feelings, but also the feelings of others. They think about the feelings of others, and they can work out how other people will react to them. They are not always correct in their analyses, but they often are when they are in familiar situations. Young infants also predict how people they know will react to events and to other people. It seems that even young children have a 'theory of mind', a schema for working out how others will feel and how they will react. Prominent researchers in this field include Judy Dunn (1988) and Paul Harris (1990; 2008). Their research is important because it throws light on the inability of children from backgrounds of emotional deprivation to understand other people's emotions, and in particular their inability to sympathise and to engage in mutual emotional interchange. This is not a far-fetched speculation, Baron-Cohen and others (Baron-Cohen *et al.*, 1993) have used a deficit 'theory of mind' to explain autism.

Judy Dunn in her book *The Beginnings of Social Understanding* (1988) points to evidence that children from 18 months on understand hurt, and that they can exacerbate, or comfort, another's pain. They also understand the consequences of their hurtful (and loving) actions for others. These toddlers comment on and ask about the causes of other people's feelings and actions. Early in the second year children grasp how certain actions will lead to anger and disapproval in people, and how other actions will lead to contentment and praise. Children in this second year can respond with sympathy to distress shown by others, and are interested in how other people feel and what motivates them. In their third year children talk about knowing, remembering, and forgetting, both as they experience these processes and as they expect others to experience them. In short they reflect on their minds and the minds of other people. They cannot yet understand shades of emotion in themselves or others, but they recognise essential feelings. In Dunn's view it is the nature of early relationships that allows, or does not allow, these developments to take place.

Paul Harris in his book *Children and Emotion: The Development of Psychological Understanding* (1990) takes Dunn's position further. His studies of infants suggest that those from backgrounds of emotional deprivation may not develop an understanding of other people's feelings. He observed such pre-school children to react with inappropriate aggression to the distress of another child.

Harris points to the possibility that children with faulty early relationships may not learn a 'theory of mind'. They have their work cut out just to survive, and don't analyse their feelings to any degree. What is more certain is that they are not concerned about the feelings of others. They cannot show sympathy. If they do not gain an understanding of the feelings of others at an early stage, they may find it more difficult to acquire it in later years. Harris postulates that the ability of young children to attribute feelings to others is developed and practised in imaginative play. Imaginative play is conducted in secure surroundings, when children have time to play and are content. Our current society does not consider imaginative vacant play important. We probably structure the play periods that we give our children to much too great a degree. Even more important is the situation of many children in adverse circumstances who have no time to play. Their energies are otherwise taken up. If they do not understand other people's feelings, and thus cannot sympathise, it is because of their social and emotional history.

Sadness and sorrow

At this point we must deal with an emotion that some authorities see as a basic primary emotion of childhood, sadness. An understanding of the reciprocal relationship clearly explains this emotion. It is a secondary emotion. In the toddler years sadness is an emotion linked to people.

The discrete (differential) emotions theory lists sadness among the basic emotions. Our experience with infants and children is that, given good nurturing conditions, infant children are not often sad. Sadness occurs in infants in their first year when frustrations and anger are so unassuaged that the child's physiology can no longer sustain the expressions of these emotions and a state of quiet dejection sets in. Protest has been displaced with despair. Later in toddlerhood developmental sadness is certainly an emotional outcome for the child when the reciprocal relationship with the caregiver does not deliver according to the child's expectations. To feel this emotion children must have expectations in the first place and be aware of their part, and that of the caregiver, in the reciprocal relationship. When a child is disappointed in the relationship, and almost all children at some time are, then a temporary sadness will occur. This emotion is different from the earlier despair or dejection of infancy. A child's disappointment with, (or sadness about), a reciprocal relationship is a secondary emotion, in that the child must have some sense of self in the relationship and an awareness of the caregiver.

When a child realises that love is lost they feel sorry for themselves. This type of sadness is thus linked with an experience of love. Thus sadness probably has a number of origins and can be seen as a mood that arises from several sources. Whereas children who are constantly frustrated and angry can become sad, sorrow is more specifically related to people and to people we love. If we disappoint them or if our relationship changes for whatever reason for the worse, then we will feel sorrow. Too much sorrow can develop into a state or mood of sadness. Where a reciprocal relationship is healthy and imbued with positive joyful emotion, but is then ended permanently, severe sadness can result. This is generally known as grief.

Grief

Grief is a secondary emotion that emerges when something is lost not temporarily but forever. It arises from love in that our most important losses are the people who loved us. If we love and lose them forever we will surely grieve. Though grief stems from love and the permanent loss of love, it is not an emotion that is greatly modified by cognitive factors. Few people can think themselves out of their grief, and certainly no toddler can do this. A child's grief may not last as long as that of an adult, but it shows clearly the most singular characteristic of emotion, its unstoppable overwhelming nature. Grief overtakes the person and against it mere cognition is no control, especially during the toddler stage.

Pride and indignation

Pride arises from a positive joyful reciprocal relationship that can be designated as loving. Pride is a more socially influenced emotion than grief. When a child does something important or worthwhile, (according to his or her culture), then the child feels that he or she is worthier than before and expects to be acclaimed and well treated by his or her caregivers. Though this may not actually happen the expectation that it will gets translated into a warm self-congratulatory feeling, pride.

Those who have not been loved find it very difficult to feel pride in themselves. Pride is a self-enhancement procedure. It adds to the self-concept. If this has never been nurtured by experiences of esteem and affection, then further personal achievement has nothing to build on. To put it another way, pride must have an audience or an imagined audience, people who will acclaim and whose acclamation is important to the child. If there is no audience, or no one whose opinion matters to the child, then pride will not grow. Pride is self-conscious.

Pride not only requires a child to have a concept of self and of others but is, when formed, an emotion closely related to self-perception. Thus pride can be hurt or injured. When pride is challenged and hurt, a type of anger can form, *indignation*. Indignation is a secondary emotion that evolves from love via pride, but is also influenced by anger. It occurs after the toddler stage. The ontogeny of the later secondary emotions such as indignation is very complex, but they retain nevertheless that essential uncontrollable element. Anyone who has experience of an indignant partner or spouse will know this to be true!

Embarrassment

Embarrassment is a secondary emotion related to shame and therefore also has its origin in an experience of love. It also derives from anxiety concerning what others may think of us. This makes it a self-conscious emotion that arises when the influence of peers becomes important in a child's emotional development. It is not indicated in Figure 5.1 because toddlers are rarely embarrassed. This secondary emotion occurs later in childhood when self-consciousness is fully rather than partly acquired. It is a very frequent feeling for those going through periods of change and is a very common emotion in early adolescence.

When we are embarrassed we are in the public gaze but we have not done anything shameful in the public's eyes. Rather we find that we are uncomfortable because of the possibility that we may err and become shameful or even laughable in the eyes of others. This is especially true if we are in a new or unexpected situation. We react to public situations with an uncomfortable feeling that has no real justification in the eyes of our audience. We have done nothing shameful; the emotion is self-generated. The public aspect of this emotion is what differentiates it from guilt.

The importance of love

The emotions formed in the second and third years, are considered as forming under socioemotional influences by Brownell and Kopp (2007) and are often referred to as self-conscious emotions by Lewis (1992) or sociomoral emotions by Tangney (2002). They depend for their development on those earlier secondary emotions that have already formed out of social interactions in the first year of life. This is rarely recognised in academic psychology. The development of a mutual love between carer and child in infancy is a key feature and a guide as to the more advanced self-conscious emotions that will appear in toddlerhood. If warm care and attendance to essential needs was not given in infancy love as a secondary emotion may not form and those emotions stemming from love will not develop. Rather their place will be taken by secondary emotions derived from anger (due to frustration) and anxious fear. This point is not often made because psychologists have a reluctance to use the word love somewhat akin to their earlier reluctance to recognise the importance of emotion in human life. This is slowly changing and three neurologically oriented psychiatrists have been in the vanguard in recognising the importance of love as a basis for appropriate emotional development (Lewis *et al.*, 2000).

We also have no reluctance in referring to love as an emotion of crucial developmental importance. We place the development of love in the child, which arises from warm loving nurturance and human interactions, at the centre of our account of the development of human emotions. The presence or absence of mutual love between caregiver and child is critical to future secondary emotional development as the next two sections will show. Not all secondary emotions are self-conscious and the mutual love that arises from good circumstances in the first year under social influences is not self-conscious but nevertheless is the most important secondary emotion for future positive emotional development in the toddler period.

When things go right

How does Figure 5.1 relate to children who have received loving nurturance in their second and third years and who have had their dependency needs met?

Such children by three years will show a wide range of emotions. They will still experience satisfaction and frustration. We trust that they are not predominantly angry, though they can be angry from time to time. They feel generally secure, though they will show some fears from time to time. They may even be shy in the presence of those they do not know very well. However, most of their emotions grow from the affectionate links that they forged in their first year. They may feel jealous particularly of newcomers. They feel shame when they are found transgressing. They may even accuse themselves of guilt. None of these emotions is pleasant, yet they all arise from the mutual love developed in a warm nurturing reciprocal relationship.

These children feel pity for others, and can show respect, sympathy, and concern. They are proud of their successes and grieve their losses and failures. They are learning to love a range of people and their open affection can be very touching. All in all, these children are happy adjusted children who fit into their families without too much trauma and into their society and culture. They are not always happy of course, jealousy, shame, and guilt see to that, but such is life even for the fortunate.

When things go wrong

Fogel (1982) suggests that emotional development is not invariant. It does not necessarily occur in a predictable sequence. If we do not have certain experiences, particularly social experiences, emotional development may be changed or diverted or limited.

Children, who have not had a loving nurturing reciprocal relationship in their first year and whose dependency needs have not been met, or only met in part and then inconsistently, probably enter their second year of life with a mixture of angry and anxious fearful feelings. These feelings, if not counteracted by loving nurturance and consistent care during the second year, lead, for the most part, to negative emotions. Such children by three years may already have inner feelings of deep inferiority and dislike others with considerable intensity. They show little respect for anyone, and may be angry/aggressive, or anxious, or both by turns. If they have had a little inconsistent loving they can be very jealous indeed. More importantly they will show little or no shame, and almost certainly no guilt feelings. They find it easier to despise the weak and unfortunate than to sympathise with them. Some of them will find it difficult to sympathise with anyone in any circumstances. They have no true pride in themselves though they may be full of boasts and brags. What they lack in this respect is self-confidence. You need consistent loving to be self-confident and these children have not had it. All in all these children are not happy. More often than not they are sad, though some of them are so used to their condition that open signs of sadness are hard to find. These children are to be admired in certain ways, primarily because they have survived. They have adapted and survived. The problem is that this survival is not admired or recognised by society, and the adaptations that these children have made to get this far are neither understood nor valued. As time goes on these adaptations will come to conflict with what society expects. This conflict is visible even at three yrs and it is a conflict that should be understood by those who have to care for these children.

Many children who have missed out on a satisfying reciprocal relationship, or relationships, have difficulties in learning to control their emotional expression. In particular they have problems in controlling their anger. It seems as if control of the expression of emotion is first learnt in the reciprocal relationship in respect of fun, joy, and satisfaction. Where control of the expression of positive feelings has not been developed, the control of the expression of negative emotions appears to be particularly difficult. There is not, as yet, much experimental evidence for this process whereby the control of positive emotion comes first, but a survey of clinical cases can easily lead to this speculation. In addition there is some developmental neurological evidence to suggest that the control of positive emotional expression and the control of negative emotional expression involve different areas of the frontal lobe of the brain (Eliot, 2001).

Children from adverse emotional circumstances do not lack emotion, even the most deprived of them will show the innate basic emotions. They often have developed secondary emotions but these tend to be negative. Those who have had a little inconsistent loving care may in toddlerhood have developed positive secondary emotions that arise from love. However, as we shall see in later years these emotions are easily suppressed by other psychological factors and are not therefore very motivating. Children from backgrounds of poor and inconsistent affection can feel things deeply, but they may not have differentiated their feelings, they may not have thought about them, and they may never have considered that other people also have feelings. This emotional picture combined with the effects of constant frustration and constant change can produce a child whose emotional motivations and behaviour are very difficult to tolerate and understand. Yet we must understand these children if we are to act in their best interests.

The early years summarised

Two points must be emphasised in connection with what we have written about emotional development in both infancy and toddlerhood. The first is that emotions evolve in complex ways and new secondary forms emerge. However, earlier emotions and proto-emotions remain and are not replaced by the newer forms. We do not lose the power to be frustrated because our frustration has evolved into anger, and further into hatred. We do not lose primitive satisfaction when from it we develop the ability to love, and subsequently the ability to feel shame or pride. We also retain the instant basic emotional reactions that were first shown in the instinctive emotional expressions present from birth or shortly afterwards. Our complement of emotions grows in childhood and we have many more emotions at three years than we had when we were one.

The second point to be emphasised is the importance of positive secondary emotions in a child's development. In some ways these positive emotions have been neglected in research, in favour of negative, problematic emotions like fear and anger (Fredrickson, 1998). Positive secondary emotions spring from satisfaction and the pleasure it brings. Satisfaction can be as calm as contentment, or as ecstatic as joy, but, in whatever form, recent neuropsychological approaches identify positive emotion as the crucial factor in the development of certain essential brain connections. Without positive secondary emotions equitable civilised social life would be impossible. It is very significant for families and for society that many children miss out on positive emotional experiences.

Though this chapter has emphasised the importance of positive emotional experience we must not undervalue the function of some negative emotions in the development of normal well-nurtured children (Bradley, 1989). Children are dependent and the impetus to seek a resolution of their dependency may well arise in children from negative emotions such as basic fear and developed anxiety. The resolution of dependency needs and the role of negative emotion in this process are among the significant topics in the next chapter.

This next chapter covers the psychological mechanisms that underlie the development of emotions in infancy and toddlerhood. We have already described these emotional developments using a description of a child's social interactions, from the earliest months onwards, to explain how these developments have taken place (Chapter 6 and this chapter). The term we have used in this chapter to describe the explanatory social interaction is *the reciprocal relationship* which is a close relationship of care and affection between a carer, usually mother, and a child. In these two chapters we have concentrated on social relationships when they were effective and only later in each chapter did we refer to situations where things go wrong. We now need to consider other ways to describe the relationships that a child needs for emotional and cognitive development and also consider the innate genetically determined qualities that the child and the carer may bring to such relationships. By doing so we will get a more theoretically informed picture of the complexities of emotional development in infancy and toddlerhood.

Questions to think about

1. What, in general terms, is a child's 'theory of mind'?
2. Why is a sense of self necessary for the development of secondary social emotions?
3. Describe the reciprocal relationship.
4. Explain how a pleasant experience of mutual love and affection in the first year of life can lead to secondary emotions in the second and third year that frequently embody unpleasant and disturbing feelings.
5. Why are pity and sympathy absent or weak emotions in children who come from adverse circumstances? Why do these children often react with aggression to other unfortunate and deprived children?
6. What is the importance of play in a child's emotional development?
7. Name three self-conscious secondary emotions.

Suggested for further reading

Tronick, E. Z. (2005), Why is connection with others so critical? The formation of dyadic states of consciousness and the expansion of individual states of consciousness: Coherence-governed selection and the co-creation of meaning out of messy meaning making. In: *Emotional Development*, ed. J. Nadel & D. Muir. New York: Oxford University Press, pp. 293–315.

Lewis, M.(2008). The emergence of human emotions. In M. Lewis, J. M. Haviland-Jones & L. Feldman Barrett (Eds), *Handbook of Emotions* (3rd edn). New York: The Guilford Press, pp. 304–319.

Harris, P. (2008). Chidlren's understanding of emotion. In M. Lewis, J. M. Haviland-Jones & L. Feldman Barrett (Eds), *Handbook of Emotions* (3rd edn). New York: The Guilford Press, pp. 409–427.

Dependency, attachment and temperament

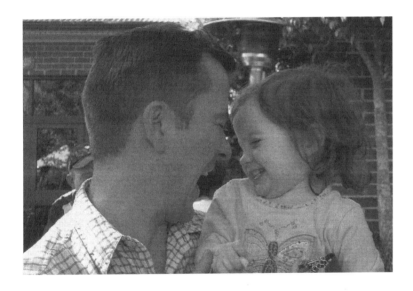

- This chapter looks at the psychological dynamics involved in emotional development in childhood. These dynamics occur within the child and carer relationships and are a central aspect of the child's social environment impacting upon secondary emotions.
- Dependency is the starting point which evokes the development of instinctive attachment.
- Attachment type dictates possible emotional development and is also a strong predictor of overall child development and wellbeing.
- Temperament plays a role in emotional development as it forms a genetic base for the behaviour and social interactions of the child. It is

> important to consider temperament in relation to the carer child relationship.
> - Different temperaments in the child and carer may challenge the reciprocal relationship and require the adult carer to be more flexible.

THE ACCOUNT OF EMOTIONAL development given in the last two chapters has been one where certain emotions evolve as the child develops. What emotions evolve in a particular child depends on the circumstances of that child, in particular his or her social surroundings. The theoretical foundation for such an approach rests ultimately on the new theories of the development of the brain in childhood. These theories point to environmental influence on actual neural connections, and it is presumed that the emotions are as dependent as any other psychological function on the development of such connections.

We have given a picture of emotions changing and developing in the child from what was there before. This picture is in harmony with the way neuroscience now views the developing brain. We have also suggested that as children grow older their emotional repertoire also grows. The first secondary emotions, or the proto-emotions from which they form, are not eliminated in this developmental pathway, nor are the basic instinctive emotional reactions. As new secondary emotions develop the more 'primitive' emotions and proto-emotions continue to be part of a child's emotional compliment. This means that certain basic emotions such as fear may exist throughout development in a 'primitive' instinctive form, as well as more complex feelings such as anxiety.

Is it possible to identify the behavioural and psychological dynamics that govern the interaction of an infant or toddler with his or her social environment? Is it possible to explain the course of the development of emotions in an individual by reference to these processes? Yes, there are factors which can explain the relationship of the child to his or her social environment and are therefore closely related to the development of the secondary emotions. The first of these factors is dependency which is catered for by a process called attachment. We all have used these words before but now we will look at these dynamics in more detail as explanatory processes behind emotional development and the reciprocal relationship(s) that is central to such development.

Dependency

We have already referred to dependency as the defining feature of childhood. For many generations of humanity the most appropriate and convenient way a child's dependency needs could be satisfied was through the child-mother relationship. Today this relationship remains, in most circumstances, the best and easiest way to cater for the child's dependencies. But there is nothing sacred about it. Equally effective relationships can be made with father or other consistent caregivers, and, if the infant's dependency needs can be satisfied by joint or multiple care-giving, then infants will still thrive and develop into adaptable emotionally secure children. Unlike an animal mother, the human mother acts largely in a cultural rather than an instinctive context, and human cultures vary considerably. We cannot be certain about mothering practices when they vary considerably from culture to culture, and we cannot value natural mothering when a caregiver, who is not the child's natural mother, can rear a child in a perfectly adequate manner. We are led to the view that the key factor is not the mother as such, or even sole care-giving, but the satisfaction of the child's dependency needs.

Earlier we introduced the concept of dependency and discussed an infant's dependency needs. We now need to look more closely at dependency in order to understand how it fuels the development of emotions. To do this we will distinguish between two forms of dependency.

Instrumental and emotional dependence

Dependency falls into two broad categories instrumental and emotional dependence.

1. *Instrumental dependence* where a child gains help from adults or caregivers in order to survive or in order to achieve goals that the child alone cannot achieve. This is not manipulative but natural. The child appeals to the caregiver and he or she responds to the child's needs. The dependence is instrumental in getting things done for the child.
2. *Emotional dependence* develops out of infant instrumental dependence when feelings associated with care and satisfaction become warm sentiments associated with people. As instrumental dependence declines in older children, emotional dependence becomes the more obvious form of dependency, though it has been an important process from the very beginning of infancy. It involves gaining emotional warmth and approval from those who are important for what the child needs and does.

A child's instrumental dependency needs must be catered for by the caregiver or caregivers. Basic instrumental care, like ensuring that toddlers have enough sleep, has been shown to have an immediate impact upon emotional responses (Berger *et al.*, 2012). However it is the pattern of how children's dependency needs are met that drives emotional development. Depending on the quality of care given to an infant, feelings will arise in the child either predominantly of satisfaction or

111

else of frustration. The association of the predominant feeling that arises from the care the infant receives with the person who delivers that care starts the process of emotional development. As we shall see later, the dependency needs of the child are so strong that even when care is inadequate the infant will persist in his or her attempt to link emotionally with the caregiver. The emotions that are developed out of inadequate care are rarely positive, but nevertheless, emotional dependency on the adult caregiver develops, and many children from adverse circumstances where care has been inadequate have great difficulty in resolving their feelings towards their initial caregivers as they grow older.

Do we need to reduce dependency?

When the child is totally dependent, the mother or caregiver should give complete care. Increasingly, however, the child learns through the reciprocal relationship to do things for themselves. The societal demands for children to grow towards total instrumental independence vary from culture to culture and across history. Emotional independence is another matter.

Emotional dependence changes in childhood but is not reduced by the developmental process. If an infant is well nurtured, in an instrumental sense, positive sentiments will form towards caregivers and others, and these feelings are often crucial in the development of secondary emotions. The process of developing secondary emotions does not, however, reduce a child's emotional dependence on other people. To be fully human adults we must retain some emotional dependence, some emotional connection with others. Rather than reduce emotional dependence, the processes of normal development change it, transform it, and widen its scope. Thus as we develop we will tend to transfer such emotional dependence from our parents to others in the environment, even if we retain love and affection for our mother and father.

As the child grows in mother's care he or she develops an emotional tie with mother (or the principal caregiver father, nanna, nanny, aunty or whoever). If we habitually refer to mothers here, it is only because mothers are the most common child rearers and usually the ones who 'carry the can'. Fathers and other caregivers can be equally as important as mothers (and as much to blame if a child's dependency needs are not adequately met). Regardless of who it is with, the child's original emotional tie in time extends to others. Often its first extension is to father, or brothers and sisters, or other relatives. This can occur quite quickly after the initial attachment is made (a matter of weeks). Young infants can be attached to more than one person. By four years of age a child's emotional ties have proliferated. Thus, in almost all well nurtured children, emotional dependence is spread over a number of people. From this age, around four, onwards emotional dependence on peers increases; though it will never quite replace dependence on family members, when family relationships are loving and stable.

A child's drive towards more independence, by which we mean a reduction in instrumental dependence and also a spreading of emotional dependence, is a powerful and natural psychological force that has much to contribute to emotional development. Sometimes, like emotion, it appears unstoppable. Mothers who cosset too much should remember this. Care for the child should be linked to and complement his or her independent actions. Problems can arise when the child is given more care than he or she needs at a particular stage, and independent action is stifled or postponed. Instrumental dependency must be catered for, but it must also be progressively reduced as is appropriate to cultural expectations. Emotional dependency must progressively be spread to others. Sudden reductions in care and concern are harmful to emotional growth, but nevertheless mothers should progressively fade into the background over the 0–18 year period. However, the time-frames for these transitions are culturally determined and may also vary slightly from generation to generation.

We must stress the slow progressive nature of the reduction in dependency, and gain in independence. Parents who wish to inculcate wide instrumental and emotional independence in their toddlers at a very early age are misguided. Such parents do not realise the link between dependence and independence. Rutter (1981) sees the key to this link as being secure attachment or bonding. We see it in relation to meeting a child's current dependency needs. One has to learn to be independent and this is a slow process. The child will take the risks of independence, but only if he or she learns to cope with such risks when mother or caregiver is there to fall back on. Mother or caregiver gives secure attachment or, in other words, caters for the child's current dependency needs.

Notice that independence is learnt while the child is still dependent; it is not learnt by being alone. Parents should realise the need for progressive incremental reduction in care for their children; care must be reduced, but slowly. Independence is given, 'when the child is ready for it', and children vary a great deal in their readiness. If a child is behind his or her peers, or the children of neighbours, or friends, it is because he or she needs more time. Parents need to be sensitive to the needs of their individual children in these processes and may take different timeframes with different children. Yet children can be unduly delayed in their drive towards independence by parents who won't change at all. Such children often 'signal' their readiness for more freedom by rebellious behaviour.

Parents have a difficult path to negotiate between giving too much independence and too little and every child is different. What should not happen is an abrogation of parental concern. Parents can give independence simply because it suits them, the parents, rather than the children. None of us, of course, ever becomes totally independent emotionally; we simply become less dependent and change our dependencies. Parents should encourage such shifts to take place.

Signs of dependency

Dependency needs and the complimentary need for independence are obviously processes linked to development. In some ways they are processes that propel development including emotional development. How do we know if children are developing correctly in terms of their dependence or independence?

Certain signs of dependence are appropriate for certain age levels. Young infants seek *physical contact*, being fed, changed, bathed and cuddled. Toddlers seek physical contact but can feed themselves. Pre-school children like *physical proximity*. When they attend pre-school some don't want Mum to leave (at first). Many children, including older children, do not want to be left in hospital. Who does! It is easy to realise that signs of dependence are not only related to age but are frequently *specific* to certain situations.

Seeking help to do something is a sign of instrumental dependence. Whether this dependence is normal or not depends on the age of the child seeking help and the type of help sought. As children grow they should need less and less help for common tasks. In general, children should be active and engage the environment rather than sit back and wait for assistance. A situation where a child repeatedly attempts a task, fails on each attempt, then asks for help is more acceptable and psychologically better than one where the child simply refuses to attempt a task (appropriate to his or her age) and demands instant help.

Older children show their emotional dependency by seeking attention and approval. If older children want continual physical contact or proximity (non-sexual), or help with feeding, then of course something is wrong. In later childhood approval is usually enough. Of course some adults need excess approval before they are satisfied, but on the whole, attention seeking declines as people grow up and become more confident and secure.

Dependency as a key concept

The goal of development in childhood, if indeed such a goal can be conceived, (bearing in mind our castigation of a "royal road" in development), is the creation of a mature independent adult. Independence, which in many ways is the basis of liberty, is greatly valued in our society. It is interesting therefore, and a little paradoxical, that true independence has its basis in dependence.

Dependency is not only the defining feature of childhood; it is the first characteristic of an infant, the first noticeable thing about a newborn child. A child's dependency needs govern a child's progress through early life, and can explain other mechanisms that are used to describe infant and child development. In particular dependency, as a concept, explains a child's need to attach himself or herself to an adult (or adults) who gives care and emotional attention. It also explains the attachment of children to each other because, though little care may be involved, and no instrumental dependency needs assuaged, the attachment of children to each other satisfies certain elements of emotional dependence.

Attachment is the result of dependence and some of the difficulties with attachment theory may be resolved if this is kept in mind. Attachment is a mechanism whereby dependency needs are met. It is not some romantic force that automatically binds natural parents to their children, though it has often been described in terms that would suggest a type of enchantment on the part of the parties involved. Not that the attachment of a caregiver and a child cannot create sublime feelings in both parties; it certainly can, but these important emotions are a consequence of the attachment rather than its cause. They may come with the process rather than initiating it.

One of the basic dependency needs in infancy and childhood is the need for security and safety. Infants and children will feel secure and safe if conditions are not only nurturing but also stable. As already discussed, anxious fear, and eventually anxiety, will arise when children develop a perception of change and find that they cannot predict when dependency needs will be met. These emotions will be particularly noticeable in infants who receive inconsistent nurturing. However, all children, once they develop a perception of change, will to some degree feel that the world is threatening and unpredictable. So why not fly to mother!

What we are suggesting is that negative emotions such as basic fear and secondary anxiety may have their place in the creation of attachments between children and their caregivers. The pre-conscious fear that dependency needs may not be met, even in situations of good nurturance, may drive infants and children into the arms of their parents or other caregivers. The fact that attachment behaviours persist in the face of abuse (Rutter, 1981) would lead to this conclusion. However, before we explore this further we should look at the process of attachment; seen by many as the key to development particularly emotional development.

Attachment

Looking at dependency it becomes clear that infants depend as much on sensitive and affectionate handling as they do on food. Indeed it appears that affectionate treatment is *more* important than mere sustenance for a child's development, though, if a child is not fed, then of course, warmth and affection are not much use. An affectionate warm emotional relationship between a child and a caregiver, to whom the child returns again and again for help and comfort, is called a secure attachment. In a secure attachment the caregiver acts as a secure base for the child as the child explores the environment

In earlier chapters we considered the growth of emotions in the early years, and the importance of a mutually affectionate interchange between caregiver and infant came to the fore. This relationship between child and caregiver can also be called an attachment. Thus we have already alluded to attachment in several contexts. What then exactly is an attachment? Are attachments the key to infant development, indeed to all development?

What is attachment?

For the child but not the parent attachment is *instinctive* (Bowlby, 1982). Attachment originates with the infant and develops into a reciprocal interchange between the child and his or her caregiver that satisfies the child's most basic dependency needs and allows the child to explore his or her surroundings. The attachment relationship is the baby's first emotional relationship and if satisfactory is the one from which the child draws *emotional comfort* and *security*. Children will seek out the caregiver to whom they are most closely attached whenever they need comfort or when they are injured.

Attachment has very close links with a child's sense of security. Security for the child is based on predictability. The child and the caregiver have had a long period of reciprocal interaction, and they know each other intimately. This allows the child to be able to predict what will happen in the caregiver's presence. This ability to predict creates a sense of security in the infant and allows the child to explore his or her environment with confidence using the caregiver as a secure base. A sense of security counters anxiety, the emotion that is fuelled by unpredictability.

According to Bowlby, the founder of attachment theory, attachment is an enduring emotional tie between infant and caregiver (Bowlby, 1982). Bowlby saw attachment as a way in which infants can reconcile their desire to explore with their wish to be secure and safe. The child uses the caregiver to whom they are attached as a secure base from which to venture into the world, but also as a person to whom they can run whenever danger or strangeness (we would say unpredictability) threatens.

Attachment and bonding

Bonding is a word used in the literature in several senses. Sometimes it is used to mean attachment. At other times bonding is used to mean the attraction that the adult feels for the child, more specifically the feelings of attraction that a mother has towards her newborn infant. This is *not* the same as attachment which is essentially the *reciprocal* relationship between the child and caregiver originating in the child. The word reciprocal in this context means a two way interaction, caregiver to child, *and* child to caregiver. It does not mean that the interactions are balanced in any way. The feelings a mother has for a newborn are very variable but if even if they are strongly positive there is no real reciprocation on the part of the newborn infant. Such reciprocation comes later when the child seeks it and it develops slowly over time. Many people make a fuss about the initial feelings that a mother has for a baby

116

and how these feelings can be enhanced, but, though it is a good thing if a mother has positive initial feelings towards her baby, this does not constitute attachment.

In the beginning attachment is an instinctive drive on the child's part to enlist help in order to meet essential dependency needs. Even when care is not forthcoming attachment behaviours will persist. Mutual attachment only comes about during the long care process particularly when the caregiver and the infant develop affectionate and enjoyable interchanges. Attachment is not so much to the person who feeds us as it is to the person who interacts with us to instruct, amuse, and comfort. These 'persons' are of course often, but not always, the same person, mother. Normal attachment is not dependent on maternal bonding at the time of the child's birth. Infants who spend their first weeks in a humidicrib can later attach totally successfully with their caregivers.

Michael Rutter (1981) uses the term bonding in yet another way. He sees bonding as attachment that is internalised by the child, usually the older securely attached child. Such bonding is an inner feeling of security, a feeling that you can rely on someone for security and support even when that someone is not physically present. This is the ultimate form of attachment and is a development seen in older secure children. It is a positive attribute that children can carry into adolescent and adult life.

When does attachment occur?

The origins of attachment lie in the developing relationship between a child and his or her caregiver that usually starts shortly after birth when the adult or adults begin a care relationship with the infant. 'Clear cut' attachment begins at about six to eight months of age. By this time many child-caregiver interactions have blossomed into a mutual emotional relationship involving enjoyment and comfort for both participants. In the best of circumstances this gives the infant the feeling of security that he or she is seeking.

Attachment seems to occur in all cultures, though there are some cultural differences. Attachment occurs with children who are disabled and even children who are abused seek attachment. Attachment seems such a powerful instinct in the lives of children that they will even seek attachment with those who abuse them. Rutter (1981) says that attachment can develop, at least to a weak insecure degree, in abused children, but bonding (in his sense of the word) or secure attachment never develops in circumstances of maltreatment.

Attachment and dependency needs

Here we reiterate the link between dependency and attachment. Essentially secure attachment is an arrangement within which the child can have his or her dependency needs met. If we survey the area of infant development, it seems that, in the vast majority of cases, attachment to a single caregiver is the most efficient way in which the child can satisfy these needs. Thus in many situations it appears that the sustaining relationship with mother is the most important element for the child's optimal, ordered, and calm development.

However, this may simply be the most efficient and common way for a child to have needs satisfied. Considerable evidence exists to show that children can become attached, at a very early stage in the process, to more than one person (Sagi et al., 1994). In most cases infants are usually attached to mother, though they may also have an attachment to father and other family members. Mother may not, however, be the principal caregiver or the person who interacts most frequently with the child. In this case the child will not attach to his or her biological mother but to the person (or persons) who gives sustenance and, much more importantly, interacts most frequently with the child especially in relation to emotional comfort. What is certain is that because a child needs others to satisfy basic needs, attachment to a person who can fulfil these needs (in full or in part) will take place. You do not meet children who have not made some type of appeal to adults for help in meeting their basic needs. When dependency needs are met in full by a secure attachment (or attachments) the child has no need for a further insecure attachment.

The measurement of attachment

Attachment in infants can be classified into two main types, one of which is further divided into three sub-types. It is possible to observe different patterns of attachment if one observes caregiver-child interactions. It was, however, a laboratory procedure that first classified attachment into types. This was the "strange situation" test or procedure, developed by Ainsworth and others (Ainsworth et al., 1978).

In this procedure the infant to be tested is first left in an observed room with his or her mother (or caregiver), then mother and child are joined by a stranger, then the child is left by him or herself with the stranger, then alone, then mother returns. At each stage the infant's reactions and behaviour are noted. Observations of infants can be classified into four types.

Secure attachment

This is shown by 70 per cent of the infants tested by this procedure in the USA. Securely attached infants use mother as a secure base from which they will explore and to which they will return for reassurance. In secure attachment the infant can rely on the caregiver both physically and emotionally. This is because the caregiver responds sensitively to the infant's dependency needs both instrumental and emotional. This reliance and assurance allows the child from time to time to venture away, exploring new and interesting things, while knowing that mother (or caregiver) is ready and competent to deal with difficulties should the child encounter them.

Insecure attachment

Insecure attachment is one where the child cannot rely on the caregiver for help and emotional support, or is only given these things on an inconsistent unpredictable basis. The infant may feel anxious, or fearful, or angry, or all of these things. This attachment type is divided into *three* subtypes.

1. Insecure-resistant attachment (sometimes called ambivalent attachment)
In this pattern of attachment the child cannot rely on the caregiver for consistent care because the infant cannot predict when care will or will not occur. The infant may become clingy and be very reluctant to be separated from the caregiver in any way. Thus these infants refuse to explore. When the caregiver is absent they whine until the caregiver returns, yet upon her return they are still not satisfied, and may not respond to the caregiver's approaches. They can even respond to her advances with physical resistance and anger. These infants are like those who have had a little affection only to have it taken away, or like those infants whose care is delivered on an inconsistent and unpredictable basis. The best words to describe their reactions are ambivalent and neurotic. When they get what they want (mother's return) they don't want it.

2. Insecure-avoidant attachment
Infants who show this type of attachment correspond to those children who have had very little affectionate nurturance in their lives. They may have had some of their instrumental needs attended to, but warm nurturance for them has been very limited. These children explore quite readily in the experimental situation. When mother returns they avoid her or become angry if she interferes with them. Chiefly they ignore her, as if she is of no consequence to them. Indeed she may be of little consequence to them. These children will readily ignore or make up to the stranger. The key observation is that they are not wary of the strange person. These infants do not have any security with the caregiver, and to some extent at least, have given her up as a bad job. Yet they are neither settled nor competent children. Their emotional dependency needs have not been met and they remain preoccupied with basic instrumental survival needs. They may see little place for mother. Fortunately such children, in our experience, are not very common.

3. Disorganised-disoriented attachment
This type of attachment was added to the classification by Mary Main (Main & Solomon, 1990). These infants appear confused in the experimental situation. They can freeze and not move at all, or they may move slowly and without purpose.

119

These infants appear stunned or disoriented. These children are at the end of their tether. Many are depressed and inactive (as you may recall from earlier chapter inactivity is not normally in the nature of children). Some are hypervigilant. So something has gone badly wrong. These infants may well be victims of abuse from which there is no escape.

The "strange situation": comments and criticism

Attachment behaviour as measured by the "strange situation" test varies somewhat from culture to culture (Levine & Miller, 1990). This fact supports some of the current criticism of the technique. Many infants in today's society will be a lot more used to separation from their caregiver than the subjects tested by Ainsworth. Day care for infants has accustomed many of them to separation and indeed taught them that such separation is only for a short time. When these infants are placed in the "strange situation" they may not respond to short separations from mother as Ainsworth would expect, yet they may be securely attached children.

Nevertheless, the strange situation test is, on the whole, a stable and reliable measure (Sroufe, 1985; Friedman & Boyle, 2008). The experimental situation may be artificial for children but it reflects the types of attachments that can be observed in the community, and agrees with other lines of thought that investigate the relationship between infants and those who care for them. In general, studies have found that insecure attachment is associated with various forms of child maltreatment. Insecure resistant attachment tends to be associated with inconsistent care (Sroufe, 1988), while insecure avoidant attachment is associated with parents who are usually indifferent or frequently unavailable (Isabella, 1993).

Attachment as a key to development

There is no doubt that investigation or observation of attachments in infancy helps us to understand the developmental process, and to understand this process when conditions for children are adverse or far from optimal. Attachment is one of the mechanisms that can be evoked to explain the development of emotions. Attachment itself is, however, not the initial impetus for emotional development, but rather a means of satisfying that impetus. The impetus is the child's need to survive and have contact with other beings, in other words the impetus arises from the child's dependent state and the need to satisfy and reduce dependency needs. It appears from both animal experiments (Harlow and his monkeys; Harlow & Harlow, 1962), and from studies of children, that a warm and affectionate caregiver is needed for normal development in the emotional sphere. When infants are dependent they are very sensitive as far as development is concerned. Actions taken during this dependent sensitive period can have both immediate effects and effects that may last for many years even into adolescence and adulthood. This is particularly true where circumstances early in infancy and childhood have been particularly adverse, for example when children have been reared in certain institutions. The work of Michael Rutter (Rutter, *et al.*, 1990; Kreppne, *et al.*, 2007) brings this home as does other work in Eastern Europe (Dubrovina & Ruzska, 1990; Hoksbergen, 2005).

However, we need to be careful not to stipulate the details of the warm affectionate relationship that satisfies and reduces a child's dependency. Children do not need to be reared by their biological mother, though she usually does a good job. Indeed children can be reared well by more than one person. Children can form a number of attachments that satisfy their dependency needs. Indeed it is the satisfaction of dependency needs that is the crucial issue, not to whom the child is attached, or the number of people to whom he or she is attached. In very adverse circumstances the adaptable nature of children has led to strange but enduring attachments, and people have grown emotionally and in other ways in spite of everything. Read Facey's *A Fortunate Life* (1981) as an example of what we mean. Siblings, friends, grandparents, teachers, and others, can serve attachment functions and in doing so satisfy the child's dependency needs.

Many children of course do not have these needs fully serviced by others and they bring themselves up fully or in part. However, they do so at a cost. Children in childcare, for example, may be securely attached to their mothers despite long hours of separation; however this is dependent on the quality of the reciprocal relations with the child care workers, the hours of contact with the mother and the sensitivity of the mothers interaction in that time (Friedman & Boyle, 2008). If this equation does not add up to overall quality experiences for the child insecure attachment may develop with subsequent poor emotional outcomes. There is no doubt that an understanding of attachment processes will help us to understand infants, children, adolescents, and adults, and the development of their emotions.

Temperament

So far in this chapter we have discussed concepts and processes that can explain, in part at least, the development of secondary emotions in infants and children. The underlying force behind the creation of a range of positive and negative secondary emotions in any person is that person's dependency in infancy and childhood and the degree to which his or her needs are satisfied by care. Thus children vary in their emotions largely because they have had different emotional histories. The quality of this care and its effect in producing (or not producing) secondary emotions both positive and negative in a child can be described, and to some degree explained, by reference to the attachment patterns that children show.

Yet children who receive, what, on the face of it, is the same quality of care, for example brothers and sisters in a family, often turn out to be quite different emotionally and in other ways. Or so it seems. What may be seen as a difference in emotion by some observers may well be seen only as a difference in emotional expression by others. It is often the case that outsiders may view family members as very similar people emotionally and in other ways, yet the members of that family may feel they have very distinct differences that distinguish them one from another. Anyone who has reared a number of children is usually impressed by the differences between them, irrespective of what outsiders may think, especially when the rearing which each child received is judged to be the same. Given very similar environmental circumstances why are children still notably different one from another?

Despite different viewpoints many people are convinced that there must be more to the development of emotion than differences in environmental circumstances. The answer may be that infants are born different one from another. What we are referring to are *genetic differences*. Most of these differences are inherited. This brings us to innate physical attributes. There are obvious physical features of people that are largely genetically determined and cannot be affected to any great degree by environmental effects. But what about emotions? We know that there are innate basic emotions and these probably have a strong inherited component. As regards secondary emotions the question is whether they also have genetic determinants. As we have already stated genetic and environmental effects *always* interact and this is true of emotional development. There is no way that genetic inherited effects can express themselves in a child or a person independently of the environment of that child or person. However, the fact that these effects always interact with the environment does not rule out the existence of differences between children reared in the same environment. There are such differences and they can to a major degree be explained by genetic inheritance. However, the picture is complicated; let us explain further.

Where the environments of a number of children are the same (or as similar, in terms of nurturance, as can be achieved) we may presume that the differences seen between these children stem from the different genetic inheritance that each child shows. Or, to put it more accurately, because genetic inheritance on its own cannot express itself, the differences between these children stem from the different patterns of interaction given by the different genetic inheritance of each child with the same environment. There is no such thing in nature as a genotype; a genotype is the genetic plan for an individual posited in his or her DNA. However, without interaction with the individual's environment, which turns genes on and off, a genotype remains a blueprint, a theoretical abstraction. All living things are phenotypes; they are expressions of genetic/environmental interactions.

Nevertheless, because phenotypes are always due to genetic/environmental interaction, we can, when the environmental part of the interaction is constant, observe differences between children that can be construed to be chiefly genetic in nature. To make such a construction, however, we must be sure that children with such differences have indeed been subject to identical or at least almost identical environmental circumstances. Because early infant development is so rapid and the changes wrought in the brain of an infant so extensive, so profound, and so subject to external effects, we often cannot be sure of the constancy of environmental effects. This is what brings in complex arguments about early subtle environmental differences before, at, and after birth.

What interests us is whether children are born with certain differences that affect their emotional development and produce variations between them in this sphere. Many people suspect that this is so, but quantifying the degree to which it is true is hard to achieve.

The problem is that human beings always exist in an environment. This is true even in the womb, and certainly after birth. This environment will always affect the child be it foetus or infant. Thus to separate and quantify inherited genetic influences from other influences is very difficult. Psychologists have attempted to do this by means of studies involving twins, both identical and non-identical. Identical twins have the same genetic inheritance whereas non-identical twins are no more alike genetically than any two other siblings. However, comparative studies of identical and non-identical twins have given no clear finding on the relative contribution of genetics and environment. All we can say for certain is that both are involved. It has become clear that even identical twins reared together do not share exactly the same environment. If they did they would have exactly the same neural connections and this is not so (Edelman, 1992). Idiosyncratic elements can affect one identical twin and not the other, even if they are reared in the same place. Those of you who have worked in child protection may well have come across the relatively common situation in abuse cases where one identical twin in a household is abused and scapegoated while the other is not. Many researchers believe that *non-shared environmental influences* are important in determining a child's characteristics. These influences can vary between identical twins reared together as they can between siblings. So there may be non-shared environmental influences on people in general and on twins, who were brought up together and share identical genetic codes. This does not, however, deny the fact that twins are very similar in many ways. Early non-shared environmental influences do not exclude stronger genetic ones.

Let us not pursue these nature/nurture arguments further but fix our attention on differences between children that can to a large degree be seen as inherent and due, as far as we can determine, to the influence of genetic inheritance. Obviously these differences will have some effect on a child's emotional development and must be considered when we look at the emotional history of an individual. *"These differences are biologically based and are linked to an individual's genetic endowment"* (Posner, *et al.*, 2007, p. 207). They are referred to as differences in temperament.

Temperament is therefore an influence on emotional development, though we would not call it an important process or a determining feature, the neural history of the newborn is too environmentally influenced for that. Nevertheless, let us expand on the idea of temperament and its possible influence on emotional development.

What is temperament?

Temperament is about genetic difference especially difference in how we react to the world. We are all different. Each of us is unique. All parents of more than one child can give testament to the fact that each child has their own personal qualities that are obvious very early in life. In particular our distinct contributions to family life are observed early, and it is our distinctiveness in social and emotional spheres that is commonly referred to as our temperament. Are we born different? Most of us believe so. Does temperament then refer to these inborn differences? The word temperament implies a genetic foundation for individual differences in *emotional and behavioural style*. Though this implication must be heavily considered as we discuss temperament it cannot be absolutely relied upon. What we mean by temperament may originate in innate genetic qualities but these will undoubtedly be mixed with early environmental influences. Indeed Bates (1987) stated that studies showed some equivocation as to whether there was a pure concept of biologically rooted temperament that could easily be measured.

To sum up, infants do not all react in the same way to the same degree of frustration, or satisfaction, or change. They vary considerably. Some children will respond to these influences with a great deal of activity, others will be more placid. Some will quickly engage their social surroundings; others will take more time to do so. Perhaps these variations in reaction are, at the very least, *partly* genetic, *partly* inherited. Whatever they are they reflect that particular child's style of response. Temperament is in fact *a style and a degree of responsiveness*.

If we consider the nature of emotion and its components we will realise that a style of responding will influence emotional expression much more than the other two components of emotion, the subjective feeling and the physiological concomitants. It is therefore in the area of emotional expression where temperament has most effect and this is true whether we are considering basic emotions on the one hand or secondary emotions on the other. Let us now consider the major studies of temperament.

The studies of Thomas and Chess

Thomas and Chess (1977; 1984) defined temperament as the consistent pattern in the way in which an individual performs an action. *How* they perform the activity rather than *why* they do it or *what* they actually do. Thomas and Chess picked out nine dimensions of temperament as follows:

1. *Approach versus withdrawal* from new experiences. The type of initial reaction a child has to a new person or a new situation.
2. Eventual *adaptation* to changes. The extent to which approach or withdrawal (see above) is modified with time.
3. Positivity versus negativity of *mood*.
4. *Intensity* of emotional reactions.
5. *Rhythmicity* of biological functioning. Extent to which biological functions, eating, sleeping, eliminating, etc., are predictable and regular.
6. *Persistence* in the face of environmental counterforces. The degree to which the child can ignore interruptions.
7. *Distractability* (this includes soothability when upset). The extent to which the child changes behaviour when interrupted. Inverse of persistence.
8. *Activity* level. Degree of movement, speed of movement, plus degree of other activity.
9. *Threshold* of stimulation necessary for a response.

Using the first five of these dimensions Thomas and Chess classified infants as follows, the *easy* infant; the *difficult* infant; and the infant who is *slow to warm up*.

The *easy infant* sleeps well, eats well and copes easily with change. The difficult infant has irregular sleeping, may be colicky, eats inconsistently and withdraws from change (i.e. new objects and people). The *"slow warmer"* infant has a low activity level and adapts slowly to change.

Thomas and Chess *suggest* that these temperaments are obvious from birth. These researchers found that temperamental types in infants can be traced into later childhood and adolescence. Thus older children showed signs of their earlier temperament. This may be so but the question arises whether the temperament is innate or partly due to learning in the very early days of life. The questions remain as to whether a child's temperament is completely inherited or completely learned or, as we believe, due to a combination of innate factors *and* very early experience.

That there is *a strong* hereditary component involved is suggested by the fact that Thomas and Chess found these temperamental differences to exist across cultures and child rearing practices. They found no sex difference in temperament. Whether these temperamental differences are due to heredity or learning or a combination of both is in the end not pertinent. Such differences are observable and real and must be taken into account when working with children. A child's temperament, easy, difficult, or whatever, is a factor in the way a child reacts emotionally and also, very importantly, in the way a parent reacts to the child. Both a child's temperament and a caregiver's reaction to it must be thoughtfully considered by those who try to understand the child's emotional history.

Many studies have supported Thomas and Chess. Korner (1967) had earlier found considerable differences between infants in respect of their ease of satisfaction after feeding and the degree to which they wanted to be cuddled. Nevertheless, we must recognise the difficulty in examining young infants with regard to inherited disposition when very early experiences, even pre-natal experiences, may also have a definite effect.

The studies of Buss and Plomin and Bates

Buss and Plomin

These researchers (Buss & Plomin, 1975; 1984) emphasise that temperament arises from genetic inheritance. They picked only three factors arising from such inheritance.

- *Emotionality*. The degree to which a child becomes negatively aroused.
- *Activity*. The degree of energy shown by the child.
- *Sociability*. The degree to which the child seems to need people.

Buss and Plomin suggested that these factors have a physiological basis, the base of which is in turn genetic. Physiological processes can of course, like neural or psychological processes, also be influenced by environmental factors.

Our experience with children in adverse circumstances suggests that a better explanation for a display of negative emotion or negative mood is the way a child is treated. We also feel that sociability is greatly affected by the child's environment. However, it is possible that a child's tendency to be distressed (negative arousal) is *in part* inherited. Nevertheless, most of the negative arousal that we have witnessed has had an easy environmental explanation. Even if children inherit a tendency to be sociable (and there is no direct evidence that they do), an adverse early environment will easily subdue this tendency.

Bates

In a later survey of the field Bates (1989) identified three dimensions of temperament:

1. General activity level.
2. Quality of mood.
3. Reactivity to new situations.

What can we deduce from an amalgamation of the studies listed above? It seems that a child's style of response is governed by two main factors (that are present, or can be inferred, in all these studies). The first of these is the *degree of activity* that a child habitually shows. Is the child an active or a placid child or somewhere in between? The second factor that we can deduce from all of these studies is the degree to which the child relates to people; how *sociable* he or she is. There may be other factors that refer to a child's emotional style but these two are, in our experience, undoubtedly the most obvious and the most important. They are important because they affect the adult's reaction to the child and this forms part of the child's social environment.

Stability of temperament

If temperament is to be a useful concept it must indicate some enduring qualities in the child, qualities that remain stable over the years. Can we trace stable temperamental qualities through childhood adolescence and beyond?

Researchers have found most difficulty in tracing temperament through the first year of life. It seems that temperamental characteristics are more stable the further we proceed into childhood. It is particularly difficult to prove the stability of temperament from birth to one year (Sroufe *et al.*, 1996; Worobey & Blajda, 1989). Perhaps this is because so much happens so quickly in that first year. Whatever the cause, indications of temperament in the early months of life are not very valid predictors of temperament when the child reaches one year. Temperament is more stable later, and this in itself is interesting, but the problem of the first year suggests that we may not be measuring genetically determined traits but those formed on a genetic base and then greatly influenced by early experience. The influence of early experience may be so profound, and so fixed and stable at one year, that it appears to resemble a physiological genetic disposition.

We are not sure of the details of the relationship between inborn traits and the effect of early experience. Most researchers feel there is a significant interaction between the factors that produce temperament. What we are confident about is the relative stability of temperamental traits from one year onwards. Indeed as age increases so does the stability of temperament. Temperament at one year is a good predictor of temperament at pre-school entry (three to four years). Thomas and Chess traced temperamental characteristics from infancy into adolescence. There is no doubt that the *way* in which children approach tasks and other challenges (*how* they do things), remains fairly stable for most children for long periods in childhood. In some cases this stability may extend into adolescence and adult life.

Temperament and attachment

If we now turn again to attachment patterns that lead to distinct differences between children in terms of their emotional growth, we may well ask the following question. Are attachment patterns, that is secure and insecure attachment, anything

127

more than a reflection of the interactions of temperaments between the children and the adults involved? This question has been investigated by Bates and other researchers and the conclusion reached was that attachment and temperament are two different things (Bates *et al.*, 1985). Temperament is the child's way of doing things, while attachment is a measure of a relationship that can or cannot be relied on. Temperament is a style of behaving that does not vary even when the child interacts with different people, while attachment has a particular reference to a specific caregiver or other person. Observations of children in, say, secure attachment situations show that they can be of any temperamental type. Some are active, others are passive, some react strongly, others do not, etc.; yet all have security in the relationship and use it as a base for exploration. In the same way infants with insecure attachment, of whatever sub-type, show a range of temperaments. No matter what their temperament they show no real faith in the relationship. How they manifest this lack of security may, however, be related to their temperamental characteristics (Belsky & Rovine, 1987).

A child's temperament does affect the way he or she interacts with carers, and an adult's temperament affects the way that the adult reacts to the child, but if the adult services the child's dependency needs on a consistent basis, then secure attachment will be achieved. If the temperament of the adult and child are at odds, then this will make the relationship more difficult but not impossible. This is good news for parents who have a highly reactive child who does not settle easily. Though things may be difficult, if the parent persists in satisfying the child's dependency needs consistently, then a secure attachment will occur. Of course if a parent has support in dealing with a child with a difficult temperament then the period and the intensity of the stress in the relationship will be less. These dynamics between the carers' and the infants' temperaments are explained in a '*goodness of fit*' model, where the degree of difference in temperament is influential in the amount of accommodations that the parent has to make for the child. In other words parents with children whose temperaments are different to their own must be flexible, adaptive and sensitive to the child's different needs.

This is where the provision of adequate supports for parents through extended family and social services comes in. Some parents have difficulty in accommodating their child's different needs. Where no support is forthcoming things are more difficult for longer, though if the parent does not give up or withdraw emotionally, things will come right in the end.

All in all, the important factor in the child-caregiver relationship is the caregiver. Infants who are difficult can cause the caregiver some problems, but most deeply troubled children and adolescents are products of parental lack of care not their own temperaments. It is not necessary for parents (or caregivers) and children to be suited to each other in emotional style for satisfactory outcomes to be achieved.

Overview of psychological dynamics

In this chapter we have looked at processes and influences in development. The most powerful force influencing development is the child's need to survive and the negative emotion of fear is prominent in this process. A child's dependency needs are therefore central to his or her emotional development. Perhaps the most common way in which a child's dependency needs are satisfied is through an attachment to a single caregiver. However, multiple attachments and other arrangements may well be satisfactory providing they give the child support, not only in areas of instrumental dependency, but also in the sphere of emotional dependence. Any arrangement will suffice if it allows the child to survive physiologically, and also gives him or her positive warm and stable emotional contact.

Children will react differently and express their emotions differently depending on their temperament which is largely an inherited feature. Temperament may well be a very influential factor in emotional expression. However, the issue of whether or not a child develops certain emotions, and the degree to which these secondary emotions are developed, does not depend on temperament. Rather it depends on those factors that impinge on the infant's early environment (or later factors in the young child's environment) particularly those factors influencing the child's relationships, especially those relationships that bring satisfaction, comfort, and joy.

Where an infant or toddler has little satisfaction comfort or joy emotional deprivation may occur. Our next chapter examines care and parenting and the way in which secondary emotional development may be affected by poor regimes of care.

Questions to think about

1. Why should mothers/principal caregivers fade into the background over the 0–18 period?
2. What is bonding?
3. Distinguish between secure and insecure attachment.
4. What is the relationship between dependency, attachment, and emotional development?
5. Name the three sub-types of insecure attachment and describe each.
6. Describe parental behaviours related to insecure attachment.
7. Discuss stability of temperament.
8. What can modify temperament?
9. What divisions did Thomas and Chess use to classify the infant temperament of young infants?

Suggested further reading

Eisenberg, N. (2006) Introduction. In W. Damon, R. M. Lerner, & N. Eisenberg (Eds). *Handbook of Child Psychology, Social, Emotional, and Personality Development* (Vol. 3) (pp. 1–23). Wiley. com.

Bernier, A., Carlson, S. M. Deschênes, M., & Matte-Gagné, C. (2012). Social factors in the development of early executive functioning: a closer look at the caregiving environment. *Developmental Science, 15*(1), 12–24, seminal attachment articles.

Graziano, P. A., Calkins, S. D. & Keane, S. P. (2011). Sustained attention development during the toddlerhood to preschool period: Associations with toddlers' emotion regulation strategies and maternal behaviour. *Infant and Child Development, 20*(6), 389–408.

Parenting, care and the development of secondary emotions

chapter 7

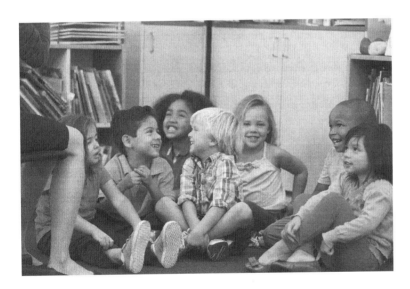

- Usually the central factor in care for children is the quality of parenting that they receive. The reciprocal relationship between the child and parents is highly influential here; more so than later parenting style.
- Warm affectionate contact is needed to develop effective communication and mutual respect between parent and child. This is the core of a

- strong reciprocal relationship which is needed for healthy emotional development.
- Authoritative parenting style is the most efficacious and helpful for healthy emotional development.
- Research shows that approximately 35 per cent of abused children go on to abuse their children. Intergenerational abusive parenting appears frequently in case work practice, but there are many who escape this pattern.
- Not good-enough parenting occurs in three ways: through general neglect of the child's needs; through inconsistent care; and through over-parenting and failure to develop the child's independence.

A CHILD'S EMOTIONAL DEVELOPMENT is closely related to the satisfaction of that child's dependency needs in infancy. The fulfilment of these needs and especially the fulfilment of the need for warm emotional contact is the basis of a child's first relationship and it is this relationship or attachment that leads to other relationships and a child's social life. It is out of social experience in association with growing cognition that secondary emotions develop and it is the quality of these social experiences that dictate the nature of the secondary emotions that are formed and the degree to which they are developed.

We refer to secondary emotions when discussing emotional development but we must not forget that children will possess from birth the universal quick basic emotions which will only change to a minor degree throughout life. All people have basic emotions but not all children will develop all of the secondary emotions. It depends on their circumstances of rearing and the quality of care given to them during infancy and toddlerhood. There are both positive and negative secondary emotions and children from circumstances of emotional deprivation whose need for warm emotional contact and communication has not been met may well develop strong negative feelings from their early social contacts. Such children may also fail to develop positive secondary emotions that develop from an experience of mutual love. Where love has been intermittent children may develop secondary emotions that are weak and do not motivate them. Many children from emotional deprivation, as they grow older, find it difficult to fit with society's expected standards of behaviour. In short they have not been appropriately socialised and this is because they lack the appropriate secondary emotions or only have these emotions in a weakened form. Secondary emotions such as guilt, shame and empathy are necessary for a peaceful and considerate society and, where these emotions are largely absent or are not prominent motivators of social attitudes and action, social harmony will break down. We need therefore to develop regimes of care for children that provide for the development of pro-social secondary emotions. To do this we need to understand those other regimes of care that lead to poor or absent development of these secondary emotions. Usually a central factor in care for children is the quality of parenting that they receive.

The nature of parenting

What is parenting and how much of it is required? Parenting is the most common type of care that exists in human societies. It is essential for the survival of children who are all born helpless and is usually delivered by a child's natural mother and father though in exceptional circumstances it can be delivered by other people. Because of the helpless nature of the newborn baby parenting is most important in the early years of life especially in the infant and toddler stages when much neurological, psychological and physical development takes place. It is the influence of parenting in these periods which give it great importance in the development of individuals. In the early years the environment of the child can change the child's brain structure and because children are cared for by parents or parent substitutes during these periods parenting can physically affect the brains of children and therefore their subsequent behaviour. There are other influences on a developing child, including their inherited temperament that can influence their current and subsequent behaviour but there is no doubt that parenting is the major environmental influence and probably outweighs genetic effects especially when the parenting is inadequate and does not fully cater for the child's dependency needs.

How much parenting is needed? The younger the child the more he or she needs care. Infants need the full care regime because they cannot do anything for themselves. As children develop they need less physical care and they become more independent and learn to do things for themselves. All of this seems self-evident and obvious but a child's ability both to develop independence and to conform to the rules of society comes from elements delivered (or not delivered) by the parent or carer during the crucial infant and toddler stages. In infancy the most important of these elements is the child's need to communicate and feel warmly valued by the parent. This need on the child's part for emotional warmth and recognition as a psychological being is crucial for the development of secondary emotions, and if this need in infancy and toddlerhood is not catered for the development of these emotions will be affected. Parenting therefore must deliver warm emotional care to the infant. If parents do not deliver such care they are inadequate parents and will affect the child's future adversely. Parental care must also insure that the child survives. These are the two essential elements of successful parenting. Research has borne out these essentials. Sharp and Fonagy in 2008 wrote "The importance of parenting practices for children's psychosocial adjustment has been an undisputed tenet of developmental psychology" (p. 737). They back up this statement by referring to the work of Gottman, Katz and Hooven in 1996. Sharp and Fonagy emphasise the importance of the parent's ability to recognise the child as a psychological

133

agent in need of warm affectionate care. For example, an infant's first cry should be seen by a parent as the child's first communication and the parent should respond immediately to the cry. For most children direct eye contact between parent and infant is also of crucial importance if the child is to be regarded as a psychological being (Hoffman, 1987; Panksepp *et al.*, 1985; Schore, 2003). According to some researchers the child has an inbuilt response to the human face (Cassia *et al.*, 2001; Cassia *et al.*, 2004). For seeing children this response and eye to eye contact is central to the establishment of a warm psychological relationship between parent and child and if this eye contact is obstructed or does not occur for whatever reason then developmental difficulties of an emotional kind will lie ahead. Blind children do not seek this eye contact and in their case tactile and auditory experiences may service the warm emotional and communicative contact that is essential between parent and child. It is the contact that is important not the sensory mode through which it is delivered.

So it appears that effective parenting in the first year must attend to all the infant's dependency needs particularly his or her need for emotional contact and warmth. Is there any evidence of a physiological mechanism that points to the importance of warm parental care? Here the new science of epigenetics is informative, see Roth and Sweatt (2011). We have no real account of the physiology behind warm parental care but we have evidence of the physiological consequences of early childhood abuse. Hyman (2009) states that evidence from animal studies suggests that epigenetic regulation of receptors in the hippocampus area, the memory area in the mid-brain, mediate early experiences into adult life. McGowan and others (2009) substantiate Hyman's suggestion and state that childhood abuse increases stress responses and later in life increases the risk of suicide and therefore confirms that parental care has an epigenetic regulation of hippocampal receptor expression.

Is care in the first year sufficient and what of later years? In the 1950s and 1960s Donald Winnicott, a paediatrician and psychoanalyst gave a very helpful explanation of parenting (Rodman, 2003). Winnicott pointed out that parents are never perfect and children can inherit difficult temperaments. How can parenting be perfect in such circumstances? The answer is that it need not be perfect. Somehow the vast majority of children in all kinds of circumstance seem to develop adequately and do not suffer the effects of emotional or cognitive deprivation. Winnicott explained that even with imperfections in the parent and genetic difficulties in the child it still is very possible, providing a few conditions are met, for parents to deliver care that is "*good-enough*" to allow for full normal development in the child. Winnicott's conditions are, however, very important riders on this idea. He believed that infancy is the most important stage and that it is necessary during this stage for a parent in order to be "*good-enough*" to attend fully and promptly to all the needs of the infant. The parent is providing what Winnicott called *the holding environment* for the infant. After infancy according to Winnicott it is necessary for a parent to very gradually withdraw this total care and slowly introduce the toddler to what Winnicott called *objective reality*. Thus after infancy the parent does not do everything for the child and does not always respond immediately to the child's demands. In this way the parent gradually introduces the child to the idea of the parent as a separate being from the child. This gradual modification of care begins to develop ideas of self and agency in the toddler. If parents begin with a total care in infancy but then gradually introduce objective reality, parents are, according to Winnicott, *good-enough* and other issues in parenting including parenting style do not matter; the child will develop in a normal way. Winnicott thus first spelt out the essentials of parenting and pointed to a threshold of care that must be reached if parenting is to be effective. His approach allows for parental imperfections and for all kinds of combinations in parenting that are due to the different inherited genetic qualities and developmental experiences of both parent and child. Providing both his conditions are met parenting will be "*good-enough*" and other influences will account for differences between children and how they develop. However, if parenting is not *good-enough* then it becomes a major influence in a child's development and the major factor in the adjustment of that person to adult life. All of these ideas emphasise the importance of care and parenting in the early years and Winnicott's ideas are supported by modern approaches, research and our clinical experience.

When parenting is not good-enough

The first way in which parenting may be ineffective is when parents neglect the dependency needs of their infants. These parents often put their own needs first and do not attend fully and promptly to the dependency needs of their infant. They are therefore in Winnicott's terminology *not good-enough*. This neglect can be total, all needs can be neglected, but more frequently the physical needs of the children are marginally and grudgingly catered for and delivered without emotional warmth. This insensitive parenting involves a lack of a positive emotional response on the part of the parent towards the infant and such a parent generally spends as little time as possible with the child. Sroufe (2002) calls this type of maltreatment *psychological unavailability* and states that it is a devastating form of care.

If this insensitivity is total children in their first year can develop a lot of anger from frustration and little else (see Figure 4.3). They have no experience of mutual love because they have had no warm psychological interaction with people. In their second and third year therefore, they will fail to develop the first signs of secondary emotions such as pity, shame, pride, guilt and empathy and these emotions will not appear in future years (see Figure 5.1). These children may become survivors in spite of their parents and because they lack emotional connection to anyone often become uninhibited. One cannot have inhibitions if emotional approval or disapproval for actions is missing. Many of these children are also hyperactive. They move continually and are unmanageable. Hyperactivity can frequently be a symptom of unhappiness, that is, of emotional deprivation. Though these children have no subjective feelings corresponding to the positive secondary emotions, if they are intelligent, some of them, but by no means all, may come to understand that, by contriving the expression of these emotions, they can manipulate people and gain their own objectives. In this behaviour they express not emotions but pseudo-emotions. Children in this position do not know what positive emotions are, never having been loved, and though they recognise the outward trappings of positive emotion (i.e. the expression), they have never experienced the inner subjective feelings of contentment that are the essence of positive emotion. Thus some of these children indulge in positive emotional expression but do not experience inner joy. They may well experience inner anger. They can be very manipulative in their affectionate behaviour, and are glib and shifting in their friendships. These children can kiss and hug people on scant acquaintance. Kisses and hugs have less meaning for them so they are randomly given. Many of these children will not express positive secondary emotions at all.

If the emotional insensitivity of the parents is not total and some emotional care is given at random the child gains emotional contact with the parent but only on an inconsistent basis. This child cannot predict when the emotional contact will take place. The psychological insensitivity on the parents' part is only partial and the child does receive some warm emotional attention on unpredictable occasions. In this case secondary emotions will form but their power to motivate the child will be limited. This is because the child's attention and energy will be taken up with a consuming and neurotic search for more consistent attention and affection. Children who are given this type of poor care taste attention and approval only to have it withdrawn. This usually leads the child on an anxious quest, inappropriately pursued, for love and recognition. In these circumstances the child continually seeks contact with the parent, most of which is not reciprocated, in order to gain emotional relief. However, unpredictably, every so often, the parent will respond with appropriate affection. The inconsistency of this emotional satisfaction, where the child is rewarded randomly for seeking attention, simply causes more attention seeking. This regime of random emotional reward is a most powerful reinforcer and the child's attention seeking becomes chronic whenever the child is with parents or other people. The development of this unfulfilling neurotic behaviour is most likely to occur if a child has had inconsistent psychological attention. It is less likely if a parent has never had much psychological contact at all with the child.

The continual attention seeking of these children explains why the secondary emotions, though present, are of limited motivational power. The children are too busy seeking attention and affection. The exception to this is the development of envy and jealousy. These secondary emotions are particularly strong and motivational in these children because in their development they combine a little insecure love with a strong development of anxious fear that arises from the unpredictability that the children face. Such a child greatly fears the loss of the little amount of love given and cannot see that there is enough love for all thus becoming jealous and, perhaps later, envious.

Winnicott stated that parents should attend fully and promptly to the needs of their infants. If parents did not attend to these needs, or only did so inconsistently, then parenting was *not good-enough* and the child would suffer emotional problems in later years. Was this the only way in which Winnicott saw parenting as being *not good-enough*? Could his concerns about the second year of parenting and his ideas of what should be introduced at this stage be relevant? Winnicott believed that toddlers should be slowly introduced to what he called *objective reality*, that is to the idea that the toddlers' parents were not servants of the toddlers catering for their every desire but were separate persons who had to be taken account of as the toddlers tried new experiences.

This second way in which parenting can be ineffective is, in some aspects, the opposite of the first. It is possible for parents to continue to fully and promptly serve their children's needs, meeting every eventuality, when such complete care is no longer necessary and is counterproductive to the child's best interests. These parents cosset too much and smother the first signs of instrumental independence or exploration in their children. Such parenting is also *not good-enough* and can have long term consequences for the child. This type of parenting for a toddler can create over-dependence in that opportunities for independence are not given. The lack of these opportunities to exercise independence causes the child to lose confidence in him- or herself. To compensate for a lack of confidence and an ability to proceed independently the child seeks further dependence. This pleases the parent who does not want, for whatever reason, the child to become independent. The flight into unnecessary dependence further reduces the building of self-confidence, and a vicious circle is commenced. Children who are over-parented in this way are protected but they are often anxious and unhappy. We can only be happily dependent if we have successfully tested our independence. Thus children test parents. As thinking toddlers they emphasise their dependency needs to see if they will be met. Are they loved and cared for? But they also test their independence. Are they allowed to be themselves? For most toddlers such testing achieves the positive results they require for further development. Their parents have slowly introduced them to the real world, to *objective reality*, and to ideas of waiting, control and restraint. Sometimes clashes between parent and toddler may be severe but if parents passively resist undue toddler demands *objective reality* is reinforced in the toddler's mind and it is only by knowing the true nature of the outside world that toddlers can commence the long road to genuine independence.

But what if parents do not passively resist ridiculous toddler demands and instead cater for every toddler need as if the child was still an infant? The psychological and emotional development of such a child will be hindered. These children fail to develop a psychological distinction between themselves and their parents. Their sense of self is hindered and their ideas of how other people think may be dysfunctional. In other words they will not have developed the beginnings of an accurate 'theory of mind'. Many over-cosseted children attempt to break their parents' suffocating care and some succeed, but others lose the will to explore and become over-dependent on their carer. This type of parenting is not common as most parents take a delight in their children's independent accomplishments but it can occur and it is *not good-enough*.

Another form of parenting that is *not good-enough* is when parents fear that the child's development will give them more difficulty than the previous stage and therefore they restrain the child physically (and psychologically) to prevent the occurrence of crawling and walking. This restraint on development is in fact physical abuse and often these parents may lock their children in rooms in order as they say 'to get some peace'. This and other forms of abuse, of course, come under the title of *not good-enough* parenting.

Finally Sroufe (2002) points out that parenting should be suited to the level of maturity of the child involved. He singles out over-stimulation of children as ineffective parenting. Infants and toddlers need stimulation for mental and physical growth but they should not be over-stimulated by parents who wish to accelerate their child's development. Sroufe states that such intensive and intrusive parenting involving over-stimulation in infancy and toddlerhood may well produce behaviour problems in later years.

Intergenerational influences on parenting

How do parents learn to parent? Are they instructed in what to do with this new life that has suddenly become their responsibility? Most new parents are not given lessons in parenting. Historically though many girls were given preparation for mothering through experience with younger siblings, or nieces and nephews from their older siblings; changing family structure means that this no longer the case. Today there are advisory agencies and books that can help but most parents proceed with their parenting on the basis of their own experiences from their childhood and how they and their siblings were cared for. Parents may remember the quality of their own care when they were young though they will not be able to recall infancy and they may have observed how their parents dealt with subsequent children. In many conscious and unconscious ways they may imitate their own parents in the care they deliver to their children. This is a satisfactory situation where the previous generation of parents has been good-enough in parenting and where sensitive care is thus delivered to the latest generation. But can it also cause inadequate care and not good-enough parenting to be transmitted from one generation to the next? Is poor parenting intergenerational?

Studies have examined mothering in animals especially in primates and other mammals where care of the young is well developed. These studies show that when the natural mother is unable to care for the infant animal and the young animal is reared instead by human intervention then that hand reared animal when faced with mothering herself tends in many instances to be an inadequate mother. Harlow's experiments (1962) with rhesus monkeys clearly indicate that young monkeys who are deprived of maternal care while young find great difficulty in caring for their own infant monkeys. Yet mothering in animals is generally regarded as instinctive and under hormonal control; though from Harlow's results it would seem that early infant experience of the mothering process is also of importance at least in highly evolved mammals.

Humans are less hormonally controlled than animals and personal social and cultural influences are important in parenting processes. However, as with animals, those people who were reared by insensitive parents who did not care adequately for their dependency needs are liable to be poor parents themselves. The key element in the last sentence is the use of the word *parents*, a plural. Humans usually have two parents and when one may be insensitive to the infant's needs the other parent may compensate for this lack of concern and care. In this situation, though not ideal, parenting will be good-enough.

When both parents are not good-enough and do not attend to the infant's dependency needs especially the need for warm comforting care then the infant must learn to survive without such care and in some way comfort him- or herself. When infants do survive lack of care, and not all of them do, they develop survival mechanisms that usually do not relate to warm human interactions. In particular these children miss out on mutual affection and therefore they have little ability to defer their own needs and cater for the needs of others. Putting another's needs before one's own is the essence of sensitive parenting and very essential when the child is a completely dependent infant. When children from psychological deprivation become parents themselves they may still put their own needs first, as they have done throughout their childhood in order to survive, though now that they are adult survival is not usually an issue. It is in this way that poor inadequate parenting bridges the generations.

Sroufe (2002) and others have investigated the parent-child boundary and especially those cases where the parent violates this boundary. The parent-child boundary separates the role of a child from that of a parent. Sroufe is particularly interested in situations where a parent does not act like a parent and abandons the parental role and the duties and obligations that go with this role. Sroufe refers to work by Levy (1999) which found that such role violations persisted across the generations. Though boundary violations are only one form of insensitive parenting nevertheless this work shows that not good-enough parenting can indeed be repeated from one generation to the next.

When insensitive parenting is considered as wilful abuse other studies reveal a complex picture. Do parents who themselves were abused as children and subsequently had great difficulty in forming emotional relationships, constitute a real risk factor in the abuse of children? This certainly appears so if we look back. In many cases of children abused by their parents it will be found that the parents themselves were abused. The problem seems *intergenerational*, victims creating victims, by means of modelling, social learning, and inner identification. However, though this is easily seen looking back (in retrospect), it is much less clear looking forward (in prospect). Egeland (1989) quotes Kaufman and Zigler estimating that approximately 30 per cent of abused children become abusing parents. Thus more than two-thirds of abused children do not abuse their own offspring. In Egeland's (1989) consideration of this issue the most important factor that separated abused children who became abusers, from those who as adults did not abuse, was that the latter group had a close and supportive relationship with someone, usually a spouse, later in life. Egeland's estimate of 30 per cent of abused children going on to be abusers themselves was supported in 1997 by Dodge, Pettit and Bates who found that only 35 per cent of children who were physically abused in their early years went on to become abusers in later years.

Nevertheless, being abused as a child undoubtedly is a risk factor for later abuse of your own children. Again risk is increased but there is nothing inevitable. If you have had little positive emotional life how can you take part in that enjoyable mutual interaction that forms the basis of attachment and the reciprocal relationship? If you have not been loved and nurtured how can you learn to love and nurture others? Thankfully many abused children have gained some affection in their childhood or later and this proves a significant barrier to intergenerational abuse.

The cycle of intergenerational poor parenting may be broken by human factors particularly by the advent of one parent in the next generation who parents well. It may also be broken by the involvement of another sensitive carer in the childhood of the younger generation or a supportive friend or spouse later in life. Insensitive parenting in one generation is not therefore a particularly good predictor of future insensitive parenting. Yet for all that it is important to realise that poor parenting can often be seen across the generations.

Parenting styles

In 1971 Baumrind outlined three main ways in which parents could relate to their children. Since then these styles of parenting have been much investigated. Each style centres around three interactions between parent(s) and child. The first interaction is the degree to which the child is *accepted* by the parent and this extends to the degree of *involvement* shown by the parent with the child. The next interaction is the *degree of control* exercised by the parent over the child's behaviour. The third issue is the *degree of autonomy* that the parent allows the child.

In *authoritative* parenting the parent is warmly accepting of the child and his or her needs which are usually catered for in a sensitive fashion. In this style the parent makes reasonable demands of the child to be socialised and explains the need for such control to the child while consistently enforcing the parental requests sometimes using non-coercive discipline when required. The same parent, however, will allow the child autonomy to make his or her own decisions when the parent believes the child is sufficiently mature to make such decisions. In general this granting of autonomy is gradual and increases as the child matures until full independence is reached.

In contrast the *authoritarian* style of parenting can be seen to be cold in its consideration of the child and though the child's needs may be met there is a lack of warm emotional expression towards the child though the underlying subjective feeling may be warm. This style concentrates on adult control of the child. Children are expected to behave totally in accordance with parental demands and to do so without question. Punishment is used if the child does not comply and sometimes this can be severe. In this style of parenting little or no autonomy is given to the child, the parent makes all the decisions and does not consult the child.

A third style of parenting is called *permissive*. In this style the child is warmly accepted and his or her needs are catered for, indeed sometimes overindulged. However, no control is placed on the child who is seen as responsible for making their own decisions regardless of age or maturity. Thus autonomy is totally granted from the outset with no real understanding that true independence in a child is related to adult guidance.

Research shows clearly that the most successful style of parenting is the middle way *authoritative* approach. On the whole it produces children who have good relations with their parents, their peers and society. Can we then take this style as the standard for good parenting? We can but nevertheless other styles of parenting can be *good-enough*. Effective adults have come from both *authoritarian* and *permissive* families. While not desirable, both these styles of parenting can deliver the essentials of *good-enough* parenting. Such parents can service an infant's needs fully and promptly and in their own ways can introduce children to objective reality and the world of other people. The *authoritarian* and *permissive* parents can transmit problems to their children but nevertheless parents using these styles can be sensitive to the child's needs.

The key issue in parenting is not parenting style but whether the parents place the child's needs before their own. In other words do the parents love the child? Permissive parents can do this, they can love their child and authoritarian parents can also love their children and act in the child's interest rather than their own. It is also possible for authoritative parents who explain things in detail to the child, and grant gradual autonomy, to put their own interests first and neglect those of the child. This is not likely with this style but it can occur though one could then argue that if this happens the parents have not warmly accepted the child.

Parenting styles are a complex matter because like any typology few parents fall neatly into a distinct category and some parents can change their style of parenting over time. Styles of parenting reflect strengths and weakness in the care of children but in the end it is the loving relationship or lack thereof between the parent and child that really counts. This relationship must fully service infant needs and thereafter act first in the child's interest as it introduces the child to the world. If it does these things it is *good-enough* and the style by which it operates is of secondary importance.

There is a fourth parenting style. It is called the *uninvolved* style and entails no parental concern for the child's needs and no interest by the parents in the child's growth, control or autonomy. This style amounts to neglect, a category of child abuse. The parents who have this approach to parenthood are insensitive and will be psychologically unavailable for their children. Such a style is obviously *not good-enough* and will be a major influence in the lives of children who are unfortunate enough to suffer it.

Our emphasis on the basic *good-enough* qualities of parenting helps to make sense of the recent criticism of parenting as the major influence in children's lives. This emphasis allows us to both accept some of the criticism while not denying the immense importance of parenting especially when it is *not good-enough*. It is to this rejection of parenting as an effective force in the development of children that we now turn.

Is parenting important in child development?

Earlier in this chapter we referred to Sharp and Fonagy (2008) who stated that the importance of parenting was an accepted tenet of developmental psychology. Sharp and Fonagy found it necessary to restate the importance of parenting in 2008 because for the previous decade there had been disagreement concerning the importance of parenting.

Most psychologists, prior to 1998, accepted parenting as perhaps the most important environmental influence on children and therefore a major determining factor in how children develop. Perhaps most still hold this view. In 1998 Judith Harris wrote *The Nurture Assumption,* a book which questioned the importance of parenting as a factor in the development of differences between children. Harris found that parenting influences do not account for most of the differences between children in personality, intelligence and mental health. She claimed that other influences must be at work both genetic and environmental. Rowe (1994) had earlier suggested that family influence on children was limited. Both Harris and Rowe supported the view that genetic influences in development were more important than those stemming from nurture; that is from the environment. Within environmental influences Harris stated that peer influence on children were more important than parental influence and she felt that environmental contexts outside of the home such as school were very important and outweighed home influences.

Rowe and Harris carried out their research and reached their conclusions at a time when genetic determinism was becoming an important factor in the explanation of human behaviour. This approach to humanity explains most human development and behaviour by reference to the genetic code that we inherit. The emphasis in the explanations given by genetic determinists is on the controlling influence of genes in human life and development. When this emphasis is applied to behaviour the approach is called behavioural genetics. Research which claimed that parenting was not the most important influence in the development of children and instead pointed to inherited biological factors as important determinants of development and behaviour was in accordance with the zeitgeist of the 1990s when genetic science was rapidly advancing in knowledge and human genetic engineering was seen as a widespread technique for the future. However, more recent developments have slowed the momentum of both genetic determinism and genetic engineering. In 2004 the human genome project succeeded well before its expected date of completion. It was found that humans have many fewer genes than had been expected. Instead of the expected 300,000 only between 25,000 and 20,000 genes were found in the human genetic code and most of these genes were shared with many other life forms (International Human Genome Sequencing Consortium, 2004). The number of genes that could account for all of the differences between all of the people in the world was very small indeed about 0.9 per cent of the total which works out at about 200 genes (Gibbons et al., 2004). This finding severely limited the ability of single genes to directly influence human differences including those in development and behaviour. There were simply not enough single genes to account for all the differences even though single gene effects could be seen in many illnesses. As with much in science things turned out in the Human Genome Project to be more complicated than expected.

However, 200 genes can be combined in a myriad of ways; factorial 200, which is a vast number. This means that though single genes are not a ready explanation for many human differences, combinations of genes (polygenes) can indeed account for these differences. Most differences in development and behaviour could therefore be accounted for by polygenetic inheritance. Not only have recent years emphasised genetic combinations but when development is considered it is found that genetics and environment most frequently act together rather than as separate influences. Thus to hold one of these influences constant and then try to estimate the effect of the other is a biological nonsense because they nearly always act together especially in development and the action of one is often dependent on the other. It is frequently found that genes that affect development are turned on and off by environmental triggers. A child may have a genetic predisposition to develop in a certain way but if the genes controlling this development are not turned on by environmental factors then the development will not take place. For example, if we consider autism, research appears to show that certain genes in combination give a predisposition to this condition. However, these genes are not missing or damaged in autistic children, they are present but are dormant as an influence. It is possible that these genes have not been turned on by environmental factors (Geschwind, 2011). Thus to set genetic influences against environmental ones is not a fruitful approach to development; both influences are always important and are interactive (Rutter, 2007). The spirit of scientific enquiry has moved on from simple genetic determinism to one that struggles with the complexity of nature/nurture interactions and a new science of epigenetics is emerging (Gottlieb, 2007).

We have digressed into the nature versus nurture debate and concluded that recent developments show that both are needed to explain development; indeed it can now be viewed as nature via nurture (Ridley, 2003). How does this help us to evaluate the work of Rowe, Harris and others who support the idea that genetics and other influences outweigh parenting as influences in development? Is there any value in the findings of these researchers; or should we still maintain that parenting is the major influence in child development?

Harris (2002) has a narrow view of parenting. She assumes that parenting is centrally involved with achieving obedience and appropriate social behaviour in children and she describes the change in parenting over the generations as due to changes in parenting styles. Her description of the changes over the decades is accurate but indicates that she sees the essence of parenting in the style of relationship between parent and child. Harris may therefore be correct in her view that what she considers as parenting, namely parenting style, is not a major influence in a child's development.

However, parenting, especially in the early years, involves much more than parenting style! Parenting in these years requires that parents meet a child's dependency needs, including the need for warm emotional contact. The way most parents achieve this is to place the child's needs before their own. In other words the essence of parenting is not a style of interacting with a child, but whether the parent loves the child and will sacrifice their time and energy to meet the infant's dependency needs. Harris does not appear to grasp this essence. From what we have said earlier in this chapter concerning good-enough parenting it can be seen that satisfactory parenting has to achieve certain outcomes for the child. Winnicott stated that these were the *holding pattern* of the first year when the child's dependency needs are met fully and promptly, and the later introduction by the parents to the child of *objective reality* when the child comes to understand his or her position in relation to other people. As long as these elements occur in parenting it is good-enough. The existence of good-enough parenting suggests that in parenting there is a threshold which if reached will allow the child to develop under other influences often those external to the home. This further development may well be guided by genetic influences. However, when this threshold is not reached and parenting is not good-enough then the inadequate parenting becomes a major influence in the child's life and will strongly influence most future psychological developments.

Harris does not consider this threshold effect and her research may well have considered children all or most of whom have had good-enough parenting in their early years. The effects of good-enough parenting thus being held constant it is not surprising that she finds other genetic and out of home factors to be the chief differences between children. These other influences do account for differences between children but they may be very minor effects indeed if parenting is not good-enough and does not reach a satisfactory threshold. In this case the child has been injured psychologically and may develop coping mechanisms that adversely affect future social and psychological developments. For such children much is unsatisfactory and unresolved and for some of them this may be a lifelong influence.

Harris may be correct about the influence of parenting styles but to state from her research that parenting is a relatively unimportant influence is a major mistake. When parenting is good-enough in later childhood it may be relatively unimportant but if parenting has not been good-enough in early childhood, it is a, or perhaps the, major factor in a person's life.

Other researchers have criticised Harris, Rowe and those who advocate an essentially genetic determinist approach to development that underplays environmental effects. Eleanor Maccoby (2002) in considering parenting effects points out the importance of the early years and how a warm caring environment in these years can influence future development. In these years she feels that parents influence children much more than children influence parents. While not denying the influence of genetic inheritance Maccoby points out that everything that is inherited is also influenced by environmental factors. She mentions the fact that even physical features such as height that are under strong genetic influence are also subject to environmental factors such as diet. Genetics alone do not determine height; a combination of genetic and environmental factors is required for such a determination. Rowe (2002) using correlational methods showed that genetically identical twins reared apart resembled their natural parents in intelligence more than their adoptive parents and therefore concluded that environment has a very minor place in the genesis of intelligence. Maccoby pointed out that Rowe was correct in his results but neglected the environmental context that each twin was brought up in. She pointed out that every twin who was adopted from a poor to a better environment increased his or her IQ. So even though adopted twins resemble their natural parents in intelligence more than the parents who adopt them they nevertheless increase in intelligence when transferred from a poor to a good environment. This again shows that both genetic and environmental influences on development are of importance and it is difficult to say which is more important. It is not productive to compare these influences by giving each a value based purely on correlational studies. From experimental biology we know that both genetics and environment are of crucial importance. Humans are continually in an environment and always have been in an environment. The functioning of genes in every cell of our bodies is under environmental influence (Lashley, 2007). Genes are the product of evolution and one of the chief driving forces in evolution is selection pressure exerted on a species by the environment. The genes we carry were selected for transmission to us by the successive environments of our ancestors. If genes are environmental in origin it is futile at best to draw a distinction between them and the environment.

Sroufe (2002) has also criticised the behavioural genetics approach much more directly. He states that longitudinal research carried out by him and others over many years shows clearly that nothing is more important for a child's development than the quality of care that he or she receives. Sroufe and his fellow workers found that quality of care in childhood influenced behaviour and emotional growth as well as relationships with peers and success at school. Sroufe recognised other influences on development but states that parental influence is the strongest. For Sroufe good genes in children and parents do not, of themselves, result in good parenting and happy and well-adjusted children. What happens in the process of rearing is still of paramount importance. Sroufe refers to the NICHD Study (1997) and states that later relationships in childhood are predicted by earlier sensitive care and not at all by infant temperament. He points out that resilience in children, the ability to withstand adversity, also shows a close relationship with the quality of care given to the child in the earlier years.

In conclusion, while Harris and others in 1998 caused a stir when they questioned the effectiveness of parenting in the development of children, recent evidence on parent and carer sensitivity challenges this view (Friedman & Boyle, 2008). Maccoby (2002) agrees that their critique was needed in that many psychologists have over-emphasised the importance of parenting and neglected the inherited features of the child. We are not blank slates at birth and Harris, Rowe and others have restored the importance of genetic inheritance. Harris has also forced those who consider development and parenting to further define what is essential in parenting as an important influence on children. However, though genetic influence has now been restored as a developmental feature it is wrong to conclude that this downplays the effects of a child's environment. These influences on children are inseparable. So what Sharp and Fonagy stated in 2008 namely, that the importance of parenting was an undisputed tenet of developmental psychology, remains true, though this belief has been much debated and substantially modified.

Summary of parenting and emotional development

In the first three years of life parenting that is not good-enough can affect the development of secondary emotions. This parenting can be inadequate in three main ways.

Three types of "not good-enough" Parenting	
1. **Inadequate or delayed** meeting of needs	Parents are psychologically unavailable to the child. Parenting like this is a kind of psychological abuse and results in disorganised or insecure (avoidant) attachment.
2. **Inconsistent** meeting of needs	Parents attend fully to the needs of the child at times, but not at all at other times. Child is likely to form an insecure (resistant) attachment.
3. **Too much** parental attention	Parents attend fully to the needs of the child but are smothering and do not appropriately introduce the child to objective reality. Child is most likely to be over-dependent on parents; occasionally they may reject their parents.

First the parents of the child do not cater for the infant's dependency needs fully or promptly. Such parents are psychologically unavailable for the infant and could also be described as psychologically abusive and uninvolved. The child will probably have a disorganised attachment to the parents or an insecure attachment of the avoidant kind.

Second the parents of the child may give their infant adequate care but only on an inconsistent basis. They attend fully to the dependency needs of the child sometimes. They can be prompt and psychologically warm in this attention but they only give care when it suits them and the child cannot predict when this care will be given. Such a child experiences loving care at times but neglect at others and is liable to form a resistant attachment to the intermittent carers.

In contrast to these two categories of inadequate parenting the third type of care that is not good-enough is due not to too little parental attention but to too much. This is where the parent smothers the child in continual care and especially in the second year does not gradually introduce the child to objective reality. Children parented in this way often fail to differentiate themselves and their needs from those of their carers. Thus they have a limited sense of self and a poor appreciation of others. They are delayed in developing the initial basis of a theory of mind and because of their lack of psychological separation from the parent often lack the ability or inclination to explore new contexts. They are rather difficult to classify in terms of attachment and are best described as being over-dependent.

Now we will summarise the effect of each of these not good-enough forms of care on the development of the secondary emotions.

When parents give little or no warm psychological care to their child, and the child manages to survive, positive secondary emotions are unlikely to form unless the child can make secure attachments to people other than his or her parents. Such children will develop much anger from frustration. They have not known loving care and warm enjoyable interchanges with their parents. Thus secondary emotions such as shame empathy guilt and pride may not develop at all and bitterness towards others and disdain for people in general especially the weak and unfortunate may be the most developed of the secondary emotions. These children will of course have the full complement of basic emotions and it is wrong to consider them unemotional. They have brought themselves up by developing their own survival mechanisms and thus can be very uninhibited and often antisocial. We will describe them in more detail in a later chapter.

If parents give a little warm care to their children on an inconsistent basis their children will experience the joy of mutual love. However, this experience will be inconsistent only occurring at unpredictable times. Yet the child will long for it to occur. Such children often seek adult contact and appreciation in order to be loved once again. They become attention seekers and are children who are generally unhappy because they know what they are missing. They are often anxious and unsure of themselves though they can disguise this with an outward bravado. They want their parents but are also frustrated with them and even annoyed with them because the care they deliver is not always there. These children develop positive secondary emotions such as pride, shame and sympathy in addition to the basic emotions. However, their positive secondary emotions are often weak and unmotivating because the children are more concerned with attention seeking than anything else. Their attention seeking interferes with their social interactions and this can cause them to be rejected by both adults and other children. These children often experience strong feelings of jealousy and envy. These secondary emotions can only develop if the child has experienced love. These children have had a little love at unpredictable times and to them it is a scarce commodity. Thus when love has to be shared they can be very jealous and do not realise that there is enough love for everyone.

Where children are over-parented and not slowly introduced to objective reality it is difficult for emotions that are formed by social interaction to develop. These children are spoilt in that they have not been properly introduced to the existence of other people and the need to regard others seriously. These children are self-centred and though they have received warm loving care they have not been required to reciprocate the love that has been shown to them. For such children loving care, being always available for them, is not valued and can be disregarded without consequences. The inability of these children to recognise the needs and motivations of others makes it difficult for them to develop sympathy. The lack of a strong sense of self means a limited development of shame and they may feel little guilt. Because they have not done much independently their feelings of true pride may well also be limited. Overall the inability of these children to recognise the wishes and needs of other people means that their chief emotions are the basic emotions and they show little development of secondary social emotions.

A cautionary note

We have outlined how parenting and the care it delivers to children influences the development of secondary emotions. However, human interactions are often complex and people are very varied. People can also change over time and this can apply to parents. Given this variability much parenting is not easily classifiable into the categories of good-enough and not good-enough that we have outlined above. It is also important to note that we have not discussed the societal and peer influences which can be substantial; these will be considered when we discuss middle childhood and adolescence. Nevertheless, what has been outlined is generally a reliable guide to understanding inadequate parenting and its consequences for emotional development and should enable us to sympathise with the plight of children in families that do not cater fully for their needs.

Questions to think about

1. What characterises parenting that is "not good enough"?
2. Is intergenerational abusive parenting inevitable?
3. How many parenting styles are there and which is most effective?
4. How important is parenting?
5. Summarise how parenting effects emotional development; both from what you've read and from your own experiences.

Suggested further reading

Grusec, J. E. (2011). Socialization processes in the family: Social and emotional development. *Annual Review of Psychology*, 62, 243–269.

Friedman, S. L. & Boyle, D. E. (2008). Attachment in US children experiencing nonmaternal care in the early 1990s. *Attachment and Human Development*, 10(3), 225–261.

National Scientific Council on the Developing Child (2007) *The Science of Early Childhood Development* http://www.developingchild.net.

Thompson, R. A. (2011). Emotion and emotion regulation: Two sides of the developing coin. *Emotion Review*, 3(1), 53–61.

Sroufe, L. A. (2002). From infant attachment to promotion of adolescent autonomy: Prospective longitudinal data on the role of parents in development. In J. G. Borkowski, S. Landesman-Ramey & M. Bristol-Power (Eds), *Parenting and the Child's World: Influences on Academic, Intellectual and Socioemotional Development.* London: Laurence Erlbaum Associates.

Chapter 8

Emotional development in early and middle childhood

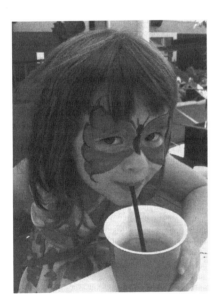

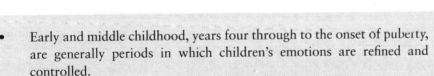

- Early and middle childhood, years four through to the onset of puberty, are generally periods in which children's emotions are refined and controlled.
- The development of emotional expression is extensive in these periods and is governed by the context the child is in, growing cognitive powers and the processes of social referencing and display rules.

- Emotional self-regulation, or control, is also developed throughout this period through the child's moderation of their subjective feelings and control of emotional expression.
- Increasingly children have an emotional history from earlier periods and this impacts upon their socialisation and their control and expression of emotion.
- Children whose dependency needs have been neglected previously may have a limited repertoire of emotions, dominated by negative emotions, which they find difficult to control.

Early childhood: the pre-school stage

By three years of age most children can experience a wide range of emotions though some will be restricted in their repertoire. Many of the basic instinctive emotional expressions of early infancy have been reinterpreted in toddlerhood by subjective experience but are still present as quick instant emotional reactions. Earlier proto-emotions such as satisfaction and frustration are still present. In the majority of children most of the early secondary and self-conscious emotions also are present by this time though the latter are often in rudimentary form.

The growth of emotion in early childhood is very much an individual development. It is subject not only to the concurrent environmental conditions, particularly the social conditions that the child experiences but also to earlier social conditions for that child. Each child will have had a different emotional history. For any child there is individual coherence across the developmental phases (DeHart et al., 2000), and even at three years the subsequent growth and development of emotions will be influenced by the emotional development, or lack of it, that has taken place in the first three years of life.

This is not to say that significant changes in the direction of emotional development cannot occur in early childhood. Such changes can occur despite the child's emotional history. The child's brain remains very flexible in this period (four to five years) and not only can certain neural circuits, already established, influence the further development of emotions, but it is also very possible for certain circuits to be pruned and new neural pathways to be established. So though there is an influence from the child's earlier emotional history, environment and social relations remain very important and new ways of feeling can be established.

Two main developments occur in relation to emotion in early childhood. First emotions that formed earlier are further refined and sometimes transformed.

Second the control of emotional expression by the child becomes a very important part of the pre-schooler's social and family life. Three main factors influence these developments. These factors are not independent and often link with and influence each other. Let us consider each of them in turn.

Expanding context

Children in this period, let us call them pre-schoolers, experience, for the most part, a wider environmental context than younger children. Their social and spatial contexts generally multiply and expand. Pre-schoolers, in short, have a wider view of the world than toddlers and are more equipped to experience and understand this wider view and the new settings they find themselves in. Perhaps this is not as true as it used to be several decades ago due to the increasing long day care experience of many infants and toddlers. However, the growing instrumental independence and cognitive development of the pre-school years generally allows children of this age deeper and more detailed experience of new environments than can be experienced by children at earlier stages.

Pre-schoolers generally have more contact with their peers than do toddlers though this is not invariably true. Toddlers are very interested in other children, and children are important to each other from the earliest ages, but in early childhood, in most instances, peers come to play a bigger part in the child's life than they did before (Hughes & Dunn, 2007). Most pre-schoolers also visit or stay in a greater number of geographical contexts than do toddlers, though again this is, of course, not invariably the case. This widening of social and spatial contexts influences the emotions that children feel and, more particularly, how they express these emotions. Children have more understanding of other people's expectations at this stage than they did and this often causes differences in emotional expression. They don't expect their parents to react in the same way as their peers and they begin to tailor their emotional expressions according to the group they are with. However, at this stage this process is far from complete. They also begin to learn to behave differently in different places. The old familiar emotional expressions they use at home they may not use in pre-school in front of the pre-school teacher and their peers (unless things get too much for them). At pre-school they often get their first experience of group emotional expression and they often respond to this new experience, as many pre-school teachers know, by modifying their own behaviour. Pre-schoolers also have more understanding of their place in a context and how their position should influence their emotional expression and that of others. In short they learn the *display rules* associated with the expression of emotion at their pre-school.

One specific aspect that they now understand is their gender position and what it implies in terms of emotional expression. Increasingly with pre-schoolers gender roles affect their emotional expressions. From the pre-school years onwards the emotional expressions of boys and girls diverge at least to some degree. All in all the expanding world of early childhood leaves room for new shades of subjective feeling and new and varied modes of emotional expression. The influence of context on emotion and its expression becomes quite noticeable at this stage and this influence, as we shall see, grows stronger as children grow older.

Growing mental powers

During the period of early childhood children develop increasing abilities in the areas of *thought and memory*. In other words their cognitive capacity increases and this directly and indirectly influences their emotional development. An example of indirect influence is the effect that developing cognition has on the understanding of the wider environmental contexts in which the child is now involved. As before, all effects work together; development is all of a piece (Thelen & Smith, 1998). This increasing mental growth in thought and memory affects the emotional development of pre-schoolers because they are now able to think clearly about their feelings and can remember them over a considerable period of time. They can also think about how they express, or have expressed their emotions, or will express their emotions. They can remember certain emotional episodes quite clearly and can reflect on them. For example: In the evening Rebecca, a four-year-old, says to her grandfather; "Grandpa I've got bad news for you". "What is it Rebecca?" he asks. "Emma hurt my feelings today". She says with a glum expression. "When did she do that Rebecca?" Grandpa asks. "At pre-school" replies Rebecca. Such processes of thought and memory can modify or intensify emotions in a child's mind particularly the secondary self-conscious emotions such as shame, pride or guilt. Emotion and cognition are again interdependent.

Another mental capacity that increases during this period is a child's *'theory of mind'*. The development of a theory of mind in some children can be seen in rudimentary form as far back as 18 months of age (Dunn, 1988), but by the pre-school stage it is well developed in most children unless they come from very adverse situations. At this stage most children can, to some degree, take into account other people's thoughts and wishes, and can infer reactions to their own behaviour. Children at the pre-school stage cannot as yet understand emotional subtleties, such as mixed feelings, but they can in a simple way take account of the straightforward emotions that they ascribe to others.

The growing mental capacity of a child during the pre-school years has a lot to do with the development of a symbolic system that can be used in increasingly effective ways to control the environment, particularly the social environment. Of course we are talking about *language* which becomes a very effective mental tool as the years progress in almost all situations. An emotional situation is no exception.

In the pre-school years, and even before, children learn the words that describe emotions. With these they can think more clearly about their own emotions and the emotions of others. Herrera and Dunn (1997) found that the more three year olds discussed emotions within their families the better they understood the emotions of others. This ability lasted into primary school where such children were good at settling disputes with their friends. It is obvious that good linguistic skill in interpreting emotions helps children cope with the wider social context they experience as pre-schoolers.

Language also helps in these years in the further development of the ability to imitate and pretend. The ability to imitate started in the earlier reciprocal relationship, as an unconscious instinctive ability to imitate present in very young infants, but is now a conscious ability and practised in many contexts, particularly with peers. Such practice in imaginative social play often involves pretend (or 'as if') emotions and it is through practice of this sort that children learn more about emotional feelings and relationships. Indeed this process is important in the internalisation by the child of family values and standards. Some of these standards and values may well apply to emotional expression. For families some emotional expressions are more acceptable than others and through practice in play situations pre-schoolers are learning the emotional expressions that are appropriate for them.

From all this you can see that the brain of a pre-schooler is indeed growing and expanding in many mental areas at once. Each of these mental developments will influence the growth or the refinement of emotions.

Growing self-awareness

The development of awareness takes place in infancy and in the second half of the first year of life subjective feeling becomes possible as myelination of the frontal lobes of the cortex takes place. By 18 months most children can recognise themselves in a mirror and distinct self-awareness has begun. However, this is not a process that stops in toddlerhood; it only begins in this period. Its further development in early childhood is a very important factor in the emotional development that takes place in this period.

As we explained in the discussion of emotional development in toddlerhood, children gain knowledge and awareness of themselves at the same time as they gain knowledge and awareness of other people. The two processes are intertwined and contemporaneous. To some extent each of us is defined by our relations with others and it is only as we get to know others that we can gain a conception of ourselves. This is certainly true in early childhood where studies of children isolated from human contact reveal children with very poor self-awareness (Newton, 2002). The development of self-awareness therefore is closely connected with the development of a sense of others; we might well say with a developing theory of mind. With increasing self-awareness in the pre-school years come expectations of the self. These expectations are often intertwined with the expectations that others have of the child. Children's expectations of themselves and also their expectations of others can influence the emotions children feel and how deeply they feel them.

Children will try to live up the expectation they have of themselves and those that significant others hold for them. This process can greatly influence certain secondary self-conscious emotions and during early childhood we see embarrassment, shame, guilt and pride become much more obvious in the emotional life of many children. These self-conscious social emotions could not develop further in early childhood unless there was a parallel growth in self-awareness.

The growth of self-awareness also allows the child of this age to see himself or herself in relation to time. Both the past and the future become clearer. Children may now ask you what they were like as a little baby. They also wonder about the future though it still seems a long time to Christmas! The growing sense of both past and future not only allows the child to gain more sense of self but also to begin to experience a sense of autonomy. Children are still very dependent at this stage and they know this. However, for the first time they can foresee a time when this may not be so. They begin vaguely to think of what it will be like to grow up. They now know that they will grow up, and this, of itself, creates a sense of autonomy. A sense of self, a sense of others, a sense of time, and a certain sense of autonomy, are all needed for that sense of self control that is necessary to curb unsocialised emotional expression. This partial mastery of emotional expression is one of the important and noticeable features of emotional development in early childhood. Before we consider this important feature we need to summarise and discuss the development of emotions in this early childhood period.

Refinement of emotions in early childhood

Most of the emotions displayed or felt in early childhood have clear predecessors in the toddler period. The instant basic instinctive emotions, fear, anger, joy, sadness, disgust, interest, and surprise persist into early childhood but are now interpreted subjectively, at least in retrospect. The initial proto-emotions of frustration and satisfaction are present in these years but, as we shall see, most pre-schoolers become able to some degree at least to control the expression of these feelings. Also present in most children of this age are the secondary social emotions. These are the emotions whose growth and expression depends on social contact. Thus love, anger due to frustration, and anxious fear all continue in the early childhood years. Secondary emotions, while they have their origin in toddlerhood, further develop in the pre-school stage.

The basic instinctive emotion of fear is an instant reaction to a dangerous situation. This type of fear originates in early infancy but continues into early childhood. However, it must be distinguished from the anxious fear that relates to insecurity and a child's inability to predict what will happen. This latter fear is developed later in infancy and is due to an association with people who are unreliable as far as the child's crucial needs are concerned. One crucial need is for a warm loving relationship. Instant anger is also a basic instinctive emotion arising from an unexpected noxious stimulus. It is different from anger developed due to frustration with people who cannot consistently service the child's dependency needs. Though the instant basic emotions are still present in early childhood, as they can be at any stage of life, it is the emotions that formed earlier due to social interaction that begin to take centre stage in pre-schoolers. In general there is a move away from the instinctive, quick emotions.

The emotions that arise from love, from anxious fear, and from anger due to frustration, the later more advanced secondary emotions of toddlerhood, all grow and develop further in early childhood. On the positive side; most pre-schoolers continue to develop sympathy and empathy for others. They can be quite touching in this regard. Most of them also now show quite clearly the secondary self-conscious emotions of pride, shame and guilt, though guilt, in particular, has some way still to go in its development. They can still be jealous of new arrivals in the family but are now probably more easily convinced than younger children that there is enough love to go around and little need to fear. On the negative side; if their frustrated anger is directed to others some of them, who have not had loving relationships, can develop distain for those more unfortunate than themselves and a general bitterness towards people. If frustrated anger is turned inwards towards the self some pre-schoolers can become depressed and withdrawn.

The expression of anger due to frustration, if directed outwards, is usually in the form of aggressive acts. We will discuss aggression in detail later but at the pre-school stage expressions of anger should be brought under significant control. At this stage children from backgrounds of adequate nurturance should be able to control their tendency to be aggressive and the tantrums of toddlerhood should have declined. If this is not the case and a pre-school child still acts out his or her fury in full measure the chances of future maladjustment increase considerably. Aggression is still essentially instrumental during the pre-school stage, that is pre-school children are aggressive to achieve a purpose. They are aggressive to get something or to achieve something. This form of aggression declines from toddlerhood but it is still the main form of aggression in the pre-school years.

Anxious fear can lead to a generally anxious pre-school child if the child remains in unpredictable circumstances. However, if the pre-school years bring more secure conditions, then an anxious child will settle to some degree, though specific fears connected to an unsure past may remain. Anxiety that arises from the fear that nurturance is unpredictable may also decline as the pre-school child becomes more autonomous. However, the anxious child is the very child for whom autonomy is most difficult. We should remember that independence grows out of secure dependence. Nevertheless, the growing mental powers of this stage of development may allow the anxious child to learn certain strategies that reduce anxiety.

Thus in the early childhood stage emotions develop evolve and change. By the end of this stage most children are quite complicated people from an emotional standpoint and have the bases for all future emotional development. Where they differ most from toddlers is in the realm of control of emotional expression and here pre-schoolers make considerable progress. This is part of the socialisation of the child; the process whereby unsocial expressions of emotion are curbed so that we can all live together in a degree of harmony.

Development of control of emotional expression

For children in good rearing conditions the control of emotional expression advances very considerably from four to five years. This control can be thought of as the control of excitement and the control of the expression of anger. These expressions arise from intense satisfaction on the one hand and frustration on the other. Children at this age, it is said, have started to learn emotional control. What is forgotten is that emotions have by definition an element of uncontrollability (the unstoppable factor we referred to earlier) and the degree to which they can be controlled is limited. Rather at the age of three years children are beginning to learn to control the *expression* of emotion rather than the subjective feeling which they will inevitably experience.

The development of control over emotional expression in the pre-school years is best seen in relation to the proto-emotions of satisfaction and frustration. Many pre-schoolers develop the ability to delay gratification; that is to postpone satisfaction and even to suffer some extra frustration in the process (Bridges & Grolnick, 1995). Many pre-school children seem able to tolerate a degree of frustration that would have disturbed and activated them at an earlier stage. Thus during the pre-school years children learn to maintain organised behaviour, at least to some degree, in the face of a strong emotional experience. This control of emotional expression is under much cultural influence. Most children at this stage find it easier to control expressions of joy and affection than feelings arising from frustration such as anger. Not that pre-schoolers are good at controlling the expressions of their feelings, they are not. They often have a charming openness in their emotional dealings, but the beginnings of control are there, and we suspect strongly that this control of expression is much more easily gained when the emotional experience is a pleasant one than when it is aversive. Perhaps it is this ability to deal with the expression of positive pleasant emotion that helps in the eventual control of expressions of emotion arising from frustration.

The ability to control emotional expression in the pre-school years is probably a development of the child's ability to limit positive emotional expression in the earlier reciprocal relationship. The ability to limit a positive proto-emotion such as satisfaction (or derivations from it such as joy and delight) seems to come first. The left portion of the frontal lobe of the cortex controls this ability (Eliot, 2001). Somehow in the pre-school years this controlling function in relation to expression spreads to the right side of the frontal lobe where negative emotions are felt and then ability to tolerate frustration is developed. It may be that early positive emotions are particularly important for the development of control, certainly they have attracted less research attention and should be investigated more (Fredricksen, 1998). In the pre-schooler the ability to tolerate and control frustration is aided by the presence of adults who can encourage and help the process. This further emphasises the connection between the control of emotional expression and positive nurturing relationships.

Pre-school children do not just learn to postpone satisfaction and to tolerate frustration. They learn appropriate control over the expression of many emotions. When in unfamiliar contexts they learn the appropriate emotional expression by copying adults or other children of importance to them, that are with them in that context. This looking to others for a guide to emotion and emotional expression begins in infancy and is called *social referencing* (Feinman, 1982). It starts as young as five months and by the pre-school years it is well developed and applies distinctly to the expression of emotion in new or less familiar contexts (Vailant-Molina & Bahrick, 2012). This process continues into adolescence and adulthood.

While copying others through *social referencing* is one way to behave appropriately, young children also eventually learn the rules that determine what is appropriate. The appropriate emotional expression for any particular context is set by *the display rules* of the culture and moderated depending on who is in the audience (Zeman & Garber, 1996). Each culture has rules concerning the display of emotion in certain situations and most children at this stage learn to conform to these rules. The display rules for each gender within a culture may be different.

Children in the pre-school years also begin to learn how to hide their feelings. They are beginning to know the difference between feeling an emotion and expressing it. As the pre-school years progress children become more able to express emotion that they do not feel (Kieras *et al.*, 2005). This ability to *deceive* is, however, not very prominent in early childhood. Pre-schoolers are usually direct, spontaneous and sincere in their emotional expressions. The ability to separate emotions from their expressions starts in this period of development but grows much more rapidly in the next period, middle childhood.

We have concentrated in describing emotional development in this period on children learning to control their emotional expression rather than the emotion itself. Nevertheless in the pre-school years not only do children learn to control the expression of an emotion but they slowly develop a degree of *emotional self-regulation*. Though emotion in our definition cannot be completely controlled it is possible for a person to control what they are feeling or will feel to some degree.

In the years four to five this ability advances. At this age children can develop the ability to anticipate and avoid situations they know will result in negative feelings (in our family this often involved hiding behind the couch to avoid sad or scary scenes on TV). They also can to some degree use positive focused thoughts to counter negative emotions that they are experiencing. Positive thoughts that are contradictory to an experienced emotion do not entirely control the emotion but they do allow the child to better tolerate the often negative experience.

Middle childhood

Middle childhood covers the period from six years to the onset of puberty. It is a period of steady rather than dramatic emotional development. Many of the processes of emotional development begun in toddlerhood or early childhood are simply continued in middle childhood but are further developed. In general development as a whole, including physical development, slows down during this period, which Freud called the latency period. However, emotional development during this period is not latent; rather it is steady and progressive. To a large extent emotional development in this period is an extension of that in the early childhood period and is subject to similar developmental influences. Let us call the children in this period primary school-children. The emotional development of a primary school-child is subject to many influences but is also coherent with the *emotional history* of that particular schoolchild, that is, with his or her history as an infant, toddler and pre-schooler. The chief influences that bear on emotional development in middle childhood are the child's growing cognitive capacity and his or her sense of context. These influences are closely linked.

Cognitive growth in middle childhood

Middle childhood is a period when children usually further refine a number of cognitive competencies that influence emotional development. Children of this age develop cognitive skills in appraising ambivalent situations, in dampening emotional expression, and in displaying emotions that they do not feel – usually in order to please others (Saarni *et al.*, 2006). Underlying these skills is the child's understanding of what emotions are and what they lead to. Children first begin to understand emotion as toddlers, however their understanding of emotion advances very considerably in early and middle childhood. In middle childhood many children can consider multiple aspects of an emotional situation simultaneously. They can consider a person's emotional history in simple terms and, at the same time, consider that person's emotional expression. Thus they can understand why someone is angry and make allowances for their behaviour. They further develop their understanding of the display rules of emotional expression and how to suit emotional display to different contexts. In order to do this they need some under-standing of the contexts they are in. Primary school-children increasingly under-stand the contexts of emotional expression and that expression can vary with context and contingencies. One of the most important contexts in this regard is the cultural context. Every culture, and sub-culture, has its own *'display rules'* concerning emotion.

This ability to understand the control of emotional expression allows primary school age children increasingly, as they grow older, to mask their emotions or feign an emotion they do not feel. Unfortunately children from adverse backgrounds seem to develop the ability to feign emotional expression just as easily as children from nurturing situations. Perhaps this is because this understanding is largely a cognitive feature rather than one based on a child's earlier emotional history.

Primary schoolchildren generally know much more about the world than pre-schoolers and their cognitive skills allow them to contemplate and manipulate this knowledge to a greater extent than before. They also generally have more ability than pre-schoolers to consider the future and future happenings. Thus most primary schoolchildren have a subtle evolved theory of mind which they can use in situa-tions involving other people.

The growing cognitive capacity of these middle years allows children to think about themselves. In this way their *sense of self* becomes more refined and they tend now to describe themselves in psychological terms rather than the physical terms which they used in earlier stages. Thinking about oneself in psychological terms helps the growth of a strong self-concept. This can be reinforced by the child's ability to do things in middle childhood. Many children at this stage are very interested in making things and then doing things with the instrument they have made. When children make things they often have considerable pride in their industry and achievement. Because they have a distinct sense of the future they begin to develop relatively long-term expectations.

These expectations influence their emotional life and their self-concept. In the historical period referred to as the Middle Ages, children grew up at about seven years of age when they became instrumentally competent. Boys often left home at this age to be apprenticed. The point being that children of this age can survive instrumentally on their own and their self-concept can be quite robust if their earlier nurturance has been good. We tend to forget this in modern society. in general we now think of children as having instrumental competence at about ten years of age.

Context and emotion in middle childhood

The emotional expressions of most primary schoolchildren are strongly influenced by the context that the children are in. Though to some degree the influence of context on emotional expression was seen in pre-schoolers it is, in middle childhood, a very distinct pervasive factor. As we have already explained, at this stage children are very aware of the context they are in and are often practised at suiting their emotional expression to that context. One might say that they have a sense of context. This sense includes an appreciation by the child of the child's own position within a context or a number of contexts. Context often interacts with a child's sense of identity and gender identity has by this time become an important factor in emotional expression. Three main contexts stand out in middle childhood. These contexts will vary to a considerable degree according to culture (Shweder *et al.*, 2008).

The context of the peer group

Peers figure prominently in the life of a primary schoolchild. By middle childhood belonging to a peer group or having a number of friends is an important issue for most children though it is not essential for appropriate emotional development. For most children group norms and peer pressure have a considerable influence on the primary schoolchild's expression of emotion in many situations. This contextual influence is heightened because, at this stage of development, most peer groups are single sex groups and their norms reflect the gender of the group. Gender is also an influence on emotional expression in other contexts such as the classroom or the family. In fact gender could be described as a major contextual influence.

The peer group is often very important to the child's growing sense of self in that, to some degree, it can contribute to identity. The child therefore conforms to the behaviour expected by the peer group particularly as far as emotional expression is concerned. It is often particularly important to a child that peers see him or her as competent. Conformity to peer norms is often strongest when other contexts in the child's life have been inadequate or where a child's history of nurturance has been poor. Thus the peer group is important for children in middle childhood as a context for relationships and the feelings that arise from these relationships. Feelings of loyalty, solidarity and mateship become prominent outside the family context for the first time, though such feelings may have started at the pre-school stage. So in the refinement, transformation and expression of emotions the peer group context is very significant. The peer group becomes even more influential in adolescence where it allows children to begin the process of identity separation from their parents or caregivers. In middle childhood this psychological process may have started but it develops full strength in adolescence. Nevertheless for most primary school-children the peer group is of great significance as far as their emotional development is concerned. What is most influenced by peers is emotional expression. This includes not expressing emotion. Von Salisch (2001) suggests that display rules among peers at this age cause a dampening down of the emotional expression that a child will show to companions. It is important at this age and also later to be 'cool' and this often means limiting emotional expression.

The school context

School becomes a very important part of life for most children in middle childhood. As a context for emotional refinement and expression it overlaps at times with that of the peer group. Many peer groups form at school but children can be connected to peers who do not attend their school. School is a context where adults figure prominently as well as peers and a child must learn appropriate emotional expression if he or she is to be accepted in school by both groups. School leads to wider experiences for the child. For example school can give a child his or her first experience of travel without parents and school camps can further widen horizons. These wider contexts give further room for new emotional experiences and further development of appropriate emotional expressions. The quality of school life is an important factor in a child's emotional adjustment. Because school frequently provides a child's peers, schools that induce properly socialised behaviour in their charges can be a very good thing as far as parents are concerned. However, peer groups formed in school may only pay lip service to official school norms of expression and, when free to do so, the latent unofficial norms of the peer group may be let loose – much to parental dismay!

The family context

For most primary schoolchildren the family remains the most important context as far as the development of emotion is concerned. A family which provides support for the child's growing autonomy, structure and warmth is important (Grusec, 2011). If family disruption occurs children can feel distinct emotional effects. The importance of the family in emotional development in middle childhood is most dramatically seen when things go wrong. When things are flowing smoothly both children and parents may take the family context for granted and concentrate on emotional issues arising in other venues.

The development of emotions in middle childhood

Emotional development in middle childhood is a direct uninterrupted continuation of the process in early childhood. Usually no dramatic developments occur. It is very much a matter of the refinement of emotions already existing before this period and their synchronisation with various contexts particularly in respect of emotional expression. All of the emotions experienced by adults can be seen to be present in this period and what happens is the adjustment of emotional expression. This is facilitated by the child's growing powers of thought. Most children in middle childhood use their increasing powers of understanding to analyse and refine their emotions and to fit their emotional expressions to the context they are in. Thus guilt is present before middle childhood, but the guilt felt with peers in the primary school playground may be very different from that felt in the classroom, which in turn may also be very different from this emotion felt at home. Likewise what makes children feel proud in their peer group may in fact make them feel ashamed in a family context.

While children continue to make progress in this period, many from good-enough backgrounds still face substantial and frequent challenges in both emotions and their expression. Within any class there are children who have considerable emotional difficulty that can be due to non-family factors, such as shyness and bullying. As we have noted cognitive development and emotional development are concurrent and mutually dependent. Therefore parents and teachers need to be sensitive and responsive to children facing these emotional challenges so as not to hinder them educationally. The significant relationship between emotions and learning is only recently an area of growing interest (Hascher, 2010).

The moral development of a primary schoolchild (in terms of moral behaviour rather than moral judgement) can be closely linked to that child's emotional development (Wilson, 1968). Children at this stage are being socialised and the tendency to 'do the right thing' is strongly associated with the development of the secondary self-conscious emotions, shame, guilt and pride. Children from adverse backgrounds may not have been given the opportunity to develop these secondary emotions in their earlier development. Their nurturing interactions with caring adults may be limited, and their sense of self and their sense of others underdeveloped. In this situation they may not develop the secondary emotions or have them only weakly developed. With weak or absent feelings of guilt shame and pride it is difficult to develop the moral sense out of which, hopefully, comes moral behaviour.

When things go wrong in early and middle childhood

In this book and this chapter we have referred several times to the emotional development of children in adverse circumstances. We have considered parenting care that is not good-enough. We will now retell the story of adversity but not from a parenting perspective dealing with infants and toddlers but from that of the child in the early childhood and middle childhood stages. If we are to understand children from adverse circumstances, who often cause us trouble at later ages, we must consider their possible emotional development in some detail. The difficulties these children suffer may well have begun in infancy or toddlerhood. In fact this is, in our experience, usually the case. However, the early and middle childhood years may well aggravate difficulties from earlier periods.

Before we consider children from adverse backgrounds we should return to a major theme of this book namely variation. Children from adversity are varied; varied in themselves and also in the degree of adversity that they have had to endure. As far as emotional development is concerned the adversity which matters most is a failure to give the infant and toddler a warm secure emotional environment. This adverse situation can extend into early and middle childhood but even if the emotional environment improves in these later stages the effects of early emotional deprivation may linger. It is also possible that a secure early and middle childhood may cancel some or all of the earlier adverse effects.

In this book we often use the words 'most children', when talking about adequate development, or use such words as 'often' or 'generally' when describing development. This is because variation is the rule. The situation is no different with regard to adversity. Many factors interact and no two cases are the same. However, for the sake of clarity and simplicity we now, somewhat hypocritically, will consider just two main categories of emotional adversity. This division is artificial but will help us to elaborate what can go wrong more simply and clearly.

Some children have *few of their dependency needs met* in infancy and toddlerhood, yet because physical needs have been met to some extent the child has survived (Neglected children group). However, the emotional dependency needs of such a child, the need for warm human contact and communication, may not have been met at all or only to a very limited degree. These children usually show disorganised or avoidant attachment.

Other children have had their *emotional needs met on occasions but not consistently* (Inconsistent care group). These children become rather attention seeking and because they cannot predict when emotional warmth will come they often show some fearful anxiety. The problem is that they are not secure in their emotional relationships. They usually show resistant attachment.

Children from adversity often correspond to one of these groups more than the other. On the other hand it may be difficult to classify a particular child. When we consider things going wrong in the emotional development of pre-school and primary school children we should try to cover the variation indicated by this division.

Let us first consider the secondary self-conscious emotions. Children from backgrounds of good, secure and consistent emotional nurturance (Normal group) already have, at three years the basic feelings of shame guilt and pride. These emotions and other secondary emotions grow and develop considerably in early and middle childhood. In early childhood when children are secure and nurtured they will internalise, into their growing sense of self, the standards that their parents (or caregivers) set for them. From then on failure to meet these standards will induce the emotions of shame and guilt in the child, while achievement of the expected standard will evoke pride.

Unfortunately children, from the neglected group, reared without any affection find it difficult to internalise standards. For those children who have not been loved at all, and thus have not had the basis for the experience of '*love lost*', there can be no subsequent development of shame and guilt. Because these children do not experience shame or guilt or pride, they cannot be induced to behave by reference to these feelings. They are not motivated by a tendency to 'do the right thing'. Indeed their motivation in general is low. They are more swayed by consequences than by conscience and this tendency has become obvious by middle childhood.

For those children for whom love has been intermittent, inconsistent group, the development of shame guilt and pride will occur but will be weak especially in comparison with the neurotic drive that these children have for attention. If we look further at motivation we see that these children from adverse backgrounds, those who have been loved only on an inconsistent basis, have little security to draw on when they face a new challenge. They have not developed a confident sense of pride in their own achievements, and success may have little inner meaning for them because they still lack emotional security. These partially loved children do not feel much shame when they fail. This diminution of shame robs failure of its aversive quality and makes it acceptable. Thus many insecure children become 'losers' and fail because essentially their minds are dominated by other neurotic mental factors. They continually seek attention and when they get what they want they don't want it because they have had to seek it.

If we now turn to the control of the expression of emotion by children from adversity in early and middle childhood we find further difficulties. Children in these stages from adverse backgrounds, both where there is a lack of loving nurturance and where it is inconsistent often do not develop the appropriate controls over their emotional expression. In particular they find it difficult to inhibit their expressions of frustration or anger. This makes both groups of these children from adversity difficult to live with, difficult to educate and difficult to control. At least these difficulties will arise if we do not understand the emotional position of these children and make allowances for it. These children often do not understand the *display rules* of emotion and have limited ability to adjust their emotional expression appropriately to the context they are in.

Why do these children from both groups of adversity have such difficulty with the control of their expression of emotion? We are not sure what the explanation is. What is clear is that children with few experiences of positive emotion, who have not been warmly nurtured or securely attached, find it particularly difficult to develop control over their negative emotional expressions. This is very unfortunate as most of their emotional life is in this negative sphere. They express negative emotions such as anger frequently. One would think that they should therefore have repeated practice in controlling these negative expressions. It seems that repeated expressions of negative emotions have little to do with their control. We suggest that the control of angry expressions is absent in these children because they have had few positive emotional experiences and few opportunities to control their positive emotional expression. If this is, as we suggest, a pre-requisite for the control of negative emotional expression then these children do not possess it and for them the control of expressions of anger may always be difficult. Rather than give them help with the direct control of anger perhaps we should give them positive emotional experiences. We should then help and encourage them to control the emotional expressions that arise from these positive experiences. If we achieve such control hopefully it will be extended in time to the control of negative expressions such as anger.

Finally children who have not been warmly nurtured (Neglected group), have limited understanding of their own emotions or the emotions of others. We could say that they have not developed a clear theory of mind. Such children may well lack empathy and Harris (1990) observed children from adverse backgrounds attacking a defenceless child who was distressed. Most children from good nurturance would try to comfort the child. Some of the children who have been subject to intermittent nurturance may also feel insecure and attack those that they see as more defenceless than themselves.

Is this rather bleak situation for children from adverse circumstances redeemable? Can we correct poor or absent secondary emotions, poor motivation arising from emotion and poor control of emotional expression? Are children from adversity redeemable in early or middle childhood? We simply do not know. However, two approaches can be taken.

We can try to *redevelop the child emotionally* in order to correct the adverse emotional history that they have experienced. This *reworking* is very difficult to achieve because in most instances we do not have, nor should we have, the power to reorder the child's emotional environment which usually means changing family circumstances. However, in extreme situations where abuse has occurred children can be transferred to new emotional environments. Where the child is young, where the new carers have insight into the child's earlier emotional development combined with warm disinterested (impartial) patient affection towards the child, and where the new arrangements are stable for many years, new emotional developments may take place. However, as Rutter pointed out in 1981 it is very rare, indeed almost unknown, for a child from adverse circumstances to proceed to a situation where conditions are optimal for the redevelopment of emotion. This approach is in reality not often possible in many standard welfare situations. Nevertheless more recent work in Britain, also by Rutter (1998), with children from Romanian orphanages, has shown some success particularly with children 'rescued' at a very young age. The approach works best with those children who have suffered early from inconsistent emotional nurturance rather than with those children who have had little emotional nurturance at all in their lives.

The second approach is to deal with the child as they are with the emotions they *have* developed. It is possible to guide these children by appealing to that which can be explained to them as being in their own interest, as well as to their well-developed sense of survival. Sometimes the child is best guided by cognitive rather than emotional motivation. This is possibly the best approach for those children who have had very little or no emotional warmth and nurturance in their lives and who, being survivors, have essentially brought themselves up.

Dealing with anger and insecurity that is developed from adversity is not easy and we will explore these approaches further when we look at emotions in adolescence. Before we go to this topic, however, it is necessary to look in more detail at the behaviour that springs from persistent anger, namely frequent aggression, and that which arises from insecurity, undue anxiety. We will also consider children who show persistent oppositional behaviour. All of these conditions arise from not good-enough parenting of one kind or another. We are interested in these feelings and behaviours because if not corrected they can further disrupt appropriate emotional development.

Questions to think about

1. Define emotional self-regulation and give two examples from your own experience.
2. What are emotional display rules? Give two examples.
3. What is social referencing? Give two examples.
4. True or false: During the preschool years children's descriptions of their own behaviour and that of other people, indicate that they have the capacity to infer intentions.
5. Explain how a child's widening contexts affect emotional development (particularly expression) in early and middle childhood

Suggested further reading

Harris, P. L. (1990). Children and emotion: *The Development of Psychological Understanding*. London. Blackwell.

Hascher, T. (2010). Learning and emotion: Perspectives for theory and research. *European Educational Research Journal*, 9(1), 13–28.

Grusec, J. E. (2011). Socialization processes in the family: Social and emotional development. *Annual Review of Psychology*, 62, 243–269.

Rutter, M. (1998). Developmental catch-up and deficit following adoption after severe global early privation. English and Romanian Adoptees (ERA) Study Team. *Journal of Child Psychology and Psychiatry*, 39(4), 465–476.

Chapter 9

Oppositional behaviour, aggression and anxious behaviour

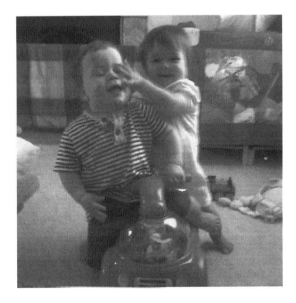

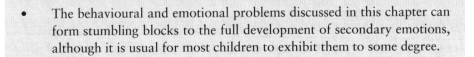

- The behavioural and emotional problems discussed in this chapter can form stumbling blocks to the full development of secondary emotions, although it is usual for most children to exhibit them to some degree.

- Some oppositional behaviour is normal and serves a psychological purpose, but unresolved it becomes a problem that can effect emotional development.
- Aggression is a natural behaviour that arises from anger, but uncontrolled aggression is the best predictor of future psychological and social difficulties.
- A modicum of anxiety is also normal, but inconsistent care can result in severe anxiety that can lead to debilitating internal preoccupation of the child.
- Oppositional behaviour and aggression provide external difficulties, while anxiety causes internal difficulties. In excess all three cause serious developmental delay and difficulties, because they preoccupy the child and distort social relations.

As CHILDREN GROW MANY parents and caregivers become concerned with certain behaviours that seem to disturb a child's smooth progression into an adjusted socialised adult. It is usual for children to show some oppositional behaviour, aggression and anxiety. Many parents wonder about the 'normality' of these behaviours and whether the child is 'on the right path'. From the standpoint of emotional development it is advantageous to look at these fairly common behaviours for two reasons. First, these behaviours can influence a child's emotional development directly, especially if they are not resolved in an appropriate way. Second, these behaviours can be a direct influence on parents or caregivers, who form a very important part of the child's social environment and thus have a considerable influence on the growth of secondary emotions in children. In development the child influences the parent and the parent influences the child. Though these difficult behaviours are issues in many instances in early and middle childhood the key to understanding them comes from the earlier toddler period. These behaviours, in altered form, often occur again after middle childhood. Because we have dealt with toddlerhood already and are about to discuss emotional development in adolescence this is an appropriate juncture to consider these behaviours in more detail and how they can influence emotional development.

Oppositional behaviour

An oppositional or negative stance is the tendency children have to defy adult advice and to oppose instructions designed to protect them or socialise their behaviour. It is expressed as oppositional behaviour and some of this behaviour is "normal" (Turner, 1991). This behaviour first becomes noticeable in toddlerhood when a child learns for the first time to resist and even to say 'no'. Oppositional behaviour in toddlers can easily lead to severe tantrums even for well-adjusted secure children. If oppositional behaviour is understood and dealt with in an adequate manner in the toddler years it will not be particularly troublesome in early and middle childhood but may well return in quite a different form in adolescence. It is, of course, important to identify these behaviours as truly oppositional and not due to persistent, severe, unhappiness; a distinction can be hard to make in children who have had inconsistent parenting. To understand oppositional behaviour and how it influences a child's emotions we must start with the toddler. Why does a toddler show such negative behaviour and what if anything can be done about it?

Understanding oppositional behaviour in toddlerhood

Nearly every child goes through a period of negativism in his or her toddler years. One of the first words that a child learns is 'no', perhaps because they have heard the word many times before they could say it. However, toddlers don't just say 'no', they fly into temper tantrums when others do not react to their commands or when things will not go their way. Temper tantrums are the most typical form of oppositional behaviour in toddlerhood and we will concentrate on them, however, toddlers can also sulk, be unco-operative, and give you the 'silent treatment' from time to time. These are other forms of negative oppositional behaviour. If we consider tantrums, more than half of all two year olds will have tantrums at least once a day (Leach, 1989). Almost all children will have had tantrums during their toddler years. Toddlers who have temper tantrums are not bad children; they will often grow into sensitive intelligent people if the response to their tantrums has been appropriate.

Tantrums and other negative behaviours grow out of an immediate need that the child has, but they also have a more deep-seated psychological function. The immediate cause of tantrums is a build-up of frustration. During toddlerhood the child becomes aware that he or she is an agent who can act on things and change things. One of the things toddlers may wish to change is what mothers want the toddlers to do. To effect this change can be difficult because toddlers are small and not very powerful. Nevertheless, toddlers wish to exert the power that they have and often attempt to resist the adult. This resistance may not work and the toddler explodes in frustration. He or she becomes out of control and a tantrum results.

At a deeper level the toddler is trying out independence. The sense of agency that the child now possesses has to be exercised to see how far it will go. The toddler soon learns that some obstacles are hard to get around and it is from the failure to move or influence these objects that the frustration comes. One of the

171

objects is mother (or caregiver) and the child's clash with this person is very important for further development. If the caregiver does not retreat or succumb to all of the toddler's demands the toddler begins to learn that the adult is an agent in his or her own right. The adult cannot be pushed around at the will of the toddler, at least not every time that the child desires something. This resistance shown by the adult helps the child define him or herself more clearly and the child learns the limitations on his or her will. When limitations on action are understood and accepted by the toddler then frustration does not arise so easily and tantrums decrease. What has happened is that the child has defined him or herself more accurately and has begun the normal and necessary psychological separation from the parent that will develop further in later childhood and adolescence.

Understanding the psychological function of temper tantrums is the key to understanding what one should do when a toddler has such a tantrum. If a parent or caregiver retreats *all* the time and *always* gives in to the angry child, the psychological function of the tantrum will not be achieved by the child. If the parent constantly retreats and acquiesces the child will gain no sense of where the adult stands and in turn no sense of the limitations on his or her own actions. Thus parents who retreat and give in to children on all occasions rob those children of an important element in their quest for self-definition. These parents are not good-enough because they fail to introduce the toddler to objective reality. Objective reality (Rodman, 2003) is when the adult is seen as separate from and not under the control of the toddler.

At this juncture three important points must be made. First, parents should themselves *avoid negativity*. Parents should not always deny requests from their children. Children who can never persuade their parents to do anything for them are deprived children. Parents should acquiesce with reasonable requests from a toddler. Indeed toddlers should learn that they can influence their parents and this will help their sense of self. Second, an *occasional* lapse when parents give in to an unreasonable demand by a toddler will do no harm. Even parents with a child who is very demanding and full of tantrums may give in *on occasions* without damaging the child's quest for self-definition. Parents must be constant in the 'war' with toddler demands, but if a certain 'battle' is lost to the child, not all is lost. If the parent does not give up the general struggle, even when certain issues are lost, but mostly persists in passively opposing the toddler's tantrums over time, the child will eventually wilt. The passage of time allows the child to become more socialised as he or she slowly recognises the separation of the persons in the conflict. Third, parents should react *passively* to tantrums, rather than respond actively. They should be calm and restrained even though they may need to be strong and restrain an active child. Parents should neither punish nor reward tantrums; rather they should resist or ignore them. However, parents should not give in, except on rare occasions, and overall they should maintain a constant calm watch over the child. Parents or caregivers should, where appropriate, allow the child to be part of the decision making process that affects the child. However, they should not leave the child alone to make all the decisions. To do so denies the nature of the child as a dependent person. Children are not miniature adults. They learn decision making from observing it and from being involved in the process at a level appropriate to their abilities. They do not learn by being hoisted with the main responsibility for the process. This approach which recognises the child's dependence is concordant with an authoritative, but not an authoritarian, type of parenting. However, even when a child is rightly considered as dependent, if authoritative parents make an error they should apologise unreservedly to the child.

All in all this approach requires the parent to remain calm, to stand firm, and to try to defuse the temper of the child. Eventually the child will come to see the parent as at least a semi-independent person in this process and this will advance the child's theory of mind and his or her understanding of other people's feelings.

Oppositional behaviour in later childhood and adolescence

Though children can be negative and oppositional after toddlerhood the intensity of extreme oppositional behaviours such as tantrums normally declines progressively in early and middle childhood. Other forms of oppositional behaviour such as sulking may not show the same decline but, on the whole, negativism decreases as the child gets older. In early adolescence most children seem to renew the earlier quest for independence with renewed vigour. They are it seems impelled into this quest by the physical changes which they are undergoing at this time.

However they no longer suffer the powerlessness of the toddler and the oppositional behaviour of this stage though sometimes bad temper cannot be described as a tantrum. Oppositional behaviour in adolescence serves basically the same purpose as it did earlier, namely to separate the teenager psychologically from his or her parents (or caregivers). It often, at this stage, involves a defiance of reasonable parental rules and a resort to peer group norms as an alternative guide for behaviour. Again the appropriate parental behaviour is to be calm passive and unmoved by silly ideas that could, in certain instances, be dangerous to the young person. In today's society this may not be enough to avoid trouble but it is all that can be done.

Hopefully the ambivalent demands for adolescent freedom will decline as the older adolescent engages with the reality of life. By later adolescence the psychological break with parents has come and gone and hopefully a new equitable psychological relationship between parent and adolescent is starting to form. The development of most children is concordant (coherent) over the age grades and many of those who have severe oppositional problems as adolescents have a long history of uncontrolled oppositional behaviour in childhood, which was never corrected by appropriate adult action. We will discuss adolescent emotional development in the next chapter. For the moment we must consider how oppositional behaviour and its control affects the development of emotions particularly those secondary emotions that first form in toddlerhood.

Relation of oppositional behaviour to emotional development

Oppositional behaviour becomes important in the development of emotions when it is not resolved and the child continues to be continually oppositional over the years. Where a child is dominated by one psychological and behavioural feature other developments can be pushed into the background. Oppositional behaviour that continues without moderation into early and middle childhood, and which becomes extreme in adolescence, will occupy the child's psychological energies.

Such children become obsessed with opposition and though the secondary emotions may form in such a child they are not very motivating. Thus the child may have some feelings of shame, guilt and pride but acts on nearly every occasion to oppose people rather than on the basis of these secondary self-conscious emotions. The emotions are overwhelmed on most occasions by the child's struggle to be oppositional. This state of affairs, where opposition by the child is un-relenting, also influences the child's caregivers who will spend a lot of their time dealing with opposition rather than contributing by other interactions to the development of the secondary emotions. Continual oppositional behaviour makes a child unpopular with both adults and peers and subverts positive social interactions. Oppositional behaviour may take up all the child's time and physical and mental energy. These are the reasons why unresolved oppositional behaviour affects the further development of emotions and their expression. It is of some importance therefore in emotional development that periods of natural negativism and opposition are resolved. This resolution allows caregivers appropriate influence, may restore the child's popularity and gives time for the development of the positive secondary emotions. In such circumstances these emotions will be exercised and can become motivating forces in the child's life. As we shall see undue aggression and severe anxiety, especially in the form of attention seeking, also form barriers to the development, and especially the exercise, of important secondary emotions.

Aggression

Aggression is usually an expression of anger; aggression is a behaviour not an emotion. When the expression of anger is not controlled we refer to the expressed emotion as rage. Anger can be greatly aided in its development as an emotion by frustrating experiences. In some instances frustration may be the source of most of the anger in a person. Thus most children who are constantly or frequently frustrated easily become angry and anger can constitute much of their emotional life.

Yet anger can arise from other causes and can be seen in most human beings including those who are not frustrated or are rarely frustrated.

Are anger and the subsequent aggression that it produces inborn characteristics of human beings? In Figure 5.1 you can trace the development of anger from frustration. Anger arises from other causes but frustration is a major contributor to its genesis. Anger can be exhibited as aggression which is largely a behaviour but one that is difficult to define without some reference to mental antecedents or concomitants.

Aggression is a well-known feature in human society even though many of us live fairly peaceful lives. The potential for aggression exists in many human interactions including those of childhood. However, this potential is not often realised, and even when it is, aggression is not always displayed. Anger and frustration can lead to aggression, but this is a chicken and egg situation, because aggression that arises from other causes can be *repressed* or *converted* into anger and frustration. Aggression can be *displaced* from one situation to another. Aggression can be *sublimated* into socially acceptable competitive behaviour. Thus all of us can be aggressive but, in terms of the total number of human interactions we take part in, we are not often openly aggressive.

Is aggression important?

If most of us are not openly aggressive very often, why is aggression an important topic for people who work in social services? Aggression is a behaviour that can cause great social difficulty even if it is displayed by only a very small section of the population. We all depend on social relationships and these are harmed or distorted by aggression. For this reason we wish to control or limit overt aggression in society. Aggressive children grow up for the most part to be aggressive adolescents and adults. Aggression in childhood is a good predictor of later aggression (Huesmann *et al.*, 1984) and is more predictive of poor academic achievement than other behavioural problems (Brennan *et al.*, 2012). Aggressive children are likely to grow up with social adjustment problems, low intellectual achievement, and a tendency to get into trouble with the authorities, be they teachers or police. Although some aggression in toddlers is to be expected, toddlers with high levels of aggression are shown to have poorer academic skills by the time they reach school (Brennan *et al.*, 2012). If we can understand aggression, we may be able to control or limit it.

What is aggression?

Aggression can be defined as, "A first act of hostility or injury" (Davidson *et al.*, 1994). Notice that the word *first* is used. Is retaliation aggression? No *not usually*. Most retaliation springs from a different psychological motivation to aggression, that of self-preservation when attacked. Though most retaliative acts are not aggression, some people use retaliation as an excuse for intentional aggressive acts. These people retaliate in response to any stimulus however insignificant or unintentional. They are being aggressive because the slight or injury received should in no way justify a response. These people hide their genuinely aggressive acts under the guise of retaliation.

What is hostility? Hostility can be a behavioural act of injury or a threat but it can also be an emotional or motivational state or a mixture of all of these elements. Hostility is usually defined as intent to hurt. Can there be aggression without overt hostility? Yes. Aggression need not have an overt display. Aggressive feelings can be transformed and transferred within the human psyche.

We can now expand the initial definition. Aggression is "a first act of hostility or injury which entails intentional harm being directed towards people or their possessions". The intentional aspect in this definition is important. It is the intention to harm that defines an act as aggressive rather than the consequences of the act. This excludes accidents from aggressive acts, though if one designs an accident then one is being aggressive and of course the incident is not an accident. If no harm results from an action, yet harm was intended, then the action was aggressive.

Aggressive acts can be *displaced* from one behavioural situation to another (Freud, 1915). Thus the Japanese factory worker strikes a large doll with a kondo sword! The doll has the face of the boss. Aggression can also be channelled into competitiveness, assertiveness, and even feelings of mastery and confidence. Aggression can be turned inwards into the psyche and can cause depression and suicidal thoughts.

All of this makes us question whether aggression is a unitary phenomenon. The motivations behind aggression seem to be as important (as defining features), as the aggressive acts themselves. We have made the point quite strongly that aggression is defined by the intent in the mind of the aggressor, an intent to be hostile and to do injury. If we do not intend to be hostile, irrespective of what we actually do, we are not aggressive. This brings us to types of aggression.

Types of aggression

It is possible to divide true, intentional aggression into two categories depending on the intent.

- *Instrumental* aggression is where the aggressor intends to be hostile in order to achieve a purpose other than the injurious one.
- *Hostile* aggression is where the aggressor intends only hostility and injury. This type of aggression is therefore 'mindless' and contributes most to the worst type of delinquency. Such aggression is often without conscience and is unlimited.

In children instrumental aggression can be observed more frequently than hostile aggression and first emerges around the first birthday and increases in the third year as a result of increased interaction with peers (Hay *et al.*, 2011). In some children hostile aggression can be turned to a more instrumental purpose when the aggressive child sees opportunity for gain. Children can also proceed from instrumental to hostile aggression particularly when the objectives of the instrumental aggression have been thwarted. In children therefore the boundary between hostile and instrumental aggression may not be clear from time to time, yet the distinction between aggression for gain and pure mindless aggression is a useful one. Where a child is being instrumentally aggressive to achieve a particular gain we can remove the child's goal and hopefully the aggression will cease. Instrumental aggression is sometimes called proactive aggression and hostile aggression is sometimes called reactive aggression.

Theories of aggression

The instinct theory of aggression

Some theorists believe aggression is an instinct, an inbuilt genetic propensity. There have been two chief proponents of aggression as an instinct. Freud (1915) saw aggression as an innate potential. The aggressive drive he postulated was part of the death instinct, Thanatos. He eventually placed this death instinct, Thanatos (aggression), on a par with Eros the life instinct. The First World War played its part in such a conclusion. Freud felt the child was born with an aggressive instinct, but the way in which this innate potential was expressed depended on the nature of the child's early developmental and environmental experiences. Thus experience and learning played a part in Freud's view of aggression. Lorenz (1966) on the other hand saw aggression as innate and totally uninfluenced by learning. His theory envisaged aggression as an innate response released when a child is subjected to certain environmental stimulus patterns. These patterns of stimuli or *triggers* release the aggression. It is instinctive. The child has little influence on the situation.

Instinct theories suggest that aggression may be periodically 'released' by catharsis or displacement. However, research indicates that there is little evidence to support the view that catharsis decreases aggression. Indeed the acting out of aggressive impulses may even increase future aggressive behaviour (Mallick & McCandless, 1966). Generally, we believe that aggression begets aggression and would advise against 'acting out' (or cathartic) methods of dealing with aggression in children. Perhaps some children, withdrawn shy individuals, need to practise their aggression but the vast majority do not need to demonstrate further expressions of anger. Instinct theories of aggression have been widely criticised. What children with undue aggression need is training to help them control aggression or transform it into other acceptable outlets rather than the further expression of aggression that they gain in 'acting out' cathartic sessions.

The frustration–aggression hypothesis

This theory (Dollard *et al.*, 1939) fits in with the picture we have already given of the development of anger in early life and how this gives rise to later feelings of inferiority, bitterness, hatred, and disgust at others. In this theory aggression is seen as a response to frustration. Thus according to this theory children who are continually frustrated will show many aggressive impulses and acts. The theory postulates that frustration is learnt from the environment. Severe potential punishment, poor school success, poor recognition by peers and/or parents, have been postulated as environmental factors producing frustration. There is no doubt that a link exists between aggression and frustration.

Frustration does seem to produce aggression in some cases. Yet much aggression occurs without obvious frustration. The link between frustration and aggression is too simple an explanation for all aggression. Frustration appears to be a facilitative but not a necessary condition for aggression. So though one can follow the process in a child, from say, severe punishment, to frustration, to aggression, not all aggression can be based on such a sequence (or similar sequence). It may be true that frustration and aggression go together in some cases, but does the frustration cause the aggression, or are they both related to other unidentified factors? For child welfare workers this link to frustration is interesting. It may be possible in many cases to remove factors that frustrate the child. Hopefully this will reduce aggressive acts.

Bandura's Social Learning Theory of aggression

It is possible to give an alternative explanation to the observation that severely punished children often become aggressive. This may not be due to frustration but to modelling. Children may imitate the people who frequently punish them. Such children may go further and identify with the punishing person. They may adopt the aggressive behaviour, the attitudes, and even the justifications used by those who punish them. Thus, in some instances, we see child abuse and wife bashing running in families from generation to generation because family members model their behaviour on one another.

Social learning theory, now sometimes referred to as social cognitive theory, was expounded by Bandura (1977) who believed that aggression was learnt from the social context in which children found themselves. Children, he believed, model their behaviour on those around them who have influence over them. Influence often stems from love or from power. When parents are aggressive, even towards their child, the child will introject this behaviour, model the parents and produce aggression on subsequent occasions. Modelling is complex associative learning and children will also model those in their environment whom they esteem. Thus modelling can take place by following TV and other public models as well as family models.

This theory postulates that aggression breeds aggression and it seems as if this is true. Thus the heavily punished child may be modelling father's behaviour rather than trying to rid him or herself of frustration. Bandura's theory of aggression is the one that explains most about this human behaviour and it has gained wide acceptance among child psychologists. Modelling and social learning depend on the social environment. This is influenced by:

(a)   the contingencies – rewards and punishments in the environment;
(b)   situational factors – who or what is in the environment;
(c)   cognitive factors – how well does the child comprehend the environment; and finally,
(d)   cultural factors.

One can see that social learning is indeed a complex operation. In our opinion, the Social Learning Theory is the most accepted and useful theory concerning the origin of aggression. It is particularly useful in child welfare practice as it explains the often observed fact that some child abuse is intergenerational occurring in succeeding generations in the same family. Perhaps such a cycle can be broken by giving the abused child an alternative non-aggressive model as a foster carer.

Developmental changes in aggression

Aggression depends on intent. How much intent does a one year old have? True intentional aggression is possible only when a child is sufficiently advanced to be able to understand how their actions will affect others. To do this the child must have a sense of self and an understanding to some degree at least that other people have minds. In short the child must have a 'theory of mind'. Children must be able to construe how a person will react to their aggressive behaviour if the behaviour is to be truly intentional. The ability to predict how others will act takes some time to develop in its full form, but as early as 18 months a child may have the beginnings of a theory of mind if they have been reared in an environment of security and affection.

Children reared in adverse circumstances where the development of a sense of self and of others is not encouraged by reciprocity and imaginative play will lag considerably in this development of intention. Indeed because the development of their theory of mind has been limited, certain of these children will show, at later ages, behaviour normally judged to be aggression but which is not true aggression. This is because, in these cases, true intention has not developed and therefore the behaviour cannot be seen as aggression but merely as assertive behaviour.

Many toddlers have learnt how to be aggressive, indeed they use aggression as a means of opposing their parents or caregivers and, as we have explained above, as a means of defining their separate identity. In toddlerhood it is the constraints of parents and others that cause frustration and the most aggressive outbursts. Aggression between peers can occur in toddlerhood but deliberate aggression in order to annoy or injure one's peers is generally a later development, beginning at the pre-school stage. Though pre-schoolers can show hostile aggression, most of the aggression of the pre-school years (early childhood) is instrumental aggression for the most part. This type of aggression declines in middle childhood. Older children do not try to get what they want by simple aggressive strategies, largely because they have discovered more effective methods to achieve their goals and have been socialised to abandon purely aggressive approaches. Where socialisation against instrumental aggression has not taken place, as happens in homes with poor discipline and nurturance, instrumental aggression may not have been inhibited and older children from this background may still indulge in inappropriate instrumentally aggressive demands.

In middle childhood though *instrumental aggression declines* in most children *hostile aggression increases*, especially in boys. In the early primary school years this may well take a physical form, but hitting declines in frequency as the school years progress and is often replaced with taunts insults and other forms of verbal aggression. Hostile aggression of whatever form, peaks in early adolescence and declines thereafter (Cairns *et al.*, 1989).

The developmental context of aggression

Aggression like any other developmental feature is subject to context. The number of children who show open aggression in schools is very small in comparison to the whole school population, yet these pupils can cause deep anxiety to a majority of other children and of course to staff members. What are the contexts from which these children come? Two contexts are important in relation to this question. The first is the family context. Social learning theory states that aggression is learned by means of complex associative mechanisms; that is by modelling. The family context is where most modelling takes place and if this is an arena of expressed aggression then this is what some of the children will unconsciously follow in their own behaviour. The second important context is culture or sub-culture. Certain cultures and sub-cultures approve of aggression (usually in males) more than other cultures do. The tendency to be aggressive in any culture (or sub-culture) will, to some degree at least, be related to the expectations of that culture (or sub-culture).

Aggression and emotional development

Aggression in children is a complex behaviour. Some children appear more aggressive than others. Aggression usually springs from an emotional base and thus it has physiological concomitants. Some of these are hormonal. As an aspect of the 'fight or flight' response aggression can cause an adrenalin rush, and some children can enjoy the feeling this brings and wish to repeat it. As an expression of underlying emotion aggression is subject to display rules. Thus aggression is under considerable cultural control and cultures vary considerable in the degrees and forms of aggression that they will tolerate (Shweder *et al.*, 2008). Aggression still varies considerably between the sexes, males generally showing more overt aggression than females, but there is no simple reason why this is so. Aggression is linked to hormone production and the sexes vary in this respect, but it is also closely related to cultural norms and imperatives and these are also, in most instances, different for men and women.

Its close links with physiology and culture mean that aggression is in some senses a natural phenomenon arising from the anger and frustration that is almost inevitable in life. Need we concern ourselves with its effect on emotional development if it is a natural inevitable factor? Will not most aggressive behaviour be socialised and controlled in a natural way as the child develops?

For the most part it will be so controlled, but when it is not, undue aggression can disrupt and limit other emotional developments in childhood. Unsocialised aggression is, by definition, out of control and because it disrupts human relationships essential for emotional development it can cause a child to develop with emotional deficiencies. Of all the problems of childhood unsocialised aggression is the best predictor of future difficulties in life. Aggressive behaviour that grows uncurbed in early childhood may well extend into middle childhood and then adolescence and adulthood. It becomes such a predominant feature of a child's development that it occupies excess time and energy on everyone's part and can easily disrupt the processes that relate to the development of the socially beneficial secondary emotions. In this it is similar to oppositional behaviour and the line between these two problems is often blurred.

The family is probably the most potent context for the development of aggression in children. We have mentioned modelling an aggressive person as a mechanism for the display of excess aggression by children. What of a child's emotional growth, dependency needs, and attachments, are these related to the development of aggression?

We would expect that those infants reared with frequent experiences of frustration and little security would become angry and therefore aggressive. This is generally true as can be seen from research on children with insecure resistant attachment patterns. These are children who have no feelings of security because they realise that their caregiver will not meet their needs in a consistent way. Pre-school children with a history of insecure avoidant attachment are often hostile and aggressive towards other children in the pre-school. These children frequently have difficulty in developing emotional relations with other children preferring instead to be vicious and aggressive towards their peers. At the same time some insecure children can be excessively clinging and instrumentally dependent on adults (Sroufe, 1983; Troy & Sroufe, 1987).

Aggression like oppositional behaviour can come to dominate a child's relationships with other people and if not resolved can limit or mask the development of some important secondary emotions. Toddlers who have suffered abuse often respond to a whingeing distressed companion with anger and aggression, rather than sympathy and concern, showing again the important effects that modelling and adverse conditions have on the development of positive secondary emotions (Main & George, 1985; Harris, 1990).

Dealing with aggression

How can we modify aggressive behaviour and limit its effect in the emotional life of a child? There is no easy method of influencing children to develop control of their aggressive impulses. The problem is that aggression is complex and each child we deal with has a different history with respect to aggression. However, there are a few rules and hints. Most approaches for limiting aggression involve one or more of the following factors. Either the aggression must be suppressed, or it must be diverted, or it must be brought under the child's inner control. The third of these approaches is certainly the most effective but it usually only obtained through the development of a long-term relationship, which is predicated on love and respect. By far the most effective time to limit aggression is early in a child's development. Passive resistance to tantrums, which often involve aggression, has already been mentioned as an important strategy. Social learning theory is useful because it gives hints on how to deal with aggression.

What can we do with an aggressive child? Several things:

1. We can analyse the child's aggressive behaviour. Is it intentional, instrumental, hostile? If it is instrumental then we may be able to remove the goal of the aggression.

2. We can, on some occasions, ignore the aggression. Some aggression will subside if ignored if, for example, it is instrumental as an attention seeking ploy. However most aggression will not just 'go away'!

3. Rather than simply ignoring aggression it is better to reinforce behaviour that is incompatible with aggression. Laughing, smiling, sharing and even simply being busy can all be, in certain situations, incompatible with aggression and thus should be reinforced.

4. We can set limits of tolerance for childish aggression. Aggression is natural and normal if kept within socialised limits. Thus children should be taught by rewards, moderate punishment, and modelling to keep their aggression within acceptable limits. Limits should be set by firm unaggressive adult control.

5. Frustration for the child should be lessened whenever possible. Frustration facilitates aggression.

6. Punishment should be moderate and non-aggressive. 'Time out' and social isolation are the best approaches for most aggressive children. Corporal punishment may lead to further aggression due to the child's social learning processes. Thus one must be a non-aggressive model for a child. Self-control can be modelled as easily as aggression and with much more positive outcomes.

7. Children should be able to understand the limits of aggression. Rules should be clear and explained when necessary.

8. Love and respect should be shown to the child who hopefully will model these positive attributes.

These eight points are hints on dealing with aggression in children. However, aggression is to be socialised, not totally eliminated. We need a little of it. Or do we? We leave the philosophical issue with you. As you consider the issue, ponder 'Is aggression natural'? In certain circumstances it appears accepted. Aggression is, as I have said, under much cultural influence. It is accepted at certain ages and with the male sex. Must this always be so? We trust this will give you a basis to cope with aggressive children whom you may meet in your practice. It should also allow you to formulate advice for the parents of aggressive children. Often the parents must change their own behaviour if the problem of aggression in a child is to be ameliorated.

Anxiety

Children, as we have learned, have an instinctive need to feel secure. Some of them, indeed many of them, will feel anxious when this need is not met. Parents can also feel anxious. Unlike aggression and oppositional behaviour, anxiety is a secondary emotion. High levels of anxiety are an inevitable part of most welfare issues where people are in trouble. Let us therefore look at it in more detail.

What is anxiety?

Sometimes people are overcome by the feeling expressed thus 'I know something is going to go wrong'. They frequently don't know what the something is but they are concerned that it will not turn out right. Children can have such feelings and if they are frequent and intense they can be quite disabling. Some children may be more predisposed to anxiety than others but children whose early history has been one of disruption may be easily affected by anxious thoughts.

Anxiety arises in most, but not all, instances from a child's inability to predict in association with that child's negative experience of change. If you turn back to Figure 4.2 you will see that it is an infant's perception of change that leads to fear and anxious fear if the changes the infant is subjected to are frequent and unpredictable. Frequent and unpredictable changes often happen to infants who are not properly nurtured. Not all children from disrupted or deprived backgrounds are anxious but many are. Some do not *appear* anxious but are churned up inside. Some show distinct signs of chronic anxiety. Some are not anxious in any way. Anxious children are obsessed with certain thoughts. They over-think (think too much) and can't get fearful thoughts out of their heads. They are not usually disruptive children. They don't want to cause trouble but something is wrong.

Anxiety and attachment

When we discussed attachment we referred to insecure attachment. There are three types of attachment that come under this category but all are characterised by feelings in the infant of insecurity and/or anger. Numerous studies have shown that there is a strong link between insecure attachment and anxiety in early childhood and through to adolescence (Colonnesi *et al.*, 2011). We must consider insecure attachment and the developments it leads to as one of the main sources of anxiety in children. This is not to say that securely attached children cannot be anxious from time to time; but anxiety as a feature of the enduring disposition of the child may well have its origins in an insecure attachment. Is there then temporary anxiety and anxiety of a more enduring kind? This leads us to the work of Speilberger.

Specific state and trait anxiety

Spielberger (1973) and other psychologists make the distinction between anxiety associated with a particular situation, or object (specific state anxiety), and that not associated with any specific element but seen as a pervasive characteristic of the anxious person (trait anxiety). Research has shown that most anxious people in most situations have anxiety levels due to both the specific situation facing them and their general level of anxiety. In fact anxiety is not situation free but neither is it totally intrinsic to any situation. Anxiety level depends both on specific and general factors.

Though it may be difficult to divide anxiety into two distinct types in practice when considering an anxious person, it is probably useful to discuss it by means of the 'specific state' and 'trait' division. Freud made much of 'free floating' anxiety which occurs when repression of ego-threatening psychic material occurs. The threat is forgotten but the anxiety lingers on! However we consider it, some people seem more anxious in general than others. Thus when we survey children we can see the anxious ones. We tend to presume that they are anxious due to trait anxiety but on investigation this may not be the case. Specific situations often of a constant nature may be contributing to their anxiety level. This is important in welfare practice because it may be possible to remove the specific irritant. Do not dismiss a child as over anxious in a trait sense without investigating the environment for specific anxiety producing factors. Collonesi *et al.*'s (2011) review of insecure attachment and anxiety showed little difference and a consistent effect between these two, regardless of the type or intensity of anxiety that was studied.

Anxiety and fear

The difference between anxiety and the basic instinct called fear parallels, or is equivalent to, the distinction between state and trait anxiety. Those who distinguish between anxiety and fear tend to view anxiety as a diffuse reaction and fear as bound to a specific object or situation. In practice it is difficult (as with state versus trait anxiety) to separate anxiety from fear in children. Children are frightened of bogey men. Such a reaction could be seen as a specific fear in childhood. In adulthood being frightened by a bogey man would be seen as a chronic anxiety state or as a schizoid delusion. Reality and fantasy are closer in childhood and this makes the distinction between fear and anxiety more difficult. Alternatively, a fear can generalise into all aspects of a child's life becoming an anxiety state.

Reactions to anxiety

If we believe 'something awful is going to happen' we can *run away* or if our anxiety resides in a social context, we can *withdraw*; or we can *avoid* an object or situation that we feel anxious about. If we are forced to remain with our anxiety it may overwhelm us and we may *breakdown*. Children and adolescents can show any of these reactions to anxiety.

Roots of anxiety in children

What causes anxiety and insecurity to arise in childhood? Insecure attachment has already been mentioned and it may well be the major contributor to trait anxiety. However more specific factors are also of interest.

Demanding parents. Demanding parents can make a child anxious. Parents who set tasks above the child's ability level can induce anxiety in the child. Even where tasks are appropriate, parents can be perfectionists, and, in the face of a creditable performance by the child, they can be ultra critical. The child comes to fear failure, or even to fear partial success, and becomes anxious. The child's self-confidence is undermined. One has only to watch the performance of parents at a football match or other junior sporting activity to see this process in action. Given such an attitude to junior sport it is no wonder that many children reject sport altogether, possibly as something that makes them anxious, and we have in much of the Western world a young adult population that is gaining in obesity and associated problems.

Over-permissive parents. Over-permissive parents can make a child anxious. Most children need to know that their behaviour has definite limits. This understanding will make them feel secure. Without such limits the child cannot predict the consequences of his or her behaviour. Lack of predictability in any situation will make people anxious and this feature is often part of a permissive treatment of children. Children with over-permissive parents can become highly anxious. Parents who are highly permissive usually tolerate the behaviours that their children produce. However, there are certain social and safety situations where even these parents are forced to act. When they do react, sometimes very vigorously, the child is taken aback and may not respond well to the parent's inculcations. If this happens frequently the child will not be able to make accurate predictions of how the carer will act and may become anxious.

Inconsistency. Inconsistency can make children anxious. Inconsistency in parental approaches to children causes unpredictability and this produces anxiety in the child. A parent must not be too demanding and should have clear, moderate and easily enforced rules for his or her children. Inconsistent treatment of children is the worst of all approaches because it causes unpredictability and thus directly raises the child's level of anxiety.

Over-pessimistic view of dangers. An over-pessimistic view of dangers, on the part of a parent, as they direct and influence a child's behaviour can cause anxiety in the child. Children can be made anxious by direct inculcation of safe behaviour and constant reference to danger.

Anxious model. Children can become anxious by copying an anxious model (Social Learning Theory). If parents are anxious, children may learn to be anxious simply by imitative observational learning. Of course this does not invariably happen and the anxious parent can have a calm sensible child.

Family difficulties. Family difficulties can cause anxiety in children. Family fights where bitterness goes unresolved can cause anxiety and divorce may do the same. (In some instances, divorce may lessen anxiety; it usually, but not invariably, disturbs children.) Children are likely to be most anxious when family difficulties split their inbuilt loyalties, where they are torn between two loved people.

Sexual demands, responsibilities and confidences. Children can become anxious if they are given too much responsibility and treated as adults. Sexual demands, responsibilities and confidences can cause anxiety. Demands of a financial nature can also cause apprehension. Children lack the psychological maturity to cope with adult problems. Of course sexual abuse causes anxiety; but not all anxiety in children is caused by sexual abuse.

Severe punishment. Severe punishment threatened or frequently administered can also cause children to be anxious.

Children can, of course, become anxious for a combination of the causes given above.

The effects of anxiety

Anxiety has very many effects (as it has causes) but we can summarise its general consequences. In this discussion we are referring to severe persistent anxiety (trait), rather than the specific anxieties that normal children may feel from time to time. There are, at least, nine detrimental effects from severe anxiety; these are outlined below.

1. Anxiety affects *intellectual performance*. When anxiety is severe it detracts from intellectual and scholastic performance. Highly anxious children score below their true ability level in IQ and reading tests. This effect decreases somewhat with age so if you are quite anxious before an examination it does not mean, at your age, that your performance will be reduced! In fact at all ages a very little anxiety can sharpen performance. Of course, even with older people, overwhelming anxiety will cause disturbed thinking. The effect of anxiety on a task also varies with the complexity of the task. Highly complex tasks suffer more in their completion from anxiety factors than simple ones.

2. Anxiety affects a *child's popularity*. Anxious children are not popular among their peers or adult acquaintances.

3. Anxious children are generally *more easily influenced* by others especially figures of authority than are non-anxious children. A raised level of anxiety makes people more susceptible to the influence of propaganda. Brainwashers take note! Anxiety can thus predispose a child to subtle exploitation.

4. Anxious children *lack confidence*, that is, true inner confidence as opposed to outward bravado, and develop *poor mental images of themselves*. Their self-concepts are lower than they need be and they exaggerate their physical idiosyncrasies.

5. Children whose anxiety stems from *their inconsistent treatment in infancy* are particularly liable to lack inner confidence. These children can at the same time be aggressive to other children and clingy and anxious with adults.

6. Anxiety in children decreases their displayed aggression against others, but may increase their covert feelings of *aggression*. Anxious children are aware of their increased aggressive feelings towards others and they fear these feelings. This increases anxiety. This fear of aggression may explain the different reactions to adults and children referred to in 5 above.

7. Anxious children are *over-dependent*. This is especially true of boys.

187

8.   Anxious children *develop many inhibitions*. In particular they become indecisive. They fear to act and can't decide which action to take. They become rigid and over-cautious. They may restrict their behaviours as they fear the consequences.

9.   Anxiety *generalises* easily from one of behaviour into another. This is one of the most damaging effects of anxiety and is most prevalent in children. The generalising effect of anxiety is an additional reason why fear and anxiety are difficult to separate in childhood. A specific fear in a child quickly generalises into a state of anxiety about everything. This difficulty in separating fear and anxiety is greater the younger the child considered.

Phobias

Fears and anxiety are difficult to separate in childhood but the term phobia is still used concerning certain childhood disorders. This can be inappropriate. Some features of childhood labelled as phobias are in fact general anxiety states, while some general anxiety seen in childhood can have its origin in fairly specific fears. Specific fears are easily developed by anxious children. In such children fear spreads easily, being generalised quickly from the feared object to other objects and situations. In this way a general state of anxiety is produced. (Generalisation of the stimulus; maintenance of the response.) A fear of arithmetic exams may become a fear of all examinations.

Fears are negatively reinforced by avoidance behaviour. Fear outweighs reason and if the feared object is avoided fearful reactions are reduced. This process is rewarding in the sense that negative reinforcement occurs (avoidance of a noxious stimulus) and so further avoidance reactions are made more likely. In this behavioural sequence both fear and avoidance are reinforced. What this creates is a situation where fears need not be tested against reality as the feared object is always avoided. Children's ability to fantasise aggravates this situation. One can see these dynamics operating as stutterers avoid threatening words. Some phobic children never find out that there is nothing to fear, in reality. So children avoid dogs and never learn that most dogs do not bite. Children may develop certain characteristic age-related fears. For example fear of strangers between say nine months and two years; fear of animals, later, 2–3 years; fear of the dark and ghosts, 4–5 years; and fear of school characteristically 5–11 years.

School phobia

This phobia is of considerable concern to parents and professionals because it is quite serious and common (3 in 1,000 pupils). School phobia, more common in girls than boys, must be distinguished from truancy, more common in boys than girls. School phobia is, in fact, a neurotic generalised anxiety disorder. Truancy is a wilful absence from school in order to do more enjoyable things. Some authorities point to two types of school phobia.

Type I where the child becomes generally anxious, especially about mother, in a home situation that appears happy and adjusted. This type of school phobia is relatively easily understood by parents who involve themselves in the remedial process. Type I tends to occur with younger (primary) children and in acute episodes. Type II is a chronic condition usually at late primary/early secondary stage. The condition is interwoven with maladjustment in the home. Father and mother lack insight into the problem and may even be hostile to solutions. Father is usually very detached while mother, though appearing cooperative, psychologically clings to her daughter.

Many school phobics suffer from a generalised anxiety condition originating in separation anxiety (from mother) but distributed over situations, including school, where parents are not present. Going to school is compulsory so a focus arises on this symptom. This focus is further developed because it often appears that a specific incident or object at school has started the fear which has then expanded to anxiety about school in general. The psychodynamics are, however, in many cases more related to the family and the child suffers from a fear of separation. This is aggravated by an unhappy friendless school existence. School phobia can be relieved by a desensitisation of anxiety process.

Cures for anxiety

As with many other things prevention is better than cure. To limit anxiety in children, parents and professionals should:

1. minimise evaluation of the child;
2. give the child realistic goals (this may involve readjusting, covertly, the child's own goals);
3. give deserved and unpatronising praise to the child;
4. use the child's peers to contribute to the child's confidence;
5. have the child overlearn certain tasks, e.g. public performances (children are easily made anxious, like the rest of us, if they don't know what they are doing);
6. be predictable;
7. give the child a routine; and
8. do not throw children into things that are beyond their competence.

Though these measures will limit and even prevent anxiety, how is it tackled once it occurs? Anxious children benefit from understanding but the most effective way of removing the symptoms of specific or phobic anxiety is a procedure known

189

as *Desensitisation of Anxiety* (counter-conditioning). This behavioural approach involves identifying the events or objects that evoke marked emotional discomfort and the arrangement of these anxiety producing events into a graded list from the least to the most disturbing. Then a seemingly incompatible association of noxious anxiety producing events is made with pleasant relaxing stimuli. This is done at each stage of the graded list. This association counters the anxiety and causes the feared situation to lose its unpleasant connotations. Once one stage is desensitised the procedure goes to the next on the graded list. School phobia treated by this procedure serves as an example.

1. School is the anxiety producing situation.
2. The associations of school can be divided, following discussion with the child, into a hierarchy of anxiety producing situations. These are listed from the least anxiety provoking to the most anxiety provoking. The hierarchy not only forms an analysis of the fear, but a step-by-step treatment plan.

    (a) Sitting in the car in front of school (empty).
    (b) Getting out of the car with welfare officer in front of the school.
    (c) Crossing the empty playground.
    (d) Going to the school door.
    (e) Going into school (empty).
    (f) Entering the classroom (empty).
    (g) Having teacher join us in the classroom.
         This sequence is then repeated but with children present in the playground, school and classroom. Thus there are 14 steps in the hierarchy.

3. At each of these steps there should be an association of the anxiety developed with pleasant consequences. The child must be relaxed and/or rewarded in some way. The child may already have been trained in relaxation techniques, or he/she can be comforted by chocolate, or other goodies, or given the welfare worker's attention and approval. In any event the pleasant stimulus must be used until the signs of anxiety, shown by the child at each step, return to normal levels. Only then does one proceed to the next step. What should happen is that the pleasant stimulus which is incompatible with anxiety will cause the anxiety to diminish. Once the child feels pleasant and comfortable in a school situation they will realise they have nothing to fear.

Anxiety and emotional development

Anxiety can be beneficial. It is natural. Without it we would succumb to danger and perhaps not be spurred to succeed. Over-anxiety, however, is a disabling disorder causing quite severe problems. One of these problems is that severe over-anxiety can interfere with appropriate emotional development. It is much the same situation as exists with severe continual oppositional behaviour and frequent severe aggression. As in these other conditions children who are continually anxious have less time to develop the human interactions that lead to the higher secondary social emotions. Over-anxious children are also less popular with adults and other children and this increases their difficulties in relationships. Human relationships are an essential element in the development of secondary emotions. Continual anxiety consumes time and energy. The child will do little else except continually seek the security of routine and predictability if he or she is over-anxious. Only when this need is satisfied can such children return to fruitful relationships that will advance emotional development.

Over-anxious children need security and predictability but they also need positive regard and affection from those around them. Many anxious children are ashamed of their anxiety and inculcations to 'snap out of it' only increase their worry. What they need is support, understanding and comfort to help them face their anxieties. We need in child welfare work to have a particular understanding of anxiety that arises from insecure attachment and to consider arrangements that produce more security for infants and children. Children need security and permanent arrangements. Decisions need to be made early in a child's life to give such outcomes.

Questions to think about

1. Why is it necessary to resist the oppositional behaviour that a toddler may show? In what way should such resistance be effected?
2. Must a parent win every psychological battle with a toddler?
3. What theory of aggression is most explanatory? Explain why?
4. True or false: boys are more aggressive than girls.
5. How stable is aggression in males from middle childhood on?
6. In what ways can anxiety be beneficial

Suggested further reading

Lemerise, E. & Dodge, K. (2008). The development of anger and hostile interactions. In M. Lewis, J. M. Haviland & L. Feldman Barrettt (Eds), *Handbook of Emotion* . New York: The Guilford Press, pp. 730–741.

Hay, D. F., Hurst, S. L., Waters, C. S. & Chadwick, A. (2011). Infants' use of force to defend toys: The origins of instrumental aggression. *Infancy, 16*(5), 471–489.

Chapter 10

Emotional development in adolescence

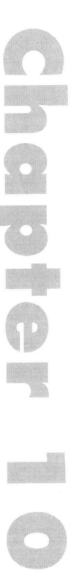

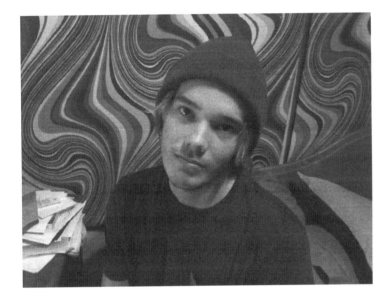

- Adolescence is both a biological and social construct.
- The child is father to the adolescent; for the range of emotions has been developed in earlier childhood and this period is really about control and expression of emotion in an increasing variety of contexts.
- Different rates of pubertal development, between and within the sexes, have an impact on emotional development.
- The influence of social referencing by the peer group, and other inputs, becomes marked during this period.
- Adolescents belong to different cultures and sub-cultures with different display rules for emotion.

A DOLESCENCE IS THE PERIOD of life between childhood and adulthood. It is during this period that the biological and maturational changes called puberty take place. These changes convert a sexually immature child into a person capable of reproduction. The teenage years are a long developmental period, a full decade, and because of the rapid physical and psychological changes that take place over this time there is a considerable difference between early and late adolescence.

What years are covered by adolescence? Generally adolescence is considered to cover the years 12 to 19. However, some individuals enter puberty as young as nine years and many have finished their major biological changes at 15 or 16 years. Why then is adolescence extended further?

The answer lies in the fact that adolescence, as opposed to puberty, is a social construct and a very important one in our society. It is the period between childhood, strictly speaking middle childhood, and adulthood that is an essential time for learning to take place in order that the individual can enter the adult world as a fully functioning autonomous person. During this period an adolescent remains, to a certain degree at least, dependent on adults. This requirement to learn in order to achieve independent adult status is subject to much cultural and social variation.

In our society adolescence has tended to get longer and longer. This is due to two effects. The age of onset of puberty in Western societies for both boys and girls had for several decades in the 1900s been getting younger probably because of improved nutrition. After 1970 this trend slowed and has now stopped (Karpati et al., 2002; Delemarre-van de Waal, 2005). Nevertheless, compared to earlier decades we are now pushing the physical start of adolescence back into what was previously regarded as childhood.

The second effect is that adolescence as a period for the acquisition of adult skills has been lengthened. People now need much more schooling to prepare them for adult life. Before World War II many people had no secondary education at all. They left school at 14 or 15 or even earlier and joined the work force. For many years after the war, until perhaps the early 1970s, this remained an option for many young people though they tended to leave at 15 from high school rather than primary school. After this time and particularly in the 1980s young people stayed on at school. The type of work they had left for earlier had simply dried up. What expanded was the need for skilled rather than unskilled labour. People stayed at school to become skilled. This staying on increased the period of dependency and thus lengthened the period regarded as adolescence, that is the transition period between childhood and adulthood. In the light of this it is interesting to speculate as to how we would classify those people who currently still leave school at an early age but do not gain work and become dependent on the state for support. Are these people still adolescents?

Thus what is called adolescence is not determined by biological factors alone. The age span that we talk of as adolescence depends on the society we are considering and on the era. The term teenager was not used to any degree before the 1950s.

The importance of adolescence in emotional development

Adolescence is a period of dramatic physical growth and change. This influences all other developments in adolescence including emotional growth. In general adolescence is a time when many earlier developments are reworked or refined into more advanced forms. The forces behind adolescent development are undoubtedly the physical changes that transform a child into an adult. These changes impel social changes in the life of the adolescent and these in turn produce both cognitive and emotional effects.

All of these developments, physical, social, cognitive and emotional feed off each other and development in one area has close links to another. In reality development is always 'all of a piece' and does not take place in compartments. Nevertheless, in adolescence physical development sets the scene for other developments and is of great importance especially in the mind of the adolescent. The sense of self is reworked in adolescence and linked to the adolescent's new physical form. As we have already seen in childhood a sense of self is very important to emotional development. This remains the case in adolescence.

The physical developments of adolescence can put young people under considerable pressure. Biologically they are capable of reproduction but because of their remaining dependency they are obliged to postpone reproduction, though they increasingly take part in sexual activity. Where young people have a reasonable degree of self-esteem and strong family and social supports (including access to contraception) this may not be an extreme dilemma. However, where an adolescent has a low self-concept and no family or social supports the biological pressure to reproduce may result in the birth of a child. The adolescent may find it difficult to cope and may not adequately meet the baby's dependency needs. Many teenage mothers or fathers are very adequate parents but others recommence the cycle of emotional deprivation.

The child is father to the adolescent

Though physical development is the driving force in adolescent development in general and also in adolescent emotional development, it is physical development on the base of what has gone before. This is particularly true of physical effects that influence social and thus emotional development. These physical effects influence both the adolescent and those people who interact with the adolescent. However, the influence these effects have depends on the distinct emotional history of the individual adolescent and the emotional repertoire that he or she has developed (or not developed) in earlier years. Thus what happened in infancy, how it changed in toddlerhood, and then in early and middle childhood, has an influence on adolescent emotional development.

Earlier development is of crucial importance in determining the course of adolescent emotion. In the USA James Garbarino has written extensively and with authority about the problems of adolescent boys (Garbarino, 1999; Bradshaw *et al.*, 2009). He has no doubt that adolescent problems frequently occur as sequels to what happened in childhood. Other researchers have shown that the experience of physical abuse in early childhood has a distinct correlation with later problems of aggression in that 35 per cent of children who were abused in their early years go on to become abusers in later years (Dodge *et al.*, 1997). Delinquency implies law breaking and serious disruption and it is our contention that though adolescence may aggravate problems related to the law in many cases such problems were apparent in the child long before adolescence began. The problem with adolescents is that they are bigger, faster, tougher and often more cunning than children. Many of us can deal with children because they offer us no physical challenge but would find the same children grown to adolescence quite difficult to control.

Thus adolescents do not start with a 'clean sheet'. They all have a considerable history. What has happened previously will have a considerable impact on the development of an individual in adolescence and on the type of adult he or she will become when adolescence is past. Garbarino feels that some issues and problems can have very deep roots. He sees human development as being cumulative, proceeding, in many instances, from the quality of the earliest attachment in the first year of life.

The purpose of adolescence

The general developmental task of adolescence is to allow for a process whereby the adolescent becomes an autonomous person in his or her own right, a separate individual while still retaining connections to family and others. Thus adolescents must establish an *identity* as a separate person, achieve a new relationship with *peers* and *family* and develop goals for their *independent operation in the world*.

As you can imagine the achievement of these tasks is highly dependent on the adolescent's previous history. If you do not know who your father was and have only brief contact with your mother while enduring repeated changes of substitute care, identity will be much more difficult to achieve than if you come from a settled and secure background. Likewise relations with peers will depend on a child's history of human relationships. Those adolescents who have not developed the ability to sympathise with the position of others and have little or no sense of guilt or shame may well find advanced flexible and sustained relationships with peers very difficult indeed. Relations with family are also affected by previous family interactions and whether the family has adequately serviced the child's dependency needs, particularly the need for warm emotional connection and the need for security.

As for independent operation in the world, those adolescents who were largely abandoned to their own devices as children will often react to the wider society in a worldly wise manner and this may gain them an initial advantage over more conventional and inhibited children. After all, the abandoned adolescents have brought themselves up and have had many years of practised independence. However, in many cases, because their long term skills with people are so inadequate and their self-centredness so great, the worldly wise demeanour of these adolescents soon loses its power to gain them any advantage and their long term prospects in the wider world become bleak.

The complications of adolescence

A period of storm and stress?

Does the achievement of the developmental tasks of adolescence as outlined above inevitably produce conflict and stress with parents and others? Is adolescence a stormy period? While physical changes are the driving force of adolescence, most young people take these changes in their stride. Adolescence is not always a period of storm and stress (Hill, 1980; Steinberg, 1990; Garbarino, 1999). Stress in adolescence tends to be associated with specific developments or contexts and is not general.

Nevertheless, a number of psychologists have suggested that adolescence is a stormy period especially in relation to parents and other figures because it is necessary for the adolescent to separate him- or herself psychologically from others, particularly parents. The conflicts generated in this stormy period, according to these authorities, allow the adolescent to come to terms with the stances of other people and in doing so define their own position. There may well be something of this type taking place in adolescence but whether the stormy component is essential is open to question (Casey et al., 2010).

Adolescents have to establish, to some degree at least, a separate identity and they must spread their emotional dependence outwards from the family. However, this process can be achieved quietly and whereas emotional dependence must be spread some emotional dependence remains with the adolescent's family of origin. Early adolescence is a more stormy period than later adolescence and in some ways relives the terrible twos. Adolescents at this stage do indeed bounce themselves off others to see where they stand. Matters of conflict between adolescent and parent at this time tend, in the majority of cases, to be about everyday matters such as dress, decorum and jobs around the house.

Adolescents do not, on the whole, question their parents' deep seated underlying values (Collins & Repinski, 1994). The degree of stress between adolescent and parent depends on the adolescent's earlier emotional history. The search for identity, for example, begins well before adolescence and is only accelerated in this period. This search will become more important and frenetic if earlier attempts to develop an identity have been thwarted.

Difficulties related to physical changes

The physical changes during adolescence produce two categories of people who may have particular difficulties. There are very different rates of change for boys and girls and within genders (Marceau *et al.*, 2011). These are *early maturing girls* and *late maturing boys*. These problem conditions can be vastly more complicated if they occur to individuals whose history has been lacking in affectionate nurturing care.

Because physical changes are the driving force behind adolescence, adolescents are very conscious of their bodies and how they are changing. Adolescents relate their bodily developments to how they are perceived socially and this in turn affects their self-concept and emotional development. This is an area of adolescent development where sex differences appear to be important. On average girls reach puberty 1.5 to 2 years earlier than boys.

Early maturing boys are more likely to have a positive body image than the average boy, or more especially, than late maturing boys. They perceive themselves as more attractive than boys who are smaller and they are generally stronger and more athletically able than less mature boys (Petersen, 1987).

Late maturing boys by contrast probably have poor conceptions of their attractiveness, at least in the short term; though it is such a touchy subject many of them deny any shortcoming. Things are difficult for them. Not only are they behind the boys of their age but they are well behind all of the girls who in physical appearance are years in advance. Much research has shown that some of these boys resort to acting out and daredevil behaviours to compensate them in the eyes of their peers, of both sexes, for their lack of inches and physical maturity.

Yet *in the long term* there is no evidence for late maturing boys showing additional psychological or behavioural problems. Though late maturing boys are less popular and less self-confident during adolescence (Petersen, 1987) after adolescence these features disappear. Indeed, by contrast, Livson and Peskin (1980) found that early maturing boys in adulthood had on average become inflexible and conventional. Perhaps they became too confident too early and adolescence was not therefore as good a lesson for them in flexible responses as it was for their smaller less mature colleagues. Further research showed that early maturing boys on average report more psychological problems related to risky behaviour than do boys who mature later (Huddleston & Ge, 2003). However, more recent work suggests no real long term disadvantage for early maturing boys, the positive effects balancing out the negatives (Lynne *et al.*, 2007). It seems that overall being a late or early maturing boy is in the long term not of great importance and in probably the majority of cases is not a significant factor in comparison to other influences.

Girls show an apparently different picture. *Early maturing girls* do not seem to have the initial advantages that early maturing boys have. Girls who mature early have the worst perceptions of their body, much worse than late maturing girls (Stattin & Magnusson, 1990). The early physical maturity of these girls, which involves extra weight, does not correspond to current conceptions of beauty in Western culture. Such girls tend to be short and heavy when eventually their companions catch them up.

Stattin and Magnusson found these girls to have increased rates of risky behaviour such as drug and alcohol use and running away from home. The problem of these early maturing girls is that they are the first children to mature, often two years before early maturing boys, and sexual interest may be taken in them by males who are very much older. Of course this does not always happen and sexual exploitation of females by males is a widespread phenomenon at any stage, but when these girls come from a background of adversity and have not even the beginnings of emotional defence then exploitation can be grave indeed. *In the long term*, though many early maturing girls have no lasting effects of their early puberty, some researchers suggest that, on average, some of the difficulties of early maturing girls linger into later years. They report more relationship problems and less satisfaction in the following years in early maturing girls than in girls who matured late (Graber *et al.*, 2004)

Late maturing girls by contrast on average develop the slender physique that is esteemed in our culture. They seem to carry no difficulties into adulthood and in this respect are like late maturing boys. So perhaps the sexes are not so unalike in maturity difficulties. Late maturity seems to have less effect in both sexes in a long term perspective.

How adolescents feel about themselves

Self-consciousness

Most people in early adolescence who have had a nurturing upbringing are to some degree self-conscious. This is contributed to by a number of factors. It is due in part to a consciousness on the part of the adolescent of a rapidly changing body. It is also due to cognitive developments. An early adolescent boy (or girl) has gone beyond the simple view taken in childhood, namely that other people have thoughts and these must be taken into account. Adolescents can specifically conceive that the thoughts other people have may well be very different from their own thoughts. In early adolescence they also realise in full measure that other people can think about them.

The desire to be adult

Adolescents do not want to be adolescents they want to be adults. Nevertheless, most of them do not want, at this stage, to be like their parents. Such a desire would be in conflict with the main psychological purpose of adolescence, the impetus to become separate autonomous adults. No, teenagers wish to become new adults, wiser and better than their parents. Their view of what constitutes an adult is often rather standard; they do not have the experience to form a qualified view and they cannot be told. It is necessary for proper autonomy that they find out for themselves. The conception of the adult world in early adolescence is often very stereotyped. Adolescents still have not realised the tremendous range of adjustments and attitudes that adults have. Because adolescents want to be adults and because they have a stereotypical view of what adults should be, they tend to be both conformist and easily influenced.

The self-concept

In early adolescence the self-concept is well advanced but fragile. This contributes to self-consciousness. Adolescents are not often inwardly as confident as they might seem. This is particularly true concerning individual differences, especially if it is the adolescent who holds the difference.

The imaginary audience and adolescent egocentrism

Because they feel that their bodily changes make them conspicuous and because they have simple views about what people think (though they now know that other people think and can think differently from them) adolescents feel, in many of the things they do, that they have an imaginary audience (Goffman, 1969). They feel people are watching them and thinking about them often in a way that the adolescent would not wish. This type of thinking is often called adolescent egocentrism. Is it truly egocentric? We would say no. Adolescents are turning towards others not away from them. The problem is that early adolescent experience is limited and adolescent at this stage must operate from a simple stereotyped view of what others might think. When people of any stage have inadequate information or experience of a topic they often resort to stereotypes to help them make sense of things.

As adolescence advances and the young person gains experience stereotypical views decline and so does so called egocentrism, the self-conscious feeling that everyone is watching you and what you do is of great concern to everyone else. As you know, adults often wish that others would notice them more and be more concerned about what they do. The shift from the idea that 'everyone is watching' to 'nobody cares' is often quite dramatic in later adolescence and can pose dangers if the adolescent has no support.

Paradoxically it is the children that have had to bring themselves up, and therefore, in a sense, have had most experience of the world that have least difficulty on this score. If you have long experience that nobody cares for you, you will not easily see yourself as the object of an imaginary audience. You cannot be brought to conform by feelings of embarrassment or shame because these emotions may be lacking due to your history with people.

Invulnerability

Many adolescents and indeed many people in their twenties feel that they are invulnerable. These young people seem to have no sense of their own mortality. They feel that nothing untoward will happen to them. This feature is also said to be part of adolescent egocentrism. Some explanations of invulnerability refer to the fragile self-concept of early adolescence. However, this type of thinking extends very frequently into the twenties and is associated with confident and secure young people rather than those from conditions of adversity. Our explanation of this feeling of invulnerability is that it is a natural and desirable consequence of lack of experience. It disappears with time but when it is felt it allows for great exploration in all sectors of life. The fact that many adolescents and young adults feel invulnerable can be exploited especially in situations where people are asked to risk their lives. War has long exploited many adolescents who feel that nothing will happen to them. However, it is probably to the benefit of the wider society that, in dangerous situations such as exploration, natural disaster, or war, many adolescents and young adults are often quite willing to take risks and feel they will not be harmed.

Adolescent brains, risky behaviour and addiction

Most adolescents are not convicted of crime; they do not become delinquents. Nevertheless, many adolescents have a tendency to take risks and do things which older people would consider unadvisable because of the consequences.

Some new light on risky adolescent behaviour is given by the findings of recent neuroscience in respect of this stage of development. We now know that the brain undergoes considerable change during the teenage period and these changes, though less marked, parallel those of infancy and toddlerhood. No wonder we have oppositional behaviour in both periods. In infancy and toddlerhood new circuits are created in excess between neurons and those which are not used and substantiated by interaction with the child's environment are pruned. They are used or lost. A similar process appears to be taking place, perhaps to a less dramatic degree, in early adolescence. We know this from brain imaging studies. Overproduction of connections between brain cells occurs in abundance just before puberty occurs and pruning of unused circuits takes place during the adolescent years. In addition there is some evidence that an imbalance between the development of the subcortical limbic system relative to the prefrontal cortex produces heightened emotionality in this period, but that this is moderated by genetic and environmental factors (stress, trauma) so that it is highly variable (Casey *et al.*, 2010).

This second period of severe pruning occurs in fairly specific parts of the adolescent brain and is particularly prominent in the prefrontal cortex. This part of the cortex is involved with subjective feeling and also with long-circuiting neural impulses so that planning reason and consideration of others can be applied before a neural command is issued to produce behaviour. The myelination of the prefrontal cortex started long before adolescence at six months of age but it is only after this growth spurt of neural connections prior to early adolescence and its subsequent pruning in adolescence and later that the prefrontal cortex can be considered as truly mature. The burst of neural connections in this region of the brain just before puberty is presumably there to give the brain spare capacity to confront and master some of the difficulties of early adolescence.

The fact that the prefrontal cortex of the brain is not in adolescence fully mature and may not reach this condition until the mid-twenties at least partly explains why risk taking behaviour and feelings of invincibility are common in these years. Adolescent behaviour is subject to social control but in situations where this control is weak adolescents may not wait to ponder their actions. They may act on impulse because their frontal cortices are not sufficiently long-circuiting their neural impulses. Their lack of considered thought especially in regard to danger may also contribute to their frequently reported feelings of invulnerability.

This new knowledge that the early teenage brain is quite flexible and indeed subject in certain specific areas to actual physical change is important because we can then realise how vulnerable the early teenage brain can be. Alcohol and drugs have more chance of causing permanent injury to a brain when it is growing and developing spare capacity and this is what the adolescent brain is doing. This sensitivity to environmental influence and neural pruning may be related to the tendency for teenagers to become addicted to drugs and other things. Such addiction is hard to remove because the circuits mediating it have been used and therefore preserved, while those that could have been involved in other more substantial mature behaviour have been pruned. Adolescents may, in fact, be more subject to addictions than mature people because they have more possible neural connections in certain areas of the brain than adults.

So adolescence may not on the whole be a period of storm and stress but brain growth in this period while allowing for the assimilation of appropriate new experiences and skills can also allow adverse risky and addictive outcomes to occur if these are not tempered by appropriate environmental control (Giedd *et al.*, 1999; Lerner, 2002; Spear, 2000).

Adolescence and dependency

Adolescence is a period where even the last vestiges of instrumental dependency should be reduced to zero. Adolescents are usually quite keen on these reductions. When they learn to drive a car they reach the pinnacle of instrumental independence, or almost, because one instrumental dependency remains and increasingly so in our society, financial dependence. Adequate employment and remuneration for young people is getting increasingly hard to get and the paradoxical situation is reached where to achieve a good long term income an extended period of financial dependence is required while the young person completes school and possibly attends university or college.

Emotional dependency in adolescence also changes considerably. Before this stage emotional dependence should have spread to peers. This change is reinforced in adolescence and in late adolescence emotional dependence may well be further spread to a specific partner.

Yet again the problems lie with those who did not, through no fault on their part, develop adequate emotional dependencies in childhood. These adolescents may find an initial freedom in the group dependency of early adolescence but the later partnering may not go well for them though they will often enter sexual relationships and characteristically do so at a very early stage in adolescence.

The dependency relationship in adolescence is complex particularly as far as emotional dependency on parents is concerned. The ambivalence that normal adolescents show is based in part in a reluctance to give up this dependency combined with a desire to do so. It is easier and safer to be a child and be looked after than it is to be independent, yet who wants to be tied to home! This dilemma is solved when total instrumental independence, including financial independence, is gained and the emotional dependency between adolescent and family is hopefully re-established on a new footing.

Adolescence and emotional development

As children develop they become more and more involved in the wider world beyond their immediate family. By the time they become adolescents it is necessary for them to aim towards totally independent operations in the world. This progressive involvement in wider and wider contexts outside their original home has considerable implications for the emotional development of adolescents. Yet the quality of their care situation throughout their childhood and the reciprocal relationships that adolescents developed in earlier years will be major influences on their emotional development as they face the world as autonomous individuals.

The wider contexts that adolescents face will affect their emotional development and their emotional expression but, in the best scenarios, their early relationships will serve as an anchor to their developing feelings and will hopefully draw them as autonomous people into the good side of society. Most societies have dark sides and where adolescents have no emotional anchors from earlier periods of development they can drift towards these dark sides. Garbarino (1999) refers to the negative influences of the street and the dark side of adolescent culture when he considers the difficulties of delinquent boys. Some societies and sub-cultures offer adolescents no alternatives that can lead to positive outcomes. In such situations all adolescents are at risk of criminal behaviour and may suffer the deleterious effects that this will have on their emotional growth and personal relationships. As youth culture becomes more commercialised and exploitive the context in which most adolescents must reach full independence becomes an increasingly negative factor in their emotional development.

Adolescent emotional expression, the influence of context

Most children as they grow older increasingly learn to control their expression of emotion if they are in a nurturing secure environment. They also learn the display rules of their culture or sub-culture concerning the expression of emotion. This involves learning the appropriate display of emotion for different contexts. This learning process continues into adolescence. The process becomes more complex because the adolescent often has the freedom to escape from the context of the family and explore new contexts where display rules are not so dictated.

In early adolescence particularly, many of these contexts are peer group contexts. These are situations where the norms of behaviour, including emotional expression, are controlled by an in-group or a clique of teenagers or even the looser assemblage called a crowd. This ability to escape from the family context to a new grouping and to 'be yourself' and express yourself how you wish in new contexts is very important to most adolescents. It is particularly intoxicating for those for whom earlier contexts, including the family, were not emotionally satisfying. For *some* of these adolescents the expression of an emotion is their main experience of this emotion. Because of their adverse backgrounds the growth of deep-seated feelings has been limited yet they have learned the display associated with an emotion. Thus, for example, for some adolescents the glib expression of love is all they know of love.

They have not experienced the deeper subjective feelings associated with this emotion. For many adolescents from backgrounds of emotional adversity the same is true in respect of other emotions, including advanced secondary social emotions such as grief. For most adolescents on the other hand there is no division between emotional display and the subjective feeling of emotion. However, even for these adolescents group pressure in certain contexts may require them to show more emotion than they really feel. It is in this light that much of the emotional acting out of adolescents in out-of-home contexts must be viewed.

We must remember that the self-concept, though fully formed, is rather fragile in early adolescence and group pressure to feel or not feel certain emotions, or to express or not express certain feelings, may be quite irresistible no matter what the young person really thinks or feels. The effects of group contexts on adolescent emotions and therefore motivations are by no means always undesirable. The wish of many adolescents to change society towards practices that are more open and honest and their frequent support of causes may well spring from emotions (and therefore motivations) that are influenced by adolescent group contexts rather than family contexts. Thus it can be seen that contexts where adolescents meet in groups may have powerful effects on an adolescent's emotional expression and even on their inner feelings and the way they react to events.

Youth culture has considerable influence though its influence should not be exaggerated. Once adolescents leave the youth culture context they may revert easily to what they really think and feel as individuals. Older adolescents with more experience are, on the whole, less easily swayed emotionally or otherwise by adolescent contexts and may even revert to the values and feelings mediated by the family context. Where an adolescent has not got a secure family context to fall back on they may well be profoundly influenced by contexts particularly associated with young people, and with the emotions and expression of emotion, that these contexts engender. As we shall see in the next section this can be good or bad.

When things go wrong: adolescents from adversity

When we talk of adversity we mean those adolescents whose previous history from their early years has been one of emotional deprivation. As children these adolescents were not nurtured properly. In particular they did not receive affection and positive regard or else they received these things on an inconsistent basis.

For those adolescents who did not receive any affection at all as children and who "brought themselves up", early adolescence at least is not such a bad time psychologically. Their peers are seeking the independence to which they have long been accustomed and to these uncritical peers they may appear mature and genuinely independent. This is especially true if these adolescents from adverse backgrounds are boys with early physical maturation. This esteem shown by their rather undiscriminating peers may well boost, temporarily at least, whatever self-concept these boys have managed to develop. Later adolescence is a more difficult time for these young people because as the self-assurance and critical capacity of their peers develop, by comparison, the difficulties these adolescents have with relationships become more obvious. Yet adolescence is a period of great change and it is possible that these children will in adolescence find a context where their way of doing things can be tolerated and even, on some occasions, esteemed.

For adolescents who as children received some inconsistent affection the teenage years can exacerbate their already clinging and attention seeking behaviour. Early maturing girls are particularly vulnerable. Their neurotic need for affection may lead them into early sexual liaisons, pregnancy, and even marriage. Most arrangements for these girls do not last and if they give birth the child may not have his or her dependency needs met on a consistent basis thus prolonging the cycle.

For late maturing boys who are anxious and insecure adolescence brings little relief. These boys are generally unpopular with their age mates and their attention seeking antics (if they show them) whilst being regarded as weird and thus interesting by their peers do not generally bring them either friends or admirers. These adolescents can be very 'uncool' because they lack control over the expression of their anxiety and insecurity. Many of these children in adolescence develop more control over the expression of their insecurities than they previously had, so great is the effect of peer pressure in adolescence, yet for all that, they usually remain lonely.

What can be done?

The adolescents we are considering in this section are those whose dependency needs were not met or were only met on an inconsistent basis. What can be done to help them? There are two approaches to such children. We have already mentioned these two approaches when considering the problems of children from backgrounds of poor nurturance in early and middle childhood. The same approaches can be taken in adolescence.

The first one we have called *reworking*. In this approach we try to connect the adolescent with a person to whom they will, we hope, become attached. This person it is hoped will be able to give the adolescent such security and affection that the inadequate developments of early years will be reworked for the better. Thus the adolescent will become attached to this person in the same way that ordinary adolescents are attached to their parents.

This reworking approach is most successful if used with younger children and the younger the better. Adolescents by comparison are quite old. Nevertheless, with those adolescents who come from adversity and have had some experience of love though on an inconsistent basis this intense emotional approach may succeed to a degree. It is most unlikely to succeed with those adolescents who are 'survivors' and have never known loving nurturance. In these cases no amount of affectionate pressure or application of secure routine will change the young person; though there may be exceptions to this; human beings are very varied.

Another problem with this approach is that no matter how loving a person is, or how consistent they will be in their dealings with the insecure adolescent, the move towards attachment and reworking of past difficulties must come from the adolescent. Nevertheless, it is possible that an insecure attention seeking adolescent will meet an older companion who, because of their consistent and loving approach, will give the attention seeking teenager an increased sense of security. It is possible to give guidance to these anxious adolescents and have them accept it. The prerequisite for this to occur is that the adolescent feel secure and loved without having to seek affection or consistency.

The second approach is *to accept the adolescent as they are*, with all their unsocialised behaviour and idiosyncrasies. By the time they reach adolescence many young people from adverse backgrounds have developed survival mechanisms. As all adolescents are changing to find their place in the world, those who already fit a wider picture could be thought to have an advantage. The problem is that the survival mechanisms of many of these deprived adolescents have not been subject to socialisation and will eventually clash with authorities. Though ordinary adolescents may question authority, because in general their behaviour is conventional, they will eventually adjust to the system. The survival mechanisms of deprived adolescents are often not easily reconciled with the system and if the adolescent operates alone then the tendency will be for them to slip towards a criminal sub-culture at odds with the rest of society.

It is possible for a deprived adolescent to be placed with a *mentor* who accepts the adolescent's coping behaviour but guides it away from deviant criminal objectives. A mentor should be aware of the emotional development of the adolescent and have feeling for his or her emotional position but should not try to rework the adolescent emotionally. Rather than a parent figure a mentor should be a friend and an adviser. Mentors can influence adolescents by appealing to the adolescent's self-interest. With some adolescents a mentor can appeal to the young person's intellectual understanding of the situation and have the young person understand the consequences of their proposed actions. Mentoring can, like a mature frontal cortex, try to long-circuit the decisions that an adolescent may take. He or she should subtly encourage the adolescent to be less impulsive, take stock and reconsider. A mentor will try to guide the adolescent into appropriate decisions in health, education, vocation and recreation with a final objective of true independent living.

Questions to think about

1. What is late maturation and what impact does late maturation have on:

   (a) boys, in the short term, in the long term;
   (b) girls, in the short term, in the long term?

2. Explain how children who have 'brought themselves up' fare when they become adolescents.
3. What two general approaches can we take to adolescent difficulties?
4. What is a mentor in the context of helping adolescents who are in difficulties?

Suggested further reading

Russell, S. T., Card, N. A. & Susman, E. J. (2011). Introduction: A decade review of research on adolescence. *Journal of Research on Adolescence*, 21(1), 1–2. doi:10.1111/j.1532-7795.2010.00710.x

Marceau, K., Dorn, L. D. & Susman, E. J. (2012). Stress and puberty-related hormone reactivity, negative emotionality, and parent-adolescent relationships. *Psychoneuroendocrinology*, 37(8), 1286–1298. doi:10.1016/j.psyneuen.2012.01.001

Pfeifer, J. H. & Blakemore, S. J. (2012). Adolescent social cognitive and affective neuroscience: past, present, and future. *Social Cognitive and Affective Neuroscience*, 7(1), 1–10.

Pfeifer, J. H., Masten, C. L., Moore III, W. E., Oswald, T. M., Mazziotta, J. C., Iacoboni, M. & Dapretto, M. (2011). Entering adolescence: resistance to peer influence, risky behavior, and neural changes in emotion reactivity. *Neuron*, 69(5), 1029–1036.

Chapter 11

Understanding children in social/emotional difficulty

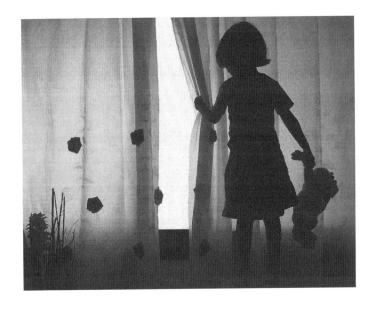

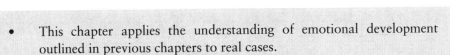

- This chapter applies the understanding of emotional development outlined in previous chapters to real cases.
- This is done by examining recent and current evidence relating to the child and inferring the probable emotional history of that child.

- This is aided by the use of three categories within a typology. However, the process is by no means straightforward.
- Gleaning evidence is often difficult and children tend not to fit neatly within one type and may have elements that fit several types.
- The case studies illustrate how the emotional histories can be inferred and used to understand each individual's emotional development. This can provide new understanding and increased empathy for the individual.

WE HAVE CONSIDERED THE development of emotions from birth to adulthood. Can this consideration help us to understand particular children especially those in difficulties? In other words, does knowledge of the emotional development of children and adolescents help parents; teachers; and health and welfare professionals, understand troubled children and youth? How does this understanding enable professionals and parents to help these children and young people? This chapter will try to answer these questions.

Our view is that it is important to comprehend variations in emotional development if we are to understand and help people who, generally speaking, are not successful in life. Children from backgrounds of adversity can develop emotions and emotional expressions that are quite different from our own. Perhaps the only way to truly understand these children, their motivations and their actions is by knowing what they feel and how they view the world. Emotion is the stuff of life; it must be foremost in our understanding of other people.

Interpretation of emotional development

If we are to understand individual children by knowing their emotional history we are faced with a number of difficulties. First among these difficulties is that we usually do not have observations or records of a child's emotional development. Most professionals see children when things go wrong and they usually do not have much information on the child's development especially in the early years. Very few of the children in difficulty that we see in our practices come with a dossier containing a full explanation of their emotional development.

In most instances the circumstances of a child's early rearing and early emotional development must be inferred from his or her current behaviour and emotional expression. How do we make such inferences concerning past emotional history? We do so by using a broad classification of current (or recent) behaviours and emotional reactions. This classification is developed from the theoretical account of emotional development given in earlier chapters and is largely based on attachment theory. It reflects possible courses of emotional development one of which may correspond with the current behaviour and emotional expression of the child.

The second difficulty is that many children do not fit classifications. Variation rules. Every child is unique. All children are, to some degree at least, exceptions to the rule. The key to the dilemma we are facing in trying to classify children who are unique lies in the words 'to some degree' mentioned in the last sentence. Every child is unique but many children share many features with many other children. So though children vary, and this must always be borne in mind, they can be classified because many of them have common characteristics.

This situation is also true for children from adversity who show social difficulties. We can therefore use a broad classification of the behaviours and emotional expressions of these children to infer what their likely emotional history was and through this process understand them better and make better arrangements for their future social integration. The classification that we use should be thoroughly grounded in theory to allow evidence-based inferences with respect to early emotional development. Our approach to using this classification must also be general enough to accommodate the individual differences that inevitably occur.

A classification of children with social/emotional difficulty

Children who are in social difficulty are usually, but not always, children who are the concern of the child welfare or educational systems. The children and adolescents in the welfare system are usually there because of issues of child protection, or alternative care, or juvenile justice. As with all human groups there is much variation among these children. However, as far as emotional development is concerned they can, for the most part, be divided into three groups. There will be certain children or adolescents who do not fit any of these groups and there will be many who overlap the groups, but on the whole, it probably induces considerable understanding of the welfare population of children and adolescents if we consider them in this way. The basis for this typology is attachment.

Three types of children with 'social/emotional difficulty'	
1. **Normal group**	Children with essentially normal early emotional development but who suffer trauma and separation from their attachment figures. They have a normal emotional repertoire and control, but are none the less deeply unhappy.

2. Inconsistent care group	Children subjected to inconsistent nurturing which leads to anxiety – as the child is unable to predict when their needs will be met. They are likely to show insecure resistant attachment and attention seeking behaviour in their quest to find more consistent love and security. They may show secondary emotions but these are overruled by the child's desire for attention.
3. Neglected group	Children who are subjected to emotional neglect and abuse. They are likely to show insecure avoidant or disorganised attachment – or no attachment. These children suffer from constant frustration and may show socially unacceptable 'survival behaviours'. They are likely to have abnormal or absent development of secondary emotions.

Normal group (Type 1)

This is essentially a 'normal' child or adolescent in that he or she had a secure attachment or attachments in infancy and toddlerhood. This attachment (or attachments) need not have been with mother, though this is often the case. Whatever the attachment arrangements may have been, and they can be quite idiosyncratic, the attachment process has satisfied the child's dependency needs early in life including the important need for emotional warmth and the need for mutual communication. Because attachment has been secure this child in early years has been able to explore the environment and has practised emotional relationships in imaginative play. Such children may have had a distinct reciprocal relationship with one person or they may have had a number of reciprocal relationships in which their emotions were socialised.

Nevertheless, these children or adolescents have gone through much trauma and separation. The protest, despair, detachment, cycle has been repeated again and again. Though their early care may have been nurturing, these children may have been distinctly frustrated at times with certain people. Because they have developed a full emotional repertoire, these children, and subsequently the adolescents they become, can be deeply hurt inwardly and often tend to detachment, anger, and withdrawal. Such a child may seem unemotional and cold in personal relations but is actually full of emotion, being continually sorrowful and unhappy because of lost love.

These emotions are usually under considerable expressive control because control of emotional expression has been learnt and life would be impossible otherwise. The person is frequently extremely guarded. Such children can be anxious though anxiety has often given way to despair. If they are anxious they can also be hyperactive. Very often such children and adolescents can suffer feelings of guilt and shame and can be socially inhibited.

Inconsistent care group (Type 2)

This is essentially a child or adolescent who has been subject to inconsistent nurturing. This inconsistency results in an inability to predict when satisfying nurturance will occur and this leads to the most noticeable feature of these children, namely anxiety. This anxiety, linked as it is to the satisfaction of the child's essential dependency needs, is usually expressed in attention seeking behaviour. These children show the features resulting from insecure resistant attachment. They want attention from the caregiver, and they seek it persistently, but when it comes they resist it, essentially because they have had to seek it. The relationship between all types of insecure attachment and later childhood and adolescent anxiety is well established (Colonnesi et al., 2011). We would argue that anxiety is particularly intrinsic to resistant attachment.

These children and adolescents have had some satisfaction in their early years but it has been inconsistent and they have suffered much frustration. Their dependency needs have been met to a degree but only on an inconsistent basis. This preoccupies their minds and causes much fantasising, which in turn leads to a situation where stories (lies) are invented to satisfy inner needs. Because their minds are preoccupied they have only limited mental opportunities for imaginative play.

This type of child is characterised by an anxious quest, inappropriately pursued, for love, recognition, attention and security. Such children have tasted a loving relationship only to have it randomly removed. They have begun to benefit from mutual affection and they know its satisfaction but only in short unpredictable episodes. Because their lives have been unstable and unpredictable they know a little about love but not much. They begin a neurotic search for affection and recognition, yet, when they get affection or recognition they feel it is bogus because they have had to ask for it. It has not been given freely or naturally.

Children and adolescents of this type usually seek attention and sometimes this can be through bad behaviour. Though most attention seeking is simply annoying, certain behaviours can be anti-social and aggressive. In general these children have not developed much control of their emotional expression when it relates to the essential attention that they seek, though they can suppress it when severe punishment is imminent. In other respects they appear to be emotional children but on further examination their emotions are seen to be somewhat shallow and transient. Most of them have little or no difficulty expressing emotion, indeed they are often excellent actors, but they seem to have much more difficulty in feeling emotion apart from their desire for attention. This desire for attention can dominate their human interactions. They hunger for recognition and, if it brings them attention, they will easily befriend strangers and spin yarns to anyone. They will use intimate terms with little thought or concern.

Such children and adolescents can be quite anxious at times and it is unfair to consider that they have no true secondary emotions. These feelings for them are simply more fleeting and changeable than those of children with a secure background. Professionals need to be aware of this otherwise they, the workers, will feel betrayed when commitment and expressions of friendship on the child or adolescent's part are not fulfilled. Of course these children possess all the basic emotions.

Children of this type are frequently hyperactive and often have a very short attention span, yet once cured of their quest for attention, can become people who can concentrate in the normal manner. Then they can show secondary social emotions to some degree. They appear to be sorry for their misdeeds and can show some signs of sympathy for others and guilt and shame. However, if the child's desire for attention returns these emotions are liable to be fleeting and easily overruled.

Neglected children group (Type 3)

There are essentially children or adolescents from backgrounds of abuse and emotional neglect who show the features resulting from insecure avoidant attachment or disorganised attachment. Indeed some of these children in their early years, though they sought attachment, may not have become attached to anyone. These children and adolescents have been subject to constant frustration and little or no satisfaction in their relations with people. Their dependency needs have not been met as far as warm emotional relationships and clear meaningful human communication are concerned. They may fortuitously have had certain instrumental dependencies cared for at a minimal level because they have survived, but warm nurturance has not been part of their experience. There has been no time in their lives for imaginative play or reflection. Their ability to fantasise and imagine is not well developed if at all.

In many ways these children and adolescents have "brought themselves up". They have survived not through our normal methods of child rearing and socialisation but through their own efforts rooted in the most basic instincts. They have been lucky; many uncared for children do not survive. These children and adolescents have their own way of doing things and getting by; they are survivors. However, their way is often very unsocialised and unacceptable. Nevertheless, in some respects, their survival has been admirable. They often have deep feelings of anger which they may temporarily suppress because of the fear of punishment. They find it hard to comprehend love and affection though many of them learn to feign such feelings in order to manipulate the people around them. In fact this may be one of their survival mechanisms.

These children and adolescents are characteristically lacking in expressed anxiety though they may hide anxiety. Usually they are quite uninhibited. They are frequently hyperactive and generally unmanageable. As already stated, as far as affection is concerned these children are pseudo-emotional. They have never experienced being loved or cared for and true love and affection remain a mystery for many of them. They may develop a glib friendliness that can be mistaken for feeling. Children of this type show little sympathy for others. They have not had the luxury of time to develop such feelings. Indeed they may distain others in weaker positions than themselves and even become aggressive to other children who are in difficulties. They have had no time for imaginative play. They have been too busy surviving.

Such children and adolescents often operate without guilt, shame, or sorrow. All of these emotions come from an experience of love. One cannot discipline these people by a resort to their conscience; they will not respond. They have never been loved even for a short period and they have had to do the best they can in the absence of this experience. Without love in their background their main emotion is often anger though many of them have learnt not to be openly angry at the powerful. They do possess the basic emotions and these can easily fit into the power based male gang culture (even if they are girls) and it is often this experience that leads them into trouble with the authorities.

Making inferences

Children who come to our attention do not classify themselves. A classification should be an aid to understanding and is imposed by us on the child. A classification or a label should be the beginning of a process of understanding the child or young person. It should not be the end point of this process. It is possible to look for certain signs and to draw inferences based on this evidence that will probably be correct. This process will give us a deeper understanding of the child and his or her problems.

The case of Jake Smith

The following article appeared in a newspaper some years ago. We have paraphrased it to a very minor degree and have used different names. This is a real case, but one on which we have extremely limited information: the newspaper article alone. Can we infer any emotional history from this?

Disturbed boy didn't want to go.

"He was very close to me and he was afraid to be taken away, that's why he jumped" -----

Mother.

A 14 year old boy plunged from the window of a Family Services building minutes after learning he was being placed in foster care, a court was told yesterday.

The Coroner's court was told Jake Smith fell to his death from the fourth floor of the department office early last year.

His mother Ms Sandra Smith yesterday said her son had been petrified of separation and was simply "looking for his mummy".

"He wanted to live," she said.

Ms Smith told the court she had agreed to place Jake in foster care because he was increasingly violent towards her and her younger son.

She said she had warned protective staff to break the news slowly because he hated being taken from her and was likely to react badly.

They also knew Jake had jumped from a building before in another state in 1991 under similar circumstances, she said.

But Ms Smith said a Family Services officer "blurted" out that Jake would be placed in residential care that afternoon. She said her son had cried: "Please, please mate, just give me one more chance, I'll be good".

"He was very close to me and was afraid to be taken away, that's why he jumped," Ms Smith told the court.

"I knew he was scared and I knew he would want to find a way out".

"He was looking around, he was scared and he was trying to get away".

The court was told Jake suffered chronic anxiety, had serious learning difficulties and reacted badly if things did not go his way.

A child psychiatrist said Ms Smith was devoted to her son but was no longer able to care for him.

The doctor said that department staff had a good insight into the case and had been trying to help Jake and his family.

The hearing is due to continue today.

Analysis

What evidence is there in this report and how can we use it to understand Jake better?

The evidence from this report is brief but it is sufficient to classify Jake into one of the categories given above. The evidence is as follows. Jake is a very anxious 14 year old who is petrified of being separated from his mother. However, he is also violent towards his mother and his younger brother. He therefore shows ambivalence towards his mother and his relationship with her resembles that of an infant showing insecure resistant attachment. He also is reported as reactive and learning disabled. Jake wants to be 'good' but when frustrated by events he reacts without control.

The significant feature is the behaviour he shows as far as his main attachment figure, his mother, is concerned. He is both *anxious* for her when separated from her and *resistant* to her when she is present. His tendency to chronic anxiety is confirmed in the report and these features allow us to classify him as a Type 2 adolescent above. The evidence is clear and the classification quite easily made, but we do not have much evidence. It may be that if more was known we would consider him differently, yet it is hard to disregard the distinct signs of an ambivalent relationship with his mother pointing to an insecure resistant attachment to her in the past that has remained unresolved. Using this evidence and the classification we have now made you should be able to some degree at least, reconstruct Jake's emotional history. See question 1 at the end of this chapter.

Jake's case shows that we can understand this boy better if we analyse his emotional history. Though the psychiatrist in the case reported that the workers concerned had good insight, this is not confirmed by the fact that workers 'blurted out' information to Jake about an attempt to isolate him again from his mother. If the workers had seriously considered this boy's emotional history the power and significance of his ambivalent and neurotic desire to be with mother might have been more appreciated. This appreciation might have given more insight into the boy's emotional disposition and the tragedy may have been averted. Who knows? In any event the best solutions follow an understanding of a child's emotional position. See the points to ponder at the end of this chapter for a task relating to Jake's case.

The case of Jo Lee

This case study is based on case history notes from a welfare agency, pseudonyms have been used and identifying information altered.

Jo Lee was born on 11/5/90. He was the first child of Ian and Marie Lee. Marie Lee was 24 years at the time of Jo's birth. In 1988 as Marie Alford she had married Ian Lee who was then aged 25 years. The couple had met in a sheltered workshop for disabled people where Marie worked and Ian was one of the maintenance staff.

Marie is a person with an intellectual developmental delay. She also suffers from a physical disability and is very short in stature and not very well co-ordinated. She is a very well intentioned person but finds it difficult to comprehend the complexities or subtleties of life. In particular her tolerance for difficult or frustrating situations is low and when confronted with even moderate difficulties she tends to withdraw. She is the product of an insecure childhood. Marie's father died in an accident when she was six. Marie had always felt rejected in her family because of her disability but when she was seven her mother married again and Marie was physically abused by her stepfather. This heightened her sense of rejection especially as her stepfather was supported in his actions by her mother.

Ian Lee is a large obese man who is also probably of limited intellect though his ability has never been assessed. He works as an odd job man and apart from being a slow worker is well considered by those who employ him. He sticks doggedly to a task and will finish his work if left alone. However, if he is hassled or interrupted he loses his temper sometimes violently. This has caused him to be fired from a number of jobs but his current employers seem to understand his difficulty and make allowances for him. It is observed that on the whole Ian tends to avoid people and is a bit of loner. He and Marie however have sustained their relationship over quite a number of years. They have a very modest income and their home is well kept.

Jo Lee had a normal birth and seemed a normal baby. His mother reports that he achieved most of his infant milestones at an appropriate age. When he was referred to a departmental psychologist at six years it was on account of wetting and soiling problems at school. The psychologist found Jo to be an obese boy of average intelligence and considered that the chief problem was that the boy had never been toilet trained.

It appeared that the stage of infant negativism (the terrible two's) had never been resolved with this boy. When an issue, such as toileting, arose between the child and his parents the boy remained stubbornly egocentric and faced with his refusals the mother withdrew. If father was present he lost his temper and then withdrew, probably driving off in his car. It seems that though Ian lost his temper he did not assault or abuse the boy. The boy was always left as the victor over his parents' reasonable demands. In this fashion the boy won every confrontation with his mother not only on toileting but on many other issues as well.

It appears that Marie could not exert any firmness or establish any boundaries for the child. By six years of age things had deteriorated because Marie had had another child Michael who had similar disabilities to her own. Michael was two and the psychologist judged that Jo was very jealous of his brother and the attention he received. The overall impression was that Jo was a fairly able child but one who was unduly obese immature and unhappy. He showed little concern for others. Apart from soiling he was progressing quite well at school. However, it seemed that, without considerable support, the family could no longer cope with the care of two children. The case was referred by the psychologist to the Family Support Service.

Family support worked with the family for two years. During this time Jo's behaviour at school deteriorated. He threatened teachers and pupils with violence and on occasions tried to deliver it. However, because he was still young (though big for his age) he could be restrained. At home he continued to lord it over his mother threatening her often and hitting her from time to time when she did not do what he wanted. He had increasingly violent confrontations with his father but, though they came to blows on occasions, Ian refrained from a full beating of his son and usually solved the issue by taking off in his car. Family support services were terminated when Jo attacked the family support worker.

The Community Services department now took a renewed interest in the family because it had received a number of notifications concerning Jo. What was provided for the family was short term foster care to give the parents and Michael respite from Jo's aggression. Twelve short (usually weekend) placements took place over two years always with different carers (those who had Jo once did not want him back again!). These foster placements may have given the family some respite but it unsettled Jo who, when returned to the family home, was more aggressive more often than before. During these aggressive outbursts he would not only be angry with his parents but would also become upset and cry. He seemed to be seeking something that his parents could not deliver. At school he did not seek much interaction with others but when he did form a friendship with a pupil or a teacher, after a short period, he terminated it in a fit of aggression again accompanied with much anguish and tears.

Jo was now eleven and was placed by the department at his parents' request in voluntary medium term foster care. Though he obviously did not get on at home with his parents, as soon as he entered the foster placement he wanted to return home. For about three weeks he tolerated the placement then he threatened the foster mother with a knife and the placement broke down. Two other placements were attempted but on each occasion they were terminated because Jo had attacked someone in the household. It seemed that this boy could not tolerate people. During these placements Jo continued to attend the same primary school as he had when he lived with his family but when he attempted to assault the school principal with a knife the school requested that he be placed elsewhere.

When Jo was 12 years his mother requested the children's court to declare him a ward of state on the grounds of an irretrievable breakdown in the relationship between parents and child. After some time the wardship order was granted for a period of two years. Jo was sent to a group home run by a foster care agency. He disliked the group home particularly because he had to live with other children. He fought with or threatened other residents.

After two days he absconded to his home blinded by tears. His mother did not welcome him when he returned home so he attacked her again (his father was at work when he arrived). When she regained her feet after his attack Marie managed to phone the foster agency who took Jo back to the group home. As soon as he had left she went to the local courthouse and took out an apprehended violence order against him. For all that Jo escaped on three more occasions and returned home where he verbally abused but did not attack his mother. This was probably because on these occasions his father was at home.

On each occasion he was retrieved by a youth worker from the foster agency. Finally Jo attacked a youth worker in the group home and was then removed by the community services department to a large fairly secure residential unit run by the department in the state capital. Here he languished, a stranger in a crowd of other children, for a year or so. During this time his mother visited him once. Jo regularly phoned home but the call always ended by his being abusive towards his mother. The one good thing about the large institution was that it had a school attached with skilled teachers and small classes. In this environment Jo's educational achievements rose and he showed a distinct interest in cookery classes.

The large institution closed when Jo had been there for about one year and after a wardship renewal he was returned by the department to his home locality and placed in the care of a second foster agency. He was now 14. At first this agency placed him in a house with two other young people. However, the agency soon realised that Jo resented company of his own age and, after a year or so, a scheme of independent living for him was developed whereby he lived in a flat but was guided in his living by a mentor. This mentor was a strong-minded mature woman who seemed to have some insight into Jo's needs. She advised him on a wide range of issues including his soiling and wetting problems (which had persisted) but insisted that in this regard he do the cleaning work himself. Jo slowly established a relationship with this mentor. He often verbally abused her but found it very inconvenient to avoid her advice. In the end he would conform to the advice because it was more comfortable for him personally to do so. The mentor also discouraged Jo from frequent contact with his home as this seemed to disturb him and gradually little by little his neurotic desire to contact his parents abated and he developed a lonely but more settled existence. He completed school work by correspondence and was introduced to work experience by the foster care agency. A particularly successful experience was a stint in the kitchen of a service club with an understanding chef.

Today (2008) Jo lives independently having turned 18 and attends Technical College. He was placed on new anti-depressant medication and this, along with his increasing maturity, seems to have reduced his aggressive outbursts in both frequency and severity. He is looking for a permanent job as a cook and has had a number of part time positions in this capacity. Unfortunately he lost some of these because he lost his temper with the kitchen staff. He still wishes to contact home but he now understands that this action upsets him. He limits his contact to occasional telephone calls. His most frequent social contact is with his mentor who, though no longer officially involved with him, gives him sound advice and support. All in all his future looks brighter than his past.

Analysis

The evidence quoted in this description of Jo comes, for the most part, from community service and other reports that have been written about him. Some of the description comes from the psychologist's observations of Jo or from records of discussions with Marie and Ian. In contrast to Jake Smith the evidence is thus quite extensive. Various professionals have regularly made detailed descriptions of this boy since he was six years of age.

In this case we have extensive evidence and therefore our inferences based on this evidence will be more secure than in the case of Jake Smith. In Jo's case the key feature that is reported on repeatedly over a number of years is his ambivalent relationship with his mother. Even more clearly than in Jake's case, Jo wants to be with mother but cannot stand her when he is with her.

Jo Lee shows the developmental picture usually exhibited by children whose dependency needs have only been partially met or met only inconsistently (Type 2 children as given above). Thus Jo's attachment is *insecure resistant*, an attachment pattern characterised by ambivalent behaviour towards the caregiver, exhibited in many cases as aggression probably in response to frustration.

Most children with this developmental picture have had care that is inconsistent because their caregivers are busy with other things and frequently neglect the child, or because the caregivers cannot maintain an affectionate attitude towards their offspring and often give mixed emotional messages. However, in Jo's case the situation was a little different from the usual circumstances that produce such a developmental picture. In his case his mother had time to care for Jo and the best of intentions towards him but simply had not the mental, or even physical, capacity to deliver secure nurturing care consistently.

This was particularly true after Jo's brother was born when Jo was four. Jo's mother had not the mental stamina to confront any of the difficulties that are bound to arise in child rearing and his father in no way compensated for the mother's lack of competence. Thus the oppositional tendencies Jo showed from toddlerhood into early childhood were not resolved until recently. Because his parents always retreated in the face of his demands, as a child Jo became more and more demanding oppositional behaviour. The processes of socialisation and emotional development were stalled by the parents' inability to give the child a firm base against which he could react and thus define himself and his position in the world. This lack of self definition confounded his social relationship with people.

He remained emotionally dependent on his parents and until recently could not spread this dependency to others. His frustration with this situation was extreme and compounded by the fact that his parents continued to retreat and never gave him a base to work from. His ambivalent relationship towards them remained though he never gained any satisfaction from it. This picture was established in infancy and toddlerhood and influenced all subsequent developmental periods.

In some other respects Jo is not a typical Type 2 child. His insecure resistant pattern of attachment shows more of the resistant elements than other elements. He does not fit all aspects of this category. His attention seeking is displayed mostly by aggression. Yet emotion is clearly involved as tears and distress often accompany Jo's aggression. Jo was jealous of his brother and, as jealousy is based, at least in part, on anxiety, he must have had anxious feelings. So though he is a child whose development has been shaped by the same attachment category as that of Jake Smith, he is, in a number of ways, quite different from Jake particularly as far as overt anxiety is concerned.

We know a deal more about Jo than we did about Jake and we can follow certain features more accurately through his developmental history. Jo is not so much neglected as frustrated by inadequate care and the aggression-frustration link is very noticeable in his case. The effects of unresolved oppositional behaviour are also quite obvious throughout his earlier emotional history. Unresolved issues tend to obscure weaken or delay other emotional developments and this was true in Jo's case.

Does this developmental history help us to understand Jo Lee better and to make better arrangement to support his future? Or was Jo simply a difficult child with an enduring difficult temperament that we cannot change? See points to ponder at the end of this chapter for a task relating to Jo's case. This task asks you to now infer Jo's emotional history under the same headings as you used for Jake. It will again be repetitious but it will be illustrative to consider his early development from several perspectives. See question 2, at the chapter's end.

Further case studies

Here are three more case studies. Each is in a condensed form. However, the outline is sufficient for us to classify the child with respect to attachment and the typology given above and to develop an understanding of the child's emotional history. We can then use this understanding to give suggestions as to what should be done in each case. For each case we will consider the emotional strengths and weaknesses that the child or adolescent has, or may have had, because of their emotional history. These case outlines are all based on real cases.

The case of Michael

This case study is based upon a personal acquaintance of one of the authors from many decades ago; names have been changed. Anna and Michael are the children of David and Rosemary Jo. Six years ago David Jo applied to join the Army. As a result of the obligatory medical examination it was discovered that he had many secondary cancers. Within five weeks he was dead. This was a great blow to what was reported to be a happy loving and stable family. Nevertheless the children remained with their mother and in two years Rosemary had remarried. Her second husband Richard had been a friend of David. The children seemed to adjust to the new relationship. About a year after their marriage Rosemary and Richard decided they must have some time together without the children. They planned a month's holiday overseas. The children, particularly Michael, were not happy with this arrangement. They were to be left with trusted friends of Rosemary. On the way to the airport Rosemary and Richard were killed in a traffic accident. At that time Anna was eight years old and Michael was nine years old. The trusted friends did not wish to keep the children on a long-term basis. Rosemary's parents were much too old to care for them and her only brother was abroad. David had been an only adopted child and his adoptive parents were even older than Rosemary's parents. The children were taken into care. At first they were placed together in a foster home. Because they stuck together and opposed the foster parents neither child adjusted to the fostering arrangements. The foster parents reported sexual activity between the children, and, without waiting for this to be investigated, much less substantiated, the department removed Michael from this foster home and placed him in another several hundred kilometres away. Michael stayed in this new situation for about six months. His school work declined dramatically in quality (he had previously been above average). After a quarrel with his foster father Michael was shifted to another foster home. Michael became withdrawn and unsociable and several changes of foster home followed. Finally it was judged that Michael might do better in a small residential care unit. He wanted to be re-united with his sister but the Department ruled against this. He has now arrived at a residential care unit. Is this the appropriate placement for him?

Analysis

Essentially Michael is a child from a secure normal background who has been affected by a series of misfortunes and separations (Type 1). Michael probably had a normal infancy and probably developed normal secure attachments. He is likely to have developed the secondary social emotions of shame guilt and pride. All in all his dependency needs were met. His troubles really started when he was nine and his current emotional reactions are probably due to the series of separations that he has suffered. He has been through the cycle of *protest, despair and detachment* several times. This is the likely reason why he is withdrawn and unsociable.

It seems as if this boy needs his sister (a real attachment). He also needs a system of care that gives him consistency and emotional space. He probably does not want anyone to bother him and perhaps he has no need of an attachment to a mother or father figure. The first new welfare measure in this case is a re-consideration of this boy's relationship with his sister. Here his sister's wishes are of paramount importance. However, if she is willing to be re-united with her brother, the alleged sexual contact between the children should be re-evaluated. It is likely that such contact, if it took place, was minor and would not therefore override the psychological need that these children have for each other. One must not be panicked into action of an inappropriate sort simply because contact between children has taken place that can be judged as sexual but may not be so.

The second welfare decision should be that this boy is quite unsuitable for a small residential group home. The boy wants to be left alone and needs emotional space. The other residents of a group home are liable to have serious emotional difficulties and will not make easy companions. They may pester others for attention or vent on them their anxieties or their aggression. A small group home is not the place for someone who wants to be left alone to recuperate emotionally.

What should be tried in Michael's case is a good boarding school with staff who understand the child's situation and spacious facilities that allow for emotional space. If a co-educational boarding school could be found that would also take his sister it would be the best option. Failing that a foster home might succeed if the two children were again fostered together and the foster carers were fully briefed about the case. It would also be essential to consult Michael and his sister about any new arrangements for their care.

The case of Nik

This case study is based upon a welfare child protection case managed by one of the authors. Nik is the son of Kylie Smith and Wayne Armstrong. Wayne it is reported died of an alcohol related liver infection before Nik was six months old. Nik's mother then lived for about five years with Ken Jardine, who by report was drug addicted and violent towards his de-facto wife. It is quite likely that Nik was also abused. Kylie and Ken had three children. On parting two of these children stayed with their father while the youngest remained with his mother. For a short period after the split in their relationship, Nik lived with Ken but soon returned to live with his mother. Kylie has now been in a relationship with Mick Dodds for six years. Mick is the father of her fifth child Bronwyn.

In 1992 Nik (7) ran away from his mother's home. He was found by the police a day later and Community Services were notified. After a few days in foster care Nik was placed in a large departmental residential institution. A few months later Nik's mother made an application for a Care Order on the grounds of an irretrievable breakdown in the relationship between her and her son. Nik was 7 years old at the time the Care Order was made. The Order was for a period of two years with a view to restoration to his mother's care thereafter. Nik was then moved to a 'preparation unit' run by an NGO (non-government organization). He stayed six months in this unit but was then restored to Kylie's care. Kylie had moved to the coast with Mick and the local Department staff gave extensive support to the restoration by means of frequent respite care and school support. Nevertheless it was reported that Nik was frequently at home without adult supervision and placed in charge of his younger siblings, or was wandering the streets. Respite care was used by Kylie and Mick to allow them to go drinking while the children were being minded. It seemed as if restoration had not worked and Nik was being neglected. Kylie and Mick agreed and Nik was again taken into care. He was now nine years old.

Over four years Nik had eight foster placements. Each one broke down because of Nik's behaviour in the foster home. Nik is hyperactive. He moves continually and struggles when restrained. In the foster homes Nik lied and stole. In particular he stole food often out of the bin. The foster carers protested that he had been well fed. His most disturbing behaviour was that he ran away. The carers could not cope with repeated episodes of this behaviour. In contrast Nik liked school and scored moderately well in most areas despite frequent changes of school. He reads quite well and enjoys books. At school he played with children much younger than he was. Nik had and still has an ambivalent relationship with his mother.

It is reported that as an infant his mother relied on him for emotional comfort and confided in him. Foster carers found him immediately affectionate providing he stopped moving for long enough to be friendly. It was frequently reported that on his wanderings he would talk to strangers and many carers were disturbed by the dangers inherent in this. Carers also reported increased stealing, lying and hyperactivity following contact with his mother. They also reported periods of sadness and withdrawal and occasional episodes of anger. It has now in 1998 at 13 years been decided to abandon foster care for Nik. Are there any alternatives for him?

Analysis

This is a child who may well have been physically abused early in his life, who has been legally abandoned by his mother, and who has been in and out of care. His history would suggest that as an infant he probably suffered an inordinate amount of frustration and insecurity. This boy has not totally brought himself up but he has largely done so. It is likely that many of his dependency needs were not properly met. His attachment to his carer in his early years was either insecure avoidant or disorganised disoriented depending on whether he suffered abuse or not. Nik has probably developed through his unstable emotional relations with his mother some secondary social emotions (shame, guilt, pride, etc.) but these are probably very fleeting feelings and are not important motivating forces.

As far as we can judge this boy lies between Types 2 and 3 as given above. He seems to have a tenuous relationship with his mother but he is largely a survivor, he has largely brought himself up. Nik has developed certain survival strategies as he has grown. He is hyperactive largely because he has never been socialised not to be, but also because it may in the past have removed him from abusive situations. Nik also finds his hyperactivity useful to avoid contact with anyone he does not want to deal with. He simply runs away. Nik has also had to learn that to survive you feed yourself when you can, even if it is out of the bin. He has developed a habit of lying to get himself out of difficulties and a technique of immediate friendship which he also uses to advance his survival.

This boy needs someone to understand him and put up with his survival behaviours. As he grows he needs someone to guide his survival behaviours away from anti-social and possibly criminal outcomes into something more constructive.

The first welfare decision in this case should be to abandon any idea of restoration of Nik to his mother. Nik does not need such restoration and it would probably upset him. It would make matters worse for him when the restoration broke down again as it inevitably would. Nik needs a person to understand him but that person is almost certainly not his mother.

The next decision to be made in Nik's case is that he would not be suitable for residential care. A large institution would not bother him much but it probably would not advance his interests. A small group home would be disastrous in his case. He does not need the companionship of other survivors or of those who are aggressive or anxious. In such a situation he may very soon run away.

The decision to abandon foster care for this boy has probably been premature. What he needs is a secure foster home that places no demands on him. This boy will not attach to a foster carer and the carer must know this. In general the carer should be educated as to the type of child that Nik is and what to expect. The carer must not believe that this boy is bad or suffering from a psychological disorder but rather understand and even admire him as a survivor.

Probably the best, least damaging, short term alternative for Nik's care is to try fostering again but this time with a properly trained, informed, and tolerant foster carer. In the long term, when Nik gets to the age (16) when perhaps he can live independently a mentor may be better than a foster carer. Perhaps with time his trained foster carer could change role into that of mentor.

The case of Eve

Eve was born in the city ten years ago and was abandoned by her mother a few weeks after her birth. Her father is unknown. The birth had been normal and no reason for the abandonment was given but it is surmised that Eve's mother was a prostitute. Eve went for a few weeks to her Aunt and then for a few months to her maternal grandmother. The quality of care she received is unknown. When Eve was seven months she went back to her mother's care. This only lasted six weeks and she returned to her grandmother. However, grandmother was now caring for three of her grandchildren and for this reason Eve returned to her mother. Two weeks later the authorities received a complaint that Eve was being neglected by her mother and she was taken into care and fostered out to John and Margo Durham. This arrangement did not last long because John and Margo's marriage broke up and Eve then aged three years was declared a Ward of State by the Department of Children's Services. Two further foster placements followed one for 12 months and then Eve was moved to a country town and fostered for two years by Ron and Edith Bayne. The Baynes reported that it was difficult for them to relate to Eve as she was given to sulking and was very uncooperative. After two years Eve was returned to the Department and the city where she stayed in a large institution. She was six years old and was put up for adoption even though she was a state ward. While waiting for adoption Eve attended school for the first time and while old for her class made good progress. She was described by her teachers and by the workers in the large institution where she lived as a quiet girl who gave no trouble.

By the time adoption formalities were concluded Eve was seven years old. She was adopted inter-state by Grace and Steven Brownlee. Grace wanted a daughter to complement her two teenage sons and hoped that Eve would become her friend and companion in feminine activities. Grace Brownlee was a very efficient mother and housekeeper who also had career ambitions. She was a very competent woman who liked a challenge and felt that she could rear any child with a regime of efficient and organised care. Neither she nor Steven had been briefed on what to expect from Eve and the only report they had was from Eve's primary school. At first they thought that Eve was just a quiet withdrawn child and she gave them no trouble for the first few weeks but, when her birthday arrived and she destroyed the dress they had given her as a present, things began to deteriorate. Eve had tried to tear the dress but failed and instead she cut it up with scissors that she took from Grace's sewing box. The Brownlees took this rebuff and tried to communicate with Eve but she sulked and would not talk to them. Over the following weeks and months Eve refused to eat appropriately at meal times but after raiding the fridge stored food under her bed where it eventually became stale and created a smell. She also would wake at all hours and despite requests she would not go back to bed or go to sleep. The Brownlees had to lock their doors to keep her from wandering off at night. The adoptive parents put up with all these difficulties as the months passed into years. What they found most difficult was that Eve would not communicate with them and gave them only a glance from time to time as they talked to her trying to cajole her towards more socialised behaviours. Eve destroyed further presents and seemed to reject the whole arrangement. She did not communicate with the boys and kept out of their way. Family events became less pleasurable because Eve had to be included and eventually it became too much for Grace.

She asked the Children's Department to take Eve into care. This was a difficult request to agree to as Eve had already been a state ward in another state before being adopted and the Department refused the request and instead offered family counselling and respite care at fixed times. This has been implemented and the Brownlees report that things are going better and Eve is not sulking as much. Whether this is true remains uncertain. The Department is still considering how to proceed and what action to take particularly as Eve is still doing well at school where she communicates and behaves well and gives no trouble.

Analysis

We do not know any details of Eve's infancy. Nevertheless from her later displays of destructive behaviour and her sullenness we can infer that infancy and toddlerhood left her with a lot of suppressed anger. Thus it is very likely that in her early infancy she had an undue number of experiences of frustration and few of satisfaction. It is also very likely that as an infant and toddler her basic dependency needs were not fully satisfied as she still has the tendency to cram herself with food whenever she can, yet refuse food at other times. This and other behaviours indicate a survivor, a child who looks after herself. The best survivors are intelligent children and Eve is probably at least of average intelligence judging from her school reports.

Though she had all the basic emotions and secondary emotions derived from anger, Eve probably did not develop the secondary social emotions of guilt, shame, and pride during her toddlerhood. She may not have had anyone available in her early years with whom she could have formed a reciprocal relationship and she may never have fully formed 'a theory of mind' to apply to other people. Thus she does not know that others think about her and she does not care if they do or not, because she does not think of them. She thinks only of herself. Indeed because she has probably not been loved, love is largely a mystery to her, perhaps even a foolishness. She does not know what it is about. Eve shows most of the signs of a Type 3 child (see above). She exhibits many of the behaviours of a survivor the tendency to move on or run away when a difficulty appears, hoarding food, being sullen and not communicating.

Eve's attachment in her infancy and toddlerhood was very probably insecure anxious-avoidant attachment. The picture appears quite clear but there is room for doubt. Two issues are worthy of consideration. First, Eve's behaviour at school is at odds with her behaviour at home and second Eve's adoptive mother had an unrealistic fantasy about Eve when she was first adopted which may well have affected their relationship. Perhaps Eve is not so much of a Type 3, as the description the Brownlees give would suggest. Given human variation and resilience there is just a possibility that Eve is not a Type 3 child and this should be borne in mind. Perhaps the earlier foster carers were also biased. Nevertheless, her destruction of presents and hoarding of food are not normally features seen in Type 1 children and strongly suggests a Type 3 classification if parental reports can be believed. But parents cannot always be believed and the uncertainty in this case convinced the Department not to take Eve back into care.

This case shows how human variation and resilience can overcome seeming disadvantage. Though the inferences made that this child was a Type 3 were correctly made on evidence from her adoptive parents Eve succeeded in confounding them as things transpired. The Brownlees continued with Eve for four more years. During that time the Department provided counselling. Grace gradually withdrew the expectations she had for Eve and their relationship improved. Eve did very well at her new high school and began to relate more easily to Steven about her studies which she took very seriously. Communication with her adoptive father seemed to please them both. When Grace and Steven divorced and moved interstate four years later Eve went with her adoptive father while the now adult boys stayed with their mother. Eve has since gone to university and, though living independently, still keeps in touch with Steven.

Concluding thoughts

What we have tried to do in this book is to lay a foundation of psychological understanding of the emotional position of children and young people, especially those who are in difficulties. Through developing insight into emotional development it is hoped that professionals working with children can further their understanding of each individual and empathise with them. Though it has not been possible to cover all the contingencies that arise in child welfare, we trust these case studies above have shown you how knowledge concerning a child's emotional development is central to the selection of the most appropriate options for that child.

There have been recent calls for more sensitive treatment of children from disadvantage, particularly children in foster care. Dozier and colleagues propose that more nurturing care is needed to help develop attachments between foster children and their carers; and they describe some intervention programmes designed to help achieve this (Dozier et al., 2013). What we have provided in this book is insight into how such children might feel and we believe that this understanding is vital to the sustainability of such efforts. Programmes with practical behavioural approaches to caring also need education on how these children feel. Empathetic understanding is needed for sustained caring interaction with children who have been reared in adversity.

At the beginning of this book we emphasised the importance of understanding how children feel and how those who wish to help them must understand the emotions of the children they deal with. We have covered a lot of ground to try and achieve this. This understanding embraces knowledge of the child's personal emotional history and emotional development; and the effects of deprivation on that development. We now know from neuroscience that emotional development is central to brain function and that, when feelings are not managed, thinking can be impaired. We also know that very early emotional development is an important foundation for future development and that it shapes the architecture of children's brains (National Scientific Council on the Developing Child, 2004; Shonkoff & Levitt, 2010). Thus early emotional difficulties, due to deprivation and abuse, can have broad and far-ranging impact upon an individual's progress.

It is possible to understand the older child in terms of the development of his/ her emotions in infancy. Were the child's dependency needs met in full in infancy, or were they only infrequently met, or not at all? Did the child develop a basis for love and security or was everything in their early life a matter of frustration and anger? We may also ask; if the child in toddlerhood developed secondary emotions, such as pride shame and guilt, or were these emotions absent or, at best, only fleeting temporary feelings?

The development of secondary emotions is very important when considering methods of behavioural control that can be used with the child (conscience versus consequences). We often seem very concerned to exert control over difficult children in welfare and educational situations. In this regard do we understand the origins of their behaviour? Do we understand the origins of their aggression? Do we understand why they are anxious? Do we understand that their anxieties often fuel their aggression or lack of co-operation? Do we understand why these children also have cognitive difficulties? If we did understand these origins would it help us with systems of control? More importantly would it help us to be more relaxed with the child?

There are still no simple answers to these questions for development is fascinatingly complex. Perhaps it is progress enough that we are asking these questions and in our attempts to answer them are considering the psychological perspectives of the children we care for, live and work with. We hope that you, having read this book, have concluded that such questioning insight has great potential to help.

Questions to think about

1. Construct Jake's emotional history under the following headings. Emotional development in infancy. Dependency needs. Attachment. Emotional development in toddlerhood. Emotional development in early childhood. Emotional development in middle childhood. Emotional development in early adolescence.
2. Construct Jo Lee's emotional history using the following headings. Emotional development in infancy. Dependency needs. Attachment. Emotional development in toddlerhood. Emotional development in early childhood. Emotional development in middle childhood. Emotional development in early adolescence.

Suggested further reading

Dozier, M., Zeanah, C. H. & Bernard, K. (2013). Infants and Toddlers in Foster Care. *Child Development Perspectives.* 7(3), 166–171.

Shonkoff, J. P. & Levitt, P. (2010). Neuroscience and the future of early childhood policy: moving from why to what and how. *Neuron,* 67(5), 689–691.

Answers to chapter questions

Chapter 1

1. Because in the past psychologists wanted to create psychology as an objective experimental science and emotion is largely subjective in nature and considered uncontrollable and therefore unsuited to experiments. If they did research emotion it was focused on the constituents of emotion that could be measured and controlled namely the physiological concomitants.
2. An individual answer.
3. An IQ score is made up of scores from separate sub scales. They measure different aspects of intelligence as defined by the IQ test. The IQ test is composed of sub scales related to cognition and memory. But there are other abilities based on emotion, sociability and physical prowess. Tests of these abilities can be developed and thus we have many ability quotients like the IQ (intelligence quotient). In other words we have multiple intelligences. One of these is based on our ability to understand our emotions and those of other people and take appropriate action. This is Emotional Intelligence EI and was developed as a concept by Goleman (1995).
4. Challenging behaviours are those that are not acceptable by society. Children from adversity can lack development of certain emotions due to poor care, limited social interaction and nurturance that lacks warmth. With limited emotions these children do not behave as society expects and develop survival strategies and behaviours which challenge the social expectations of most people.

Chapter 2

1. Seven. Emotions vary by interpretation, intensity, duration, expression, function, physiology, and during development.

2. Individual answer but variation in expression due to gender should be prominent. Of course cultural factors also play a role in the expression of secondary social emotions in these contexts.

3. Individual answer but it is important to recognise the different qualities of basic primary and secondary social emotions. You should have made the main difference (between the emotions you encountered) how they felt to you as fast or slow. The fast emotions like surprise or instant fear are usually basic emotions and the slower ones are usually the secondary social emotions. Self-conscious emotions are a subset of secondary social emotions. Because you are an adult you will usually be experiencing the more advanced self-conscious secondary emotions but you may still experience anger from frustration or love or even anxious fear. See 4 below.

4. Individual answer but here is a short comparison. Basic emotions are discrete, innate, quick and universal and though their expression can be modified are generally constant through life. Secondary emotions arise in development from general feeling states like frustration or satisfaction (proto-emotions) which relate to the child's cognition care and social interaction

Though the expression of basic emotions may change with development these emotions do not arise in development, rather they are innate and universal. The secondary emotions are those that arise from social interactions during development

Chapter 3

1. Every development that is subject to genetic influence is also, to some degree, subject to an environment. We are always in an environment. Nothing that develops is purely genetic. Even the genetic code has its origin in the history of the species under environmental selection pressures and environmental producers of mutations. *But equally* environment has to have something to influence and this is always provided by genetics; by DNA and the anatomy and physiology that it leads to. So both nature and nurture are present in every development. So it is difficult to write in favour of either genetic or environmental influences.

2. The brain is the basis of development because it is unfinished at birth and of all organs is the one most influenced by the environment. It is the organ of control in the body in areas such as perception and movement and can govern other developments especially when it acts in concert with the master gland that lies in the brain – the pituitary gland.

3. (a) Pre-determination depends on genetic influence. Genetic influence only sets the general structural framework of the brain and turns genes on and off at certain points in development (that are determined in many cases by

environmental influences). In the very early growth of the brain growth cone cells lead the migration of neurons to the head end of the embryo. The progress of these cones and their following neurons is genetically controlled and thus determine the general structure of the brain. Therefore each brain has a basis in genetic influence. However, after birth most of the influence on the infant brain is environmental rather than genetic and as we said in brackets above later genetic effects are often turned on and off by environmental stimuli.

Overall genetics and environment are both important and continually interact. Perhaps in biology where one looks at other animals which do not have much cortical development in their brains genetics is then the predominant factor but in humans, though it sets the framework with growth cones, it is the post natal environment that develops or does not develop the brain. This is shown when children such as Genie, are reared without much human contact in restricted surroundings see www.feralchildren.com.

(b) and (c) Yes, the predetermination of the general structure of the brain is important to a degree but it cannot be changed and thus the other, environmental, influence on the brain is much more important as far as those who work with children are concerned.

So predetermination of the brain may be important but as far as child development goes the much more important issue for practitioners is the influence of the environment, especially the social environment, on the child.

4. This should be a debate with yourself but the short answer is yes each brain is unique. Identical twins who share identical genes can be seen on autopsy to have had somewhat different brains (to a minor degree). Every child has unique genetics and a unique environmental experience.

5. Normative development refers to population averages and there can be individual development outside these averages. For example, a child can improve in a trait while still falling behind the average child. If this individual was only interpreted by norms a distortion would occur, namely the child's positive development (improvement) would be obscured.

6. Because it is in their nature. A child's brain demands interaction with the environment so a child is naturally active.

7. Organismic implies natural activity by children; mechanistic implies only reaction or machine like behaviour.

Chapter 4

1. Satisfaction; frustration and the perception of change.
2. Because frustration, even anticipatory frustration, heightens satisfaction when it comes.

3. Anger from frustration, anxious fear, and love of caregiver(s).
4. Basic emotions are innate but after 6 months they develop a subjective feeling due to myelination of the frontal lobe of the cortex. They are all subjectively felt at one year.
5. Six months is a dividing point on average. Before six months settled infants deal with such changes quite well. But after this age they notice change much more and shifting house or town can be quite disturbing for them.
6. First they protest; then despair sets in; finally detachment occurs. This sequence can occur with any child but is most marked with the securely attached.

Chapter 5

1. When a child realises that other people have minds that he or she should take account of then that child has developed a theory of mind.
2. A sense of self is necessary for the development of most secondary emotions and essential for the development of those secondary emotions involving other people. If we are to experience other people emotionally we must be able to distinguish us from them, me from you. This distinguishing is the basis of a sense of self. It develops only in relation to other people and is absent or weak in feral children reared in isolation. Children who cannot distinguish themselves from other people will find human interaction impossible and human interaction is the mechanism that causes secondary emotions to be felt and thus develop. Where the sense of self is exposed to an audience (real or imagined) self-consciousness will arise and this is the basis of feeling for the advanced self-conscious secondary emotions such as shame guilt and pride.
3. A reciprocal relationship means a relationship that simultaneously works both ways from adult to child and from child to adult. It is of great importance in that it is the main conduit through which the infant and child experiences life language and learning through (often playful) interactions.
4. Mutual love and the experience of an affectionate caregiver are essential elements in the genesis of many of the higher secondary emotions such as shame, and guilt. Yet shame and guilt are not pleasant emotions and can disturb us considerably. So warm and pleasant satisfactions given by a caregiver in infancy can lead on to mutual love of that caregiver but also to sorrow and grief if love is lost permanently and shame and guilt if the love is lost temporarily by caregiver disapproval or self-disapproval.
5. Adverse circumstances imply, in this case, emotional deprivation and a lack of secure attachment. In short a lack of love from parent or carer for the child and a failure to fully meet the child's dependency needs. As sympathy and pity are secondary emotions arising from an experience of being loved they are

often weak and not motivating or even absent in children suffering emotional deprivation. Such children have had to learn to survive without much care and compete with others for scarce resources. This competition fuels aggression and this can become an habitual and exciting way of dealing with others even if they are weak and helpless or unfortunate and deprived.

6. Playful interaction with the caregiver in a spirit of mutual hilarity is often the driving force behind the reciprocal relationship of the early years. This relationship is an important arena for the development of secondary social emotions and certainly involves play. Imaginative play that uses the symbolic function (where something stands for something else, a piece of wood is a car for example) is important in that it can allow a child to practise emotional expressions and even through pretence the emotion itself in "as if" mode.

7. Shame guilt and pride. Also embarrassment.

Chapter 6

1. Parents are needed for infants and toddlers in quite an intense way but when children gain instrumental independence they can usually look after their basic needs to some degree and close parental care need not be provided. The child throughout this long 0–18 month period is developing both physically and mentally and gradually becoming independent. This independence springs from initial dependency and therefore is attained gradually by interaction with adults who inform the child of the challenges of life and show the child how these can be dealt with. By 18 years the child should be fully independent.

2. Bonding is generally thought to be the one way process that guides the feelings of a parent usually the mother upon a baby's birth. (The exception to this is Rutter's use of bonding to mean a very secure attachment which operates even when the object of the attachment is not physically present.)

3. Secure attachment is a two way process originating instinctively in the infant whereby the dependency needs of the child are catered for and the secondary emotion of love grows between the parties. Insecure attachment is where the instinctive drive of the infant to seek care is imperfectly catered for in terms of the satisfaction of dependency needs.

4. Dependency requires attachment to a carer as a way to satisfy the essential needs of the infant and the type of attachment achieved governs the development of the secondary emotions (i.e. emotional development).

5. (a) resistant, characterised by infant's clingy behaviour and physical resistance to carers and later by anxiety and attention seeking. (b) avoidant characterised by lack of contact with carer and easy attitude to strangers and later by uninhibited behaviour hyperactivity and anger. (c) disorganised

characterised by stunned disoriented behaviour or hypervigilance and later depression.

6. Corresponding to same categories as in Qestion (5) (a) inconsistency of care for infant, (b) little or no care given to infant by parents besides the most basic things needed for survival and even then some children will die of neglect. (c) abuse of infant or child.

7. The research of Thomas and Chess showed temperament to be relatively stable over childhood and into adulthood. It is least stable in the first year of life.

8. Early environmental experience in the first year of life is probably the most prominent modifier of temperament. At this early stage the infant brain is open to modification because it is not finished.

9. Easy, Difficult and Slow to warm up.

Chapter 7

1. First the parents of the child do not cater for the infant's dependency needs fully or promptly. Such parents are psychologically unavailable for the infant and could also be described as psychologically abusive and uninvolved. The child will probably have a disorganised attachment to the parents or an insecure attachment of the avoidant kind. Second the parents of the child may give their infant adequate care but only on an inconsistent basis. They attend fully to the dependency needs of the child sometimes. They can be prompt and psychologically warm in this attention but they only give care when it suits them and the child cannot predict when this care will be given. Such a child experiences loving care at times but neglect at others and is liable to form a resistant attachment to the intermittent carers. Finally parents may care for the infant but do not introduce the child to objective reality in the second year.

2. Certainly not inevitable. Research shows that approximately two thirds of abused children do not go on to abuse their own children. Nevertheless in practice it seems very common for abuse to be seen as intergenerational because the two-thirds who do not go on to abuse rarely come to the attention of practitioners.

3. Four. They are the authoritarian, authoritative, permissive and uninvolved styles of parenting. Authoritative is the most effective according to research but all the first three can deliver 'good-enough' parenting whereas the uninvolved style always amounts to abuse by neglect.

4. Parenting is always an important influence on children but when it is 'good-enough' other factors can come to prominence. If, however, it is not 'good-enough', parenting will be the major or even the supreme influence on children and their development.

5. A somewhat individual response is needed but in regard to what is in the chapter the following applies: When parents give little or no warm psychological care to their child, and the child manages to survive, positive secondary emotions are unlikely to form unless the child can make secure attachments to people other than his or her parents. Such children will develop much anger from frustration. They have not known loving care and warm enjoyable interchanges with their parents. Thus secondary emotions such as shame empathy guilt and pride may not develop at all and bitterness towards others and distain for people in general especially the weak and unfortunate may be the most developed of the secondary emotions. These children will of course have the full complement of basic emotions and it is wrong to consider them unemotional. If parents give a little warm care to their children on an inconsistent basis their children will experience the joy of mutual love. However, this experience will be inconsistent only occurring at unpredictable times. Yet the child will long for it to occur. Such children often seek adult contact and appreciation in order to be loved once again. They become attention seekers and are children who are generally unhappy because they know what they are missing. They are often anxious and unsure of themselves though they can disguise this with an outward bravado. These children develop positive secondary emotions such as pride, shame and sympathy in addition to the basic emotions. However, their positive secondary emotions are often weak and unmotivating because the children are more concerned with attention seeking than anything else. Their attention seeking interferes with their social interactions and this can cause them to be rejected by both adults and other children. These children often experience strong feelings of jealousy and envy. These secondary emotions can only develop if the child has experienced love. These children have had a little love at unpredictable times and to them it is a scarce commodity. Thus when love has to be shared they can be+ very jealous and do not realise that there is enough love for everyone.

    Where children are over-parented and not slowly introduced to objective reality in their second year it is also difficult for emotions that are formed by social interaction to develop properly.

Chapter 8

1. Children especially in preschool and middle childhood learn to control their emotional expression. This they can do very efficiently by the end of middle childhood even feigning an emotion they do not feel. They also learn to partially control the subjective feeling that defines the emotion so that it is at a tolerable level. These processes together constitute emotional self-regulation. Individual examples.

2. All cultures and contexts within a culture have display rules which stipulate how emotion should be expressed in a particular context. individual examples.

3. Social referencing occurs when a child or adolescent usually in a situation that is unfamiliar takes his or her cue as to what emotion to express from another person. Usually that person is an adult who is of importance to the child (or adolescent) but can be another child or adolescent. Individual examples.

4. True.

5. A child's widening experiences of the world in different contexts leads essentially to differences in emotional expressions by the child in each different context. In early and middle childhood no new secondary emotions form and the chief development in these periods is the development of emotional expression to suit differing situations each with its own display rules. This change in expression also involves the child in the further development of emotional self-regulation particularly with respect to the expression of emotion and this can go as far as a feigning of emotion.

Chapter 9

1. Toddlers show oppositional behaviour because they become frustrated with parents. This is because a toddler does not really comprehend that a parent is different from him/herself and does not necessarily bend to suit the toddlers wishes. However, if a parent passively resists unrealistic toddler demands then the toddler begins to recognise the parent's separate existence and that his/her wishes and demands will not always be met. Eventually the child realises the separate psychological existence of the parent and realises that the parent has his/her own mind that the toddler must take account of. If a parent does not passively resist the toddler's unreasonable demands this process of separation from the parent may be delayed and the child will continue to think that everything should be directed by the child's own will and desires. That is why toddler tantrums should be *passively resisted* by a parent.

2. A parent need not win every confrontation with a negative toddler. Toddlers have needs that a parent should service but even when a toddler's demands are unsuitable and a parent gives in because they are tired and want peace not all is lost. If the parent continues the next day to offer passive resistance to unreasonable toddler demands the toddler, disappointed that the parent has not learnt a lesson, will eventually drop or moderate his/her demands and become socialised. The parent needs to win the war but need not necessarily win every battle or confrontation.

3.   The social learning theory is considered the most explanatory theory because it explains how aggression breeds aggression and how aggressive behaviour runs in families. In addition, using modelling, it can explain quite varied forms of aggression which other theories cannot do.

4.   True at least as far as physical aggression is concerned. Relational and verbal aggression are often quoted as higher in girls but research has not confirmed this and the picture remains unclear.

5.   Boys who show high levels of aggression at the preschool stage are likely to become aggressive adolescents and aggressive adults. In general with boys the level of aggression they show early in development is likely to be sustained into adulthood whether it is a high or low level. Aggression in males is thus stable over the years and, if high, is a good predictor of later problems and delinquency.

6.   Anxiety is rarely beneficial and is usually deleterious. However in some tasks a very little anxiety particularly at a planning stage can be of benefit by alerting the person concerned as to important issues and dispelling complacency.

Chapter 10

1.   Some children do not undergo the physical changes of puberty until two years after the average boy or girl. This means with some girls' menses do not commence until age 14 or later and for boys sperm production does not commence until 16 years or later. This is late maturity. Late maturing boys can be four years behind average maturing girls as average boys mature two years after girls of the same age.

2.   (a) Late maturing boys could be seen to be disadvantaged by remaining physically small and immature while their male peers are already physically men. This is in the short term where the boys may resort to being larrikins by way of compensation for their physical lack. However, in the long term they suffer little disadvantage because they have by then matured and are even helped by certain skills such as verbal ability that they may have learnt during their time of immaturity.

(b) Late maturing girls show no disadvantages from their late maturity either in the short or long term. They may well mature at the same time as their average male age peers. They tend to have slim tall figures which fit with modern conceptions of female beauty and thus they tend to be esteemed.

3.   Children who have had little care and who have brought themselves up have by necessity learnt to do things for themselves. Thus when they reach early adolescence they can seem mature and independent to other more nurtured adolescents. Particularly if they are boys in the early teenage years they may appear estimable to their age peers as they are independent to a large degree

of adult control. To a 14-year-old boy it may seem desirable to be so independent but by late adolescence the same onlooker may rate the child from adversity as a loser. This is a bit less pronounced with girls but the same feelings can apply and change when well nurtured girls consider a very independent teenager from adverse circumstances. The independence learnt to survive alone is not as socialised as that gained by slow exposure to responsibility over the adolescent years. Thus the children from adversity have a slight advantage in esteem from their peers which occasionally can be worked to their advantage by a social worker. However in later adolescence this advantage fades quickly as others mature and see the world in a more realistic light.

4. We can try to *rework* the adolescent's emotional development through social interactions with sensitive caregivers. However, adolescents are often too developed in their own ways for this to work. Alternatively and preferably we can *accept* the adolescent as they are with all of their survival behaviours and try through mentoring to avoid clashes with authorities.

5. A mentor is a person who can advise the adolescent to take responsible decisions in an independent living context. Mentors can be people who the adolescent esteems, or can be just friends not particularly emotionally attached to the adolescent but who have the ability to sway the adolescent's decisions in a positive direction.

Chapter 11

1. Emotional history of Jake Smith

There is not much evidence in this case but what there is points clearly to resistant attachment and inconsistent nurturance. This clarity is not complicated by other factors and allows us to follow the guidelines for the inconsistence group in full detail. Paradoxically this makes for a long somewhat repetitive history which might be considerably reduced if other competing evidence were available.

Jake's emotional development in infancy

In Jake's case we can infer that he had *some* satisfaction and warm loving nurturance in his first year but this was delivered on an inconsistent basis and the child's perception of change made him fearful and anxious. Jake also had a considerable amount of frustration in his early life. However, he was most affected by his inability to predict when things would happen, whether he would be satisfied, or whether he would be frustrated. Jake's early environment was characterised by insecurity and not knowing what was coming next. His upbringing lacked consistency and routine dependable care. He noticed this and it dominated his early feelings. Though he had the basis for the emotion of love and mutual affection this basis was insecure. This disturbed Jake. Though he knew a little love and warmth, he was fearful of their removal, and this fear, with a deal of frustration, dominated his early feelings and was the basis for the growth of anxious fear.

Jake's dependency needs

Jakes dependency needs were only partially met. His *instrumental dependency* must have been catered for at least adequately in his early years for him to survive and he may have been forced to become instrumentally independent at a fairly early age, but his *emotional dependence* did not advance change and redistribute itself, as it should have done.

Because of inconsistent delivery of loving nurturance Jake had a neurotic need for his mother while still being dissatisfied and angry with her. Jake had tasted affectionate rearing; he knew what it was and how good it made him feel. Yet he could not rely on his mother to deliver this care and this made him reject her. At the same time he longed for her and the semi-conscious memory of the little affection he had received spurred him on. This accounts for his ambivalence towards his mother. In Maslow's terms he had his physiological needs (instrumental dependence) met, for the most part, but not his belongingness and love needs. Yet the latter must have been *partially* met, but not sufficiently to allow the spread of emotional dependence to people other than his mother. So we get an adolescent with an infantile dependence on his mother accompanied with an ambivalence towards her that on occasions turns to violence.

Jake's attachment

Jake's attachment was likely to have been *insecure*, more precisely in the *resistant* category. As an infant Jake could not predict when he would receive care. He became clingy and very reluctant to become separated from his mother. Because of this insecurity he was unwilling to explore and wasted a great deal of energy clinging to or following his mother. In the "strange situation" test he would have objected to his mother leaving and reacted with crying while she was gone, yet upon her return he would not have responded to her and might have shown signs of displeasure even to the level of physical resistance and anger. Jake's behaviour as a teenager suggests that these early attachment difficulties were never reworked. His reaction at 14 shows that the insecure-resistant attachment with its ambivalent and neurotic qualities was never corrected or ameliorated.

The explanations of Jake's early emotional development under these three headings are very repetitive. This is because they are essentially three ways of describing the same situation with some variation for each approach. The explanations are all inferences about emotional development based on Jake's more recent behaviour.

Developments in later years are relevant to Jake's emotional history but they build on, or add to the essential core information as outlined in the three headings above. We can make further inferences about later development.

Jake's emotional development in toddlerhood

Jake's emotional development in toddlerhood was based on what happened in his infancy. It is unlikely that his environment changed significantly when he became a toddler. He still got some attention and affection but in fits and starts. Things were very unpredictable and he still clung to his mother whenever he could but at the same time rejected her advances because of angry feelings that arose from his frustration at her usual unavailability. He might have put it like this, *"Why do you want me now when you didn't want me before?"*

The mother's usual unavailability detracted from the reciprocal interaction (that is so important at this stage) and when she was available Jake's angry reaction did not allow for pleasurable interchanges. For this reason Jake may have fallen behind other children in developing a sense of self and of others. The difference between him and his mother was not as differentiated as it should have been and Jake struggled with this fact continually. Though he developed some sense of self, the unresolved clinging to his mother limited this process, and this in turn limited the development of the secondary emotions. However, he had the full complement of basic emotions. We know that Jake now desires to be good; he said so. Therefore it is probable that during this earlier period Jake developed some secondary emotions such as shame, but this development gave feelings that were fleeting and of little motivational power when faced with Jake's desire to cling to and whine for his mother. An exception is jealousy. Jake was jealous of his younger brother and his feelings did not subside with time. People who have known only a little affection are often those who are most jealous. For Jake there was little love to go around and his brother was a competitor. We know that Jake was violent towards him. There are many explanations of sibling violence but this one fits the general picture.

Jake's emotional development in early childhood

The boy's emotional development at this stage continued the pattern set in infancy and toddlerhood. For reasons of necessity Jake had now learnt how to survive without his mother but he still had extreme feelings towards her. On the one hand he longed for her and her care but on the other he knew she neglected him and he was angry and resistant. His sense of self that should have been firmly established during these pre-school years was still weak and easily overruled by his desire to be physically near his mother. Jake at this stage had little control of his emotional expression. He also had little understanding of his own emotions. Thus he probably acted (as he did later) with little control and in some respects he resembled a child at an earlier stage of development.

Jake's emotional development in middle childhood.

In middle childhood Jake retained the pattern set earlier.

He still had little control over his emotional expression and he displayed his anxiety openly. This probably made him unpopular with both children and adults and he got into a lot of trouble. He did not understand himself very well and he had little understanding of the feelings of others and had little concern for them. His emotional obsessions, his anxiety, and his anger at his mother reduced the time he had available for imaginative play. This and other circumstances (that are speculative) reduced his cognitive development and ability giving him great difficulty at school. He appeared learning disabled. This did not improve his standing with his peers or his teachers. These circumstances further detracted from the growth of a clear self-concept in this boy. The boy's lack of a clear self-concept arose from his inability to free himself from his angry emotional dependence on his mother, and it also caused him to lack understanding of his place in the world. Thus he found it hard to understand and accept events when they did not go his way.

Jake's emotional development in early adolescence.

Again this followed the pattern of earlier developmental periods. There is no evidence of a favourable change in his environment and we are now confronted with Jake as described in the court report. His neurotic ambivalent emotional dependence on his mother is still present as is his chronic anxiety and his tendency to respond to events with anger and aggression which unfortunately is transformed and turned against himself in his final act.

2. Emotional history of JO

Jo's emotional development in infancy

Though Jo is reported as a normal baby by his mother it can be inferred from his later behaviour, particularly his aggression and his attention seeking from his parents, that his emotional development in infancy was characterised by experiences of frustration and insecurity.

He may have had some *satisfactions* but these probably came inconsistently. Conversely he was often frustrated and experienced more *frustration* than an average infant should expect. His *perception of change* was, to a certain degree, one of insecurity in that, due to his caregivers' inabilities, he could not predict when his satisfactions would occur.

The evidence for this picture is in his later behaviour, particularly his desire to be with his mother and his parallel rejection and aggression towards her when he is in her company. His aggressive outbursts in later years also suggest excess frustration in infancy which probably continued into the next stage.

Jo's dependency needs

Jo's dependency needs were at least partially catered for in childhood. But they were often dealt with on an inefficient and perhaps inconsistent basis. Dependency is divided into *instrumental* and *emotional dependence*. Jo may have made reasonable progress in reducing his instrumental dependence in his early years. He learnt to feed himself and dress himself. We know this from his mother's reporting him as achieving normal developmental milestones. However, one important area of instrumental dependence remained a constant problem. This was the issue of bowel control and socialised toileting. Otherwise we cannot infer much about his instrumental dependence.

What was much more problematic was his inability to develop a secure *emotional dependency* with his mother or his father. His emotional dependency did not spread to others because he had not resolved the relationship with his mother. His consistent attempts to contact then abuse her are evidence for such a lack of resolution. His toileting difficulties were probably not resolved partly because he never reached an emotional conclusion with his mother and the problems persisted into adolescence.

Jo's attachment

For many years when Jo was away from his family he yearned to return to them. Yet on the occasions when he did return, after a very brief interval, he became frustrated with his parents, particularly his mother, and became aggressive and abusive towards her. All this indicates a pattern of infant attachment that is best described as *insecure resistant*. Children with this type of attachment do not welcome mothers return but become annoyed with her even if they had craved her presence a short time before.

Jo's emotional development in toddlerhood

In toddlerhood it is likely that an unbalanced *reciprocal relationship* existed between Jo and his caregivers, particularly his mother. His mother could not effectively resist the child's contrary demands and probably, early in the relationship, the reciprocal interchange deteriorated into a series of demands from the child. The inability of the mother to take a strong part in the relationship limited the child's ability to gain a firm *sense of self*. Fairly early in the relationship when the child became negative his mother could not resist and oppositional behaviour was not resolved. The evidence for this explanation is in two parts. First it lies in the very poor social relations that Jo had with others throughout his development. Second evidence for this explanation comes from the consistently frustrating confrontations that Jo had with his mother over the years when again and again he tried to gain a resolution to their relationship.

Because of the later picture of Jo we can infer that in toddlerhood his chief emotion was anger arising from his frustration with his mother. Because anger was dominant he did not develop full feelings of love and the development of his secondary social emotions of shame guilt and pride may, on this account, have been limited. These weakened secondary emotions were also difficult for him to express in the presence of a continual oppositional conflict with his parents. Nevertheless, he did have *some* experiences of love and satisfaction however unpredictable they may have been and, for this reason, when his brother arrived he had strong feelings of jealousy which did not abate. His unbalanced relationship with his mother prevented him from resolving his emotional dependence on her. Such a resolution would have allowed him to make his first peer relationships. We can infer this because his later peer relationships were so very poor and his interactions with his peers marked by anger and aggression. Thus as a toddler he did not develop a clear *theory of mind* as to how others felt and acted. He did not develop either pity or sympathy. We can infer all of this from his later anti-social behaviour.

Jo's emotional development in early childhood

Because of the unresolved relationship with his mother Jo did not develop socially in early childhood. He had not developed a strong theory of mind in the preceding period and thus his *social referencing* was very weak. Later in this period his peer relationships were poor and he did not learn the *display rules of emotion*. These features were aggravated by not having a consistent social model to follow and imitate. He showed little *control of his emotional expression*. All this is deduced from his later anti-social behaviour. He had all the basic emotions but his secondary emotions were not strongly developed in toddlerhood and they remained weak in early childhood. However, because he knew a little of the satisfactions of love he became intensely jealous of his brother who, it seemed to Jo, might steal the little but inconsistent love that was available from the caregivers.

Jo's emotional development in middle childhood

This is the period we have most information about, yet it simply continues with little change Jo's emotional picture as we have inferred it earlier. Jo did not succeed in school largely because of the emotional problems that have been mentioned. He gained little control of his emotional expression and his social relationships were very short-lived. He did not develop emotionally to any significant degree in this period.

Jo's emotional development in early adolescence

Jo entered his teenage years as an unsocialised boy with little control of his emotional expression and an unresolved emotional dependency on his mother. This bleak picture continued until he was fourteen when his growing cognitive ability probably allowed him, for the first time, to develop a relationship with a rather emotionally detached mentor. In time this relationship has allowed Jo to have more control in his life and to develop better daily self-care. He probably still does not have strong secondary emotions of guilt or shame and still has little understanding of, or sympathy for, others. However, since turning 14 he has developed more control of himself in certain situations at home and at work and has at last resolved, to some degree at least, the emotional dependence he had on his mother.

References

Ackerman, B., Abe, J. A. & Izard, C. E. (1998). Differential emotions theory and emotional development: Mindful of modularity. In M. F. Mascolo & S. Griffin. (Eds), *What Develops in Emotional Development?* New York: Plenum Press.

Adelmann, P. K. & Zajonc, R. B. (1989). Facial efference and the experience of emotion. *Annual Review of Psychology*, 40, 249–280.

Ainsworth, M., Blehar, M., Waters, E. & Wall, S. (1978). *Patterns of Attachment*. Hillsdale, NJ: Erlbaum.

Akhtar, N. & Martinez-Sussmann, C. (2007). Intentional communication. In C. A. Brownell & C. B. Kopp (Eds). *Socioemotional Development in the Toddler Years*. New York: Guilford Press

American Psychiatric Association. (2000). Diagnostic and statistical manual of mental disorders (4th edn, text rev.). Washington, DC: Author.

American Psychiatric Association. (2013). *Diagnostic and Statistical Manual of Mental Disorders* (5th edn). Arlington, VA: American Psychiatric Publishing.

Amsel, A. (1962). Frustrative non-reward in partial reinforcement and discrimination learning: Some recent history and a theoretical extention. *Psychological Review*, 64, 306–328.

Arnold, M. B. (1970). *Feelings and Emotions: The Loyola Symposium*. New York: Basic Books.

Aronfreed, J. (1968). *Conduct and Consciousness: The Socialization of Internalized Control Over Behavior*. New York: Academic Press.

Bandura, A. (1977). *Social Learning Theory*. Englewood Cliffs, NJ: Prentice-Hall.

Bard, P. (1934). On emotional experience after decortication with some remarks on theoretical views. *Psychological Review*, 41, 309–329.

Baron-Cohen, S (1991) Precursors to a theory of mind: understanding attention in others. In A. Whiten (Ed.), *Natural Theories of Mind*, Oxford: Basil Blackwell, pp. 233–251.

Baron-Cohen, S., Tager-Flusberg, H. & Cohen, D. J. (Eds.) (1993). *Understanding Other Minds: Perspectives from Autism*. Oxford: Oxford University Press.

Bates, J. (1987). Temperament in infancy. In J. Osofsky (Ed.), *Handbook of Infant Development* (2nd edn). New York: Wiley, pp. 1101–1149.

Bates, J. (1989). Concepts and measures of temperament. In G. Kohnstamm, J. Bates and M. Rothbart. (Eds.), *Temperament in childhood*. New York: Wiley, pp. 3–26.

Bates, J., Maslin, C. & Frankel, K. (1985). Attachment security, mother-child interaction and temperament as predictors of behavior problem ratings at three years. In I. Bretherton & E. Waters (Eds), *Growing Points in Attachment Theory and Research. Monographs of the Society for Research in Child Development*, 50 (Whole No. 209), 167–193.

Baumrind, D. (1971). Current patterns of parental authority. *Developmental Psychology Monograph*, 4(1, Pt2), 1–103.

Belsky, J. & Rovine, M. (1987). Temperament and attachment in the strange situation: an empirical rapprochement. *Child Development*, 58, 787–795.

249

Berger, R. H., Miller, A. L., Seifer, R., Cares, S. R., & Lebourgeois, M. K. (2012). Acute sleep restriction effects on emotion responses in 30- to 36-month-old children. *Journal of Sleep Research*, 21(3), 235–246.

Bermond, B., Fasotti, L., Nieuwenhuyse, B. & Shuerman, J. (1991). Spinal cord lesions peripheral feedback and intensities of emotional feelings. *Cognition and Emotion*, 5, 201–220.

Bernier, A., Carlson, S. M., Deschênes, M., & Matte-Gagné, C. (2012). Social factors in the development of early executive functioning: a closer look at the caregiving environment. *Developmental Science*, 15(1), 12–24.

Boccia, M. & Campos, J. (1989). Maternal emotional signals, social referencing, and infants' reaction to strangers. In N. Eisenberg (Ed.), *Empathy and Related Emotional Responses: New Directions for Child Development*. San Francisco, CA: Jossey-Bass.

Bowlby, J. (1982). *Attachment and Loss* (2nd edn). New York: Basic Books.

Bradley, B. (1989) *Visions of Infancy: A Critical Introduction to Child Psychology*. Cambridge: Polity/Blackwell.

Bradshaw, C. P., Rodgers, C. R., Ghandour, L. A., & Garbarino, J. (2009). Social–cognitive mediators of the association between community violence exposure and aggressive behavior. *School Psychology Quarterly*, 24(3), 199.

Brennan, L. M., Shaw, D. S., Dishion, T. J., & Wilson, M. (2012). Longitudinal predictors of school-age academic achievement: Unique contributions of toddler-age aggression, oppositionality, inattention, and hyperactivity. *Journal of Abnormal Child Psychology*, 40(8), 1289–1300.

Bridges, K. M. B. (1932). *The Social and Emotional Development of the Pre-school Child*. London: Kegan Paul.

Bridges, L. & Grolnick, W. (1995). The development of emotional self-regulation in infancy and early childhood. In N. Eisenberg (Ed.). *Social Development: Review of Child Development Research*. Thousand Lakes, CA: Sage.

British Department of Health, (1995). *Child Protection: Messages from Research*. London: HMSO.

Bronowski, J. (1973). *The Ascent of Man*. Boston, MA: Little, Brown and Co.

Bronson, G. W. (1972). Infants' reactions to unfamiliar persons and novel objects. *Monographs of the Society for Research in Child Development*, 32, (3, Serial No. 148).

Brown, T. & Kozak, A. (1998). Emotion and the possibility of psychologists entering into heaven. In M. F. Mascolo & S. Griffin (Eds), *What Develops in Emotional Development?* New York: Plenum Press.

Brownell, C. A. & Kopp, C. B. (2007). Transitions in toddler socioemotional development: Behaviour, understanding, relationships. In C. A. Brownell, & C. B. Kopp (Eds). *Socioemotional Development in the Toddler Years*. New York: Guilford Press.

Buhrmester, D. & Furman, W. (1990). Perceptions of sibling relationships during middle childhood and adolescence. *Child Development*, 61, 1387–1398.

Buss, A. H. & Plomin, R. (1975). *A Temperament Theory of Personality Development*. New York: Wiley.

Buss, A. H. & Plomin, R. (1984). *Temperament: Early Developing Personality Traits*. Hillsdale, NJ: Erlbaum.

Cacioppo, J. T., Klien, D., Berntson, G. C. & Hatfield, E. (1993). The psychophysiology of emotion. In M. Lewis & J. M. Haviland (Eds), *Handbook of Emotions*. New York: Guilford, pp. 119–142.

Cairns, R. B., Cairns, B. D., Neckerman, H. J., Ferguson, L. L. & Gariepy, J. (1989). Growth and aggression: 1 Childhood to early adolescence. *Developmental Psychology*, 25, 320–330.

Cannon, W. B. (1927). The James-Lange theory of emotion: A critical examination and an alternate theory. *American Journal of Psychology*, 39, 106–124.

Carter, R. (2000). *Mapping the Mind*. London. Phoenix.

Case, R. Hayward, S., Lewis, M. & Hurst, P. (1988). Towards a neo-Piagetian theory of affective and cognitive development. *Developmental Review*, 8, 1–51.

Casey, B. J., Jones, R. M., Levita, L., Libby, V., Pattwell, S. S., Ruberry, E. J., . . . Somerville, L. H. (2010). The storm and stress of adolescence: insights from human imaging and mouse genetics. *Developmental Psychobiology*, 52(3), 225–235.

Cassia, V. M., Simion, F. & Umilta C. (2001). Face preference at birth: The role of an orienting mechanism. *Developmental Science*, 4, 101–108.

Cassia, V. M., Turati, C. & Simion F. (2004). Can a non-specific bias towards top-heavy patterns explain newborns' face preference? *Psychological Science*, 15, 379–383.

Chisholm, J. (1990). Life history perspectives on human development. In G. Butterworth & P. Bryant (Eds), *Causes of Development*. Hillsdale, NJ: Erlbaum.

Coady, T. (1999). Morality and species. *Res Publica*, 8, 2.

Cole, P., Barrett, K. & Zahn-Waxler, C. (1992). Emotion displays in two-year-olds during mishaps. *Child Development*, 63, 314–324.

Collins, W. A. & Repinski, D. J. (1994). Relationships during adolescence: Continuity and change in interpersonal perspective. In R. Montemayor, G. R. Adams & T. P. Gullotta (Eds), *Personal Relationships During Adolescence*. Thousand Oaks, CA: Sage.

Colonnesi, C., Draijer, E. M., Jan JM Stams, G., Van der Bruggen, C. O., Bögels, S. M. & Noom, M. J. (2011). The relation between insecure attachment and child anxiety: A meta-analytic review. *Journal of Clinical Child and Adolescent Psychology*, 40(4), 630–645.

Cowan, W. M., Fawcett, J. W., O'Leary, D. D. M. & Stanfield, B. B. (1979). Regressive events in neurogenesis. *Science*, 225, 1228–1235.

Damasio, A. R. (1994). *Decartes' Error: Emotion Reason and the Human Brain*. London: Picador.

Darwin, C. (1872). *The Expression of Emotion in Man and Animals*. Chicago, IL: University of Chicago Press.

Davidson, G. W., Seaton, M. A. & Simpson, J. A. (Eds) (1994). *The Wordsworth Concise English Dictionary*. Ware: Wordsworth Editions Limited.

Davidson, R. J. (1992). Anterior cerebral asymmetry and the nature of emotion. *Brain and Cognition*, 20, 125–151.

DeHart, G. B., Sroufe, L. A. & Cooper, R. G. (2000). *Child Development: Its Nature and Course, Fourth Edition*. New York: McGraw-Hill Higher Education.

Delemarre-van de Waal, H. A. (2005). Secular trend of timing puberty. *Endocrine Development* 8, 1–14.

Denham, S. (1998). *Emotional Development in Young Children*. London: Guilford Press.

Deoni, S. C. L., Mercure, E., Blasi, A., Gasston, D., Thomson, A., Johnson, M., Murphy, D. G. M. (2011). Mapping infant brain myelination with magnetic resonance imaging. *The Journal of Neuroscience: The Official Journal of the Society for Neuroscience*, 31(2), 784–791. doi:10.1523/JNEUROSCI.2106-10.2011

Descartes, R. (1649). Passions of the soul. In E. A. Haldane & G. R. Ross (Eds), *The Philosophical Works of Descartes*. New York: Dover.

Diamond, J. (1997). *Guns, Germs and Steel: A Short History of Everybody for the last 13,000 Years*. London: Jonathan Cape.

Dodge, K. A., Pettit, G. S. & Bates, J. E. (1997). How the experience of early physical abuse leads children to become chronically aggressive. In C. Cicchetti & S. L. Toth (Eds), *Developmental Psychopathology: Developmental Perspectives on Trauma. Vol. 9. Theory Research and Intervention*. Rochester, NY: University of Rochester Press.

Dollard, J., Doob, J., Miller, N., Mowrer, O. & Sears, R. (1939). *Frustration and Aggression*. New Haven, CT: Yale University Press.

Dozier, M., Zeanah, C. H. & Bernard, K. (2013). Infants and toddlers in foster care. *Child Development Perspectives*. 7(3), 166–171.

Dubrovina, I. & Ruzska, A. (1990). *The Mental Development of Residents in a Children's Home*. Moscow: Pedagogics.

Dunn, J. (1988) *The Beginnings of Social Understanding*. London: Blackwell.

Dunn, J. & Kendrick, C. (1980). The arrival of a sibling: Changes in patterns of interaction between mother and first-born child. *Journal of Child Psychiatry and Psychology*, 21, 119–132.

Dunn, J. & Munn, P. (1985). Becoming a family member: Family conflict and the development of social understanding in the second year. *Child Development*, 56, 480–492.

Edelman, G. (1992). *Bright Air, Brilliant Fire*. New York: Basic Books.

Egeland, B. (1989). Breaking the cycle of abuse: Implications for prediction and intervention. In K. Browne, C. Davies & P. Stratton (Eds), *Early Prediction and Prevention of Child Abuse*. Chichester: Wiley.

Eisenberg, N. (2006) Introduction: A focus on emotion. In W. Damon, R. M. Lerner & N. Eisenberg (Eds), *Handbook of Child Psychology: Vol 3. Social Emotional and Personality Development* (6th edn). Hoboken, NJ: Wiley, pp. 3–8.

Ekman, P. (1984). Expression and the nature of emotion. In K. R. Scherer & P. Ekman (Eds), *Approaches to Emotion*. Hillsdale, NJ: Erlbaum.

Ekman, P., Friesen, W. & Simons, R. (1985). Is the startle reaction an emotion? *Journal of Personality and Social Psychology*, 49, 1416–1426.

Ekman, P., Levenson, R. W. & Friesen, W. V. (1983). Autonomic nervous system activity distinguished among emotions. *Science*, 361, 1208–1210.

Eliot, L. (2001). *Early Intelligence*. London: Penguin.

Elster, J. (1999). *Alchemies of the Mind: Rationality and the Emotions*. Melbourne: Cambridge University Press.

Emde, R. (1992). Social referencing research: Uncertainty, self, and the search for meaning. In S. Feinman (Ed.), *Social Referencing and the Social Construction of Reality*. New York: Plenum Press.

Emde, R., Gaensbauer, T. & Harmon, R. (1976). Emotional expression in infancy: A biobehavioral study. *Psychological Issues Monograph Series*, 10 (37), 1–198.

Facey, A. B. (1981). *A Fortunate Life*. Melbourne: Penguin.

Feinman, S. (1982). Social referencing in infancy. *Merrill-Palmer Quarterly* (1982-), 445–470.

Fogel, A. (1982). Affect dynamics in early infancy: Affective tolerance. In T. Field & A, Fogel (Eds), *Emotion and Early Intervention*. Hillsdale, NJ: Erlbaum.

Fogel, A. (1993). *Developing Through Relationships: Origins of Communication Self and Culture*. Chicago, IL: University of Chicago Press.

Fox, E. (2008). *Emotion Science*. London: Palgrave Macmillan.

Fox, N. A. & Davidson, R. J. (1988). Patterns of brain electrical activity during facial signs of emotion in 10 month old infants. *Developmental Psychology*, 24, 230–236.

Fredrickson, B. L. (1998). What good are positive emotions? *Review of General Psychology*, 2(3), 300–319. doi:10.1037/1089-2680.2.3.300

Freud, S. (1915). Instincts and their vicissitudes. Partially reprinted in P. Gay (Ed.) (1989). *The Freud Reader*. New York: Norton.

Friedman, S. L. & Boyle, D. E. (2008). Attachment in US children experiencing nonmaternal care in the early 1990s. *Attachment and Human Development*, 10(3), 225–261. doi:10.1080/14616730802113570

Frijda, N. H. & Mesquita, B. (1998). The analysis of emotions: Dimensions of variation. In M. F. Mascolo & S. Griffin (Eds), *What Develops in Emotional Development?* New York: Plenum Press.

Gabriel, Y. & Griffiths, D. S. (2002). Emotion, learning and organizing. *Learning Organization, The*, 9(5), 214–221.

Garbarino, J. (1999). *Lost Boys*. New York: The Free Press.

Gardner, H. (1984). *Frames of Mind: The Theory of Multiple Intelligences*. London: Heinemann.

Gendron, M., & Barrett, L. F. (2009). Reconstructing the past: A century of ideas about emotion in psychology. *Emotion Review*, 1(4), 316–339.

Geschwind, D. H. (2011). Genetics of autism spectrum disorders. *Trends in Cognitive Science*, 15(9), 409–416.

Gibbons, R., Dugaiczyk, L. J., Girke T., Duistermars, B., Zielinski, R. & Dugaiczyk A. (2004). Distinguishing humans from great apes with AluYb8 repeats. *Journal of Molecular Biology*, 339, 721–729.

Gibson, K. R. (1991). Myelination and behavioral development: A comparative perspective on questions of neoteny, altriciality and intelligence. *Brain Maturation and Cognitive Development*, 29–63.

Giedd, J. N., Blumenthal, J. & Jeffries, N. O. (1999) Brain development during childhood and adolescence: A longitudinal study. *Neuroscience*, 2(10), 861–863.

Goffman, E. (1969). *Strategic Interaction*. Philadelphia, PA: University of Pennsylvania Press.

Goleman, D. (1995). *Emotional Intelligence*. London: Bloomsbury.

Goleman, D. (2006). *Emotional intelligence*. New York: Random House LLC.

Gottleib, G. (2007). Probabilistic epigenesis. *Developmental Science*, 10(1)–11.

Gottman, J.M., Katz, L. F. & Hooven, D. (1996). Parental meta-emotion philosophy and the emotional life of families: Theoretical models and preliminary data. *Journal of Family Studies*, 10, 243–268.

Gould, S. J. (1989). *Wonderful Life: The Burgess Shale and the Nature of History*. New York: Norton.

Graber, J. A., Seeley, J. R., Brooks-Gunn, J. & Lewinsohn, P. M. (2004). Is pubertal timing associated with psychopathology in young adulthood? *Journal of the American Academy of Child and Adolescent Psychiatry*, 43, 718–726.

Graziano, P. A., Calkins, S. D. & Keane, S. P. (2011). Sustained attention development during the toddlerhood to preschool period: Associations with toddlers' emotion regulation strategies and maternal behaviour. *Infant and Child Development*, 20(6), 389–408.

Greenspan, S. I. (1981). *Psychopathology and Adaptation in Infancy and Early Childhood*. New York: International Universities Press.

Greenspan, S. I. (1997). *The Growth of the Mind: And the Endangered Origins of Intelligence*. Reading, MA: Addison-Wesley.

Grusec, J. E. (2011). Socialization processes in the family: Social and emotional development. *Annual Review of Psychology*, 62, 243–269.

Hamburger, V. & Oppenheim, R. W. (1982). Naturally occurring neural death in vertebrates. *Neuroscience Commentaries*, 1, 39–55.

Hanson, J. L., Adluru, N., Chung, M. K., Alexander, A. L., Davidson, R. J. & Pollak, S. D. (2013). Early neglect is associated with alterations in white matter integrity and cognitive functioning. *Child Development*, 84(5), 1566–1578.

Harlow, H. F. & Harlow, M. (1962). Social deprivation in monkeys. *Scientific American*, 207(5), 136–146.

Harris, J. R. (2002). Beyond the nurture assumption: Testing hypotheses about the child's environment. In J. G. Borkowski, S. Landesman-Ramey & M. Bristol-Power (Eds), *Parenting and the Child's World: Influences on Academic, Intellectual and Socioemotional Development*. London: Laurence Erlbaum Associates.

Harris, J. R. (1998). *The Nurture Assumption*. New York: The Free Press.

Harris, P. L. (1990). *Children and emotion: The Development of Psychological Understanding*. London: Blackwell.

Harris, P. (2008). Children's understanding of emotion. In M. Lewis, J. M. Haviland-Jones & L. Feldman Barrett (Eds), *Handbook of Emotions* (3rd edn). New York: The Guilford Press, pp. 409–427.

Hascher, T. (2010). Learning and Emotion: Perspectives for theory and research. *European Educational Research Journal*, 9(1), 13–28.

Hay, D. F., Hurst, S. L., Waters, C. S. & Chadwick, A. (2011). Infants' use of force to defend toys: The origins of instrumental aggression. *Infancy*, 16(5), 471–489.

Hebb, D. O. (1980). *Essay on Mind*. Hilldale, NJ: Erlbaum.

Herrera, C. & Dunn, J. (1997). Early experiences with family conflict: Implications for arguments with a close friend. *Developmental Psychology*, 33, 869–881.

Hill, J. (1980). *Understanding Early Adolescence: A Framework*. Chapel Hill, NC: Center for Early Adolescence.

Hoffman, H. S. (1987). Imprinting and the critical period for social attachments: Some laboratory investigations. In M. H. Bornstein (Ed.), *Sensitive Periods in Development: Interdisciplinary Studies*. Hillsdale, NJ: Erlbaum, pp. 99–121.

Hoffman, M. L. (1984). Interaction of affect and cognition in empathy. In C. E. Izard, J. Kagan and R. B. Zajonc (Eds), *Emotions, Cognition, and Behavior*. Cambridge: Cambridge University Press.

Hoksbergen, R. A. C., (2005). Post-institutional autistic syndrome in Romanian adoptees. *Journal of Autism and Developmental Disorders*, 35(5), 615–213.

Huddleston, J. & Ge, X. (2003). Boys at puberty: Psychosocial implications. In C. Hayward (Ed.), *Gender Differences at Puberty*, 113–134. New York: University of Cambridge Press.

Huesmann, L. R., Eron, L. D., Lefkowitz, M. M. & Walder, L. O. (1984). Stability of aggression over time and generations. *Developmental Psychology*, 20, 1120–1134.

Hughes, C. & Dunn, J (2007). Children's relationships with other children. In C. A. Brownell & C. B. Kopp (Eds). *Socioemotional Development in the Toddler Years*. New York: Guilford Press.

Huttenlocher, P. R. (1994). Synaptogenesis, synapse elimination, and neural plasticity in the human cerebral cortex. In C. A. Nelson (Ed.), *Threats to Optimal Development: Integrating Biological, Psychological, and Social Risk Factors: Minnesota Symposia on Child Psychology*. Vol. 27. Hillsdale, NJ: Erlbaum, pp. 35–54.

Hyman S. E. (2009). How adversity gets under the skin. *Nature Neuroscience*, 12(3), 241–243.

International Human Genome Sequencing Consortium, (2004). Finishing the euchromatic sequence of the human genome. *Nature*, 21, 931–945.

Isabella, R. A. (1993). Origins of attachment: Maternal interactive behaviour across the first year. *Developmental Psychology*. 64, 605–621.

Izard, C. E. (1977). *Human Emotions*. New York: Plenum Press.

Izard, C. E. (1993). Four systems for emotion activation: Cognitive and noncognitive processes. *Psychological Review*, 100, 68–90.

Izard, C. E. (2009). Emotion theory and research: Highlights, unanswered questions, and emerging issues. *Annual Review of Psychology*, 60, 1–25.

Izard, C. E., Kagan, J. & Zajonc, R. B. (1984). Introduction. In C. E. Izard, J. Kagan & R. B. Zajonc (Eds), *Emotions Cognitions and Behaviour*. Cambridge: Cambridge University Press.

Izard, C. E. & Malatesta, C. (1987). Perspectives on emotional development 1: Differential emotions theory of early emotional development. In J. Osofsky (Ed.), *Handbook of Infant Development* (2nd edn). New York: Wiley.

Izard, C. E., Woodburn, E. M., Finlon, K. J., Krauthamer-Ewing, E. S., Grossman, S. R. & Seidenfeld, A. (2011). Emotion knowledge, emotion utilization, and emotion regulation. *Emotion Review*, 3(1), 44–52.

James, W. (1884). What is emotion? *Mind*, 19, 188–205.

Janet, P. (1928). *De l'angoisse 'a l'extase. II. Les sentiments fondamentaux*. Paris: Librairie Felix Alcan.

Janowsky, J. S & Finlay, B. L. (1986). The outcome of perinatal brain damage: The role of normal neuron loss and axon retraction. *Developmental Medicine and Child Neurology*, 28, 375–389.

Johnson, M. H. (1997). *Developmental Cognitive Neuroscience: An Introduction*. Cambridge, MA: Blackwell.

Johnson, M. H., Dziurawiec, S., Ellis, H. & Morton, J. (1991). Newborns' preferential tracking of face-like stimuli and its subsequent decline. *Cognition*, 40, 1–19.

Joseph, R. (1982). The neuropsychology of development: Hemispheric laterality, limbic language, and the origin of thought. *Journal of Clinical Psychology*, 38, 4–33.

Kagan, J. (1984). *The Idea of Emotion in Human Development*. In C. E. Izard, J. Kagan & R. B. Zajonc (Eds), *Emotions Cognitions and Behaviour*. Cambridge: Cambridge University Press.

Kahneman, D. & Tversky, A. (Eds). (2000). *Choices, Values and Frames: New Challenges to the Rationality Assumption*. New York: Cambridge University Press.

Karpati, A. M., Rubin, C. H., Kieszak, S. M., Marcus, M. & Troiano, R. P. (2002). Stature and pubertal stage assessment in American boys: The 1988–1994 Third National Health and Nutrition Examination Survey. *Journal of Adolescent Health*, 30, 205–212.

Keller, H. & Scholmerich, A. (1987). Infant vocalisations and parental reactions during the first four months of life. *Developmental Psychology*, 23, 62–67.

Kieras, J. E., Tobin, R. M., Graziano, W. G. & Rothbart, M. K. (2005). You can't always get what you want: Effortful control and children's responses to undesirable gifts. *Psychological Science*, 16, 391–396.

Kimble, G. A., Wertheimer, M. White, C. L. (1991). *Portraits of Pioneers in Psychology*. Hillsdale, NJ: Erlbaum.

Kochanska, G. (1993). Towards a synthesis of parental socialization and child temperament in early development of conscience. *Child Development*, 64, 325–347.

254

Kolb, B. & Fantie, B. (1989). Development of the child's brain and behavior. In C. R. Reynolds & E. Fletcher-Janzen (Eds), *Handbook of Clinical Child Neuropsychology*. New York: Plenum Press.

Korner, A. F. (1967). Individual differences at birth: Implications for mother and infant relationships and later development. *Journal of the American Academy of Child Psychiatry*, 6, 676–690.

Kreppner, J. M., Rutter, M., Beckett, C., Castle, J., Colvert, E., . . . Stevens, S. (2007). Normality and impairment following profound early institutional deprivation: A longitudinal follow-up into early adolescence. *Developmental Psychology*, 43(4), 931–946. doi: 10.1037/0012-1649.43.4.931

Lang, P. J. (1988). What are the data of emotion? In V. Hamilton, G. H. Bower & N. Frijda (Eds), *Cognitive Perspectives on Emotion and Motivation*. (NATO ASI, Series D, Vol, 44). Dordrecht: Kluiver, pp. 173–191.

Lange, C. (1885). One leuds beveegelser. In K. Dunlap (Ed.), *The Emotions*. Baltimore, MD. Williams & Wilkins.

Lashley, F. R, (2007). *Essentials of Clinical Genetics in Nursing Practice*. New York: Springer.

Lazarus, R. S. (1991). Cognition and motivation in emotion. *American Psychologist*, 46, 352–367.

Leach, P. (1989). *Baby and Child*. London: Penguin.

LeDoux, J. E. (1993). Emotional memory systems in the brain. *Behavioural Brain Research*, 58(1), 69–79.

LeDoux, J. E. (1996). *The Emotional Brain*. New York: Simon and Schuster.

LeDoux, J. E. & Phelps, E. A. (2008). Emotional networks in the brain. In M. Lewis, J. M. Haviland-Jones & L. Feldman Barrett (Eds), *Handbook of Emotions* (3rd edn). New York: The Guilford Press, pp. 159–179.

Lemerise, E. & Dodge, K. (2008). The development of anger and hostile interactions. In M. Lewis, J. M. Haviland & L. Feldman Barrettt (Eds), *Handbook of Emotion*. New York: The Guilford Press, pp. 730–741.

Lennon, R. & Eisenberg, N. (1987). Emotional displays associated with pre-schooler's prosocial behaviour. *Child Development*, 58, 992–1000.

Lerner, R. M. (2002). *Adolescence: Development, Diversity, Context, and Applications*. Engelwood Cliffs, NJ: Prentice Hall.

Levine, R. & Miller, P. (1990). Commentary. *Human Development*, 33, 73–80.

Levy, A. (1999). Continuities and discontinuities in parent-child relationships across two generations: A prospective longitudinal study. Unpublished doctoral dissertation. University of Minnesota.

Lewis, M. & Michalson, L. (1982). The socialization of emotion. In T. Field & A. Fogel (Eds), *Emotion and Early Interaction*. Hillsdale, NJ: Erlbaum.

Lewis, M. (1990). The development of intentionality and the role of consciousness. *Psychological Inquiry*, 1, 231–248.

Lewis, M. (1992). The self in self-conscious emotions: Commentary on Stipek et al. *Monograph of the Society for Research in Child Development*, 57(226), 85–95.

Lewis, M. (1995). Embarrassment: The emotion of self-exposure and evaluation. In J. P Tangney & K. W. Fischer (Eds), *Self-conscious Emotions; The Psychology of Shame, Guilt, Embarrassment and Pride*. New York: Guilford.

Lewis, M. D. (2005). Bridging emotion theory and neurobiology through dynamic systems modeling. *Behavioral and Brain Sciences*, 28(2), 169–193.

Lewis, M (2008) The emergence of human emotions. In M. Lewis, J. M. Haviland-Jones & L. Feldman Barrett (Eds), *Handbook of Emotions* (3rd edn). New York: The Guilford Press, pp. 304–319.

Lewis, M. & Brooks-Gunn, J. (1979). *Social Cognition and the Aquisition of Self*. New York: Plenum Press.

Linnenbrink, E. A. (2006). Emotion research in education: Theoretical and methodological perspectives on the integration of affect, motivation, and cognition. *Educational Psychology Review*, 18(4), 307–314.

Linton, J. C. & Hirt, H. (1979). A comparison of predictions from peripheral and central theories of emotion. *British Journal of Medical Psychology*, 52, 11–15.

Livson, N. & Peskin, H. (1980). Perspectives on adolescence from longitudinal research. In J. Adelson, (Ed.), *Handbook of Adolescent Psychology*. New York: Wiley.

Lorenz, K. Z. (1966). *On Aggression*. San Diego, CA: Harcourt Brace Jovanovich.

Luvmour, J. (2011) Nurturing children's wellbeing: A developmental response to trends of overdiagnosis and overmedication. *Journal of Humanistic Psychology*, 5(3), 350–368.

Lynne, S., Graber, J., Nichols, T., Brooks-Gunn, J. & Botvin, G. (2007). Links between pubertal timing, peer influences and externalizing behaviors among urban students followed through middle school. *Journal of Adolescent Health*. 40, 35–44.

Maccoby, E. E. (2002). Parenting effects: Issues and controversies. In J. G. Borkowski, S. Landesman-Ramey & M. Bristol-Power (Eds), *Parenting and the Child's World: Influences on Academic, Intellectual and Socioemotional Development*. London: Laurence Erlbaum Associates.

Main M. & George, C. (1985). Responses of abused and disadvantaged toddlers to distress in agemates: A study in the day-care setting. *Developmental Psychology*, 21, 407–412.

Main, M., & Solomon, J. (1990). Procedures for identifying infants as disorganized/disoriented during the Ainsworth Strange Situation. *Attachment in the Preschool Years: Theory, Research, and Intervention*, 1, 121–160.

Malatesta, C. Z., Culver, C., Tesman, J. R. & Shepard, B. (1989). The development of emotional expression during the first two years of life. *Monographs of the Society for Research in Child Development*, 54 (1–2, Serial No. 219).

Mallick, S. K. & McCandless, B. R. (1966). A study of catharsis of aggression. *Journal of Personality and Social Psychology*, 4, 591–596.

Marceau, K., Ram, N., Houts, R. M., Grimm, K. J. & Susman, E. J. (2011). Individual differences in boys' and girls' timing and tempo of puberty: Modeling development with nonlinear growth models. *Developmental Psychology*, 47(5), 1389.

Mascolo, M. F. & Griffin, S. (1998). *What Develops in Emotional Development?* New York: Plenum Press.

Maslow, A. H. (1954). *Motivation and Personality*. New York: Harper and Row.

Matthews, G., Zeidner, M. & Roberts, R. D. (2004). *Emotional Intelligence: Science and Myth*. Cambridge, MA: MIT Press.

Mayer, J. D. & Salovey, P. (1997). What is emotional intelligence? In P. Salovey & D. J. Sluyter (Eds), *Emotional Development and Emotional Intelligence*. New York: Basic Books.

Meyer, D. K. & Turner, J. C. (2006). Re-conceptualizing emotion and motivation to learn in classroom contexts. *Educational Psychology Review*, 18(4), 377–390.

McDowell, M. J. (2002). The image of the mother's eye: autism and early narcissistic injury. *Behavioral and Brain Sciences*, (ted).

McEntire, N. (2009). The importance of play: Why children need to play. *Childhood Education*, 85(3), 208.

McGowan, P. O., Sasaki, A., D'Alessio, A. C., Dymov, S., Labonte, B., Syzf, M., Turecki, G. & Meaney, M. J. (2009). Epigenetic regulation of the glucocorticoid receptor in human brain associates with childhood abuse. *Nature Neuroscience*, 12(3), 342–348.

Moore, C. (2007). Understanding self and others in the second year. In C. A. Brownell & C. B. Kopp (Eds), *Socioemotional Development in the Toddler Years*. New York: Guilford Press.

National Scientific Council on the Developing Child (2004). Children's Emotional Development Is Built into the Architecture of Their Brains: Working Paper No. 2. http://www.developingchild.net

National Scientific Council on the Developing Child (2007) *The Science of Early Childhood Development* http://www.developingchild.net. Available at: http://developingchild.harvard.edu/resources/reports_and_working_papers/science_of_early_childhood _development/

Neher, A. (1991). Maslow's theory of emotion: A critique. *Journal of Humanistic Psychology*, 31, 89–112.

Newton, M. (2002). *Savage Girls and Wild Boys*. London: Faber.

NICHD Early Child Care Research Network (1997). The effects of infant child care on mother-infant attachment security. *Child Development*, 68, 860–879.

Oatley, K. (2000). Social goals and emotion. Talk given to the annual conference of the British Psychological Society as reported by P. Redford. *Psychologist*, 13(6), 290–291.

Oatley, K. & Jenkins, J. M. (1996). *Understanding emotions*. Malden, MA. Blackwell.

Oppenheim, R. W. (1980). Metamorphosis and adaptation in the behavior of developing organisms. *Developmental Psychology*, 13, 353–356.

Panksepp, J. & Smith-Pasqualini, M. (2005). The search for the fundamental brain/mind sources of affective experience. *Emotional Development: Recent Research Advances*, 5–27.

Panksepp, J., Sivly, S. M. & Normansell, L. A. (1985). Brain opioids and social emotions. In M. Reite & T. Field (Eds), *The Psychobiology of Attachment and Separation*. Orlando, FL: Academic Press, pp. 3–49.

Perlman, S. B. & Pelphrey, K. A. (2011). Developing connections for affective regulation: Age-related changes in emotional brain connectivity. *Journal of Experimental Child Psychology*, 108(3), 607–620.

Petersen, A. C. (1987). The nature of biological-psychological interactions: The sample case of early adolescence. In R. M. Lerner & T. T. Foch (Eds), *Biological-psychological Interaction in Early Adolescence*. Hillsdale, NJ: Erlbaum.

Pfeifer, J. H. & Blakemore, S. J. (2012). Adolescent social cognitive and affective neuroscience: Past, present, and future. *Social Cognitive and Affective Neuroscience*, 7(1), 1–10.

Pfeifer, J. H., Masten, C. L., Moore III, W. E., Oswald, T. M., Mazziotta, J. C., Iacoboni, M. & Dapretto, M. (2011). Entering adolescence: Resistance to peer influence, risky behavior, and neural changes in emotion reactivity. *Neuron*, 69(5), 1029–1036.

Plomin, R. (1983). Developmental behavioral genetics. *Child Development*, 54, 252–259.

Plutchik, R. (1980). *Emotion: A Psychoevolutionary Synthesis*. New York: Harper & Row.

Pollak, S. D., Nelson, C. A., Schlaak, M. F., Roeber, B. J., Wewerka, S. S., Wiik, K. L., . . . Gunnar, M. R. (2010). Neurodevelopmental effects of early deprivation in postinstitutionalized children. *Child Development*, 81(1), 224–236.

Posner, M. I., Rothbart, M. K. & Sheese, B. E. (2007). Attention genes. *Developmental Science*, 10, 24–29.

Pringle, M. K. (1958). Learning and Emotion (1). *Educational Review*, 10(2), 146–168.

Radic, P., Bourgeois, J. P., Eckenhoff, M. F., Zecevic, N. & Goldman-Rakic, P. (1986). Concurrent overproduction of synapses in diverse regions of the primate cerebral cortex. *Science*, 232, 232–235.

Rakic, P. (1991). Plasticity of cortical development. In S. E. Brauth, W. S. Hall & R. J. Dooling (Eds), *Plasticity of Development*. Cambridge, MA. Bradford/MIT Press.

Ridley, M. (2003). *Nature via Nurture: Genes, Experience, and What Makes us Human*. New York: HarperCollins.

Rodman, F. R. (2003). *Winnicott his Life and Work*. London: Perseus.

Rolls, E. T. (1999). *The Brain and Emotion*. New York: Oxford University Press.

Roth, T. L. & Sweatt, J. (2011). Annual Research Review: Epigenetic mechanisms and environmental shaping of the brain during sensitive periods of development. *Journal of Child Psychology and Psychiatry*, 52(4), 398–408.

Rowe, D. C. (1994). *The Limits of Family Influence*. New York: Guilford Press.

Rowe, D. C. (2002). What twin and adoption studies reveal about parenting. In J. G. Borkowski, *Academic, Intellectual and Socioemotional Development*. London: Laurence Erlbaum Associates.

Russell, J. A. (1994). Is there universal recognition of emotion from facial expression? A review of methods and studies. *Psychological Bulletin*, 115, 102–141.

Rutter, M., Quinton, D. & Hill, J. (1990). Adult outcomes of institution reared children: Males and females compared. In L. Robins & M. Rutter (Eds), *Straight and Devious Pathways from Childhood to Adulthood*. Cambridge: University of Cambridge Press.

Rutter, M. (1981). *Maternal Deprivation Reassessed*. Melbourne: Penguin.

Rutter, M. (1998). Developmental catch-up and deficit following adoption after severe global early privation. English and Romanian Adoptees (ERA) Study Team. *Journal of Child Psychology and Psychiatry*, 39(4), 465–476.

Rutter, M. (2007). Gene-environment interdependence. *Developmental Science*, 10(1), 12–18.

Saarni, C., Campos, J. J., Camras, L. A. & Witherington, D. (2006). Emotional development: Action, communication and understanding. In N. Eisenberg (Ed.), *Handbook of Child Psychology:*

Vol 3. Social Emotional and Personality Development (6th edn). Hoboken, NJ: Wiley, pp. 226–299.

Sagi, A., IJzendoorn, M. H., Aviezer, O., Donnell, F. & Mayseless, O. (1994). Sleeping out of home in a Kibbutz communal arrangement: It makes a difference for infant-mother attachment. *Child Development*, 65(4), 992–1004.

Schachter, S. & Singer, J. (1962). Cognitive, social and physiological determinants of emotional state. *Psychological Review*, 69, 379–399.

Scherer K. R. (2000). Psychological models of emotion. In J. C. Borod (Ed.), *The Neuropsychology of Emotion* (1st edn). Oxford: Oxford University Press.

Schneiria, T. C. (1959). An evolutionary and developmental theory of biphasic processes underlying approach and avoidance. In M. R. Jones (Ed.), *Nebraska Symposium on Motivation*, 7. Lincoln, NE: University of Nebraska Press, 1–42.

Schore, A. N. (1994). *Affect Regulation and the Origin of the Self: The Neurology of Emotional Development*. Hillsdale, NJ: Erlbaum.

Schore, A. N. (2003). *Affect Regulation and the Repair of the Self*. New York: WW Norton.

Shaffer, D. R. (1999) *Developmental Psychology* (5th edn). Pacific Grove, CA: Brooks/Cole, p. 408.

Sharp, C. & Fonagy, P. (2008). The parent's capacity to treat the child as a psychological agent: Constructs, measures and implications for developmental psychology. *Social Development*, 17(3), 737–754.

Shonkoff, J. P. & Levitt, P. (2010). Neuroscience and the future of early childhood policy: Moving from why to what and how. *Neuron*, 67(5), 689–691.

Shore, R. (1997). *Rethinking the Brain: New Insights into Early Development*. New York: Families and Work Institute.

Shweder, R., Haidt, J., Horton, R. & Joseph, C. (2008). The cultural psychology of the emotions: ancient and renewed. In M. Lewis, J. M. Haviland-Jones & L. Feldman Barrett (Eds), *Handbook of Emotions* (3rd edn). New York: The Guilford Press, pp. 409–427.

Skinner, B. F. (1989). *Recent issues in the Analysis of Behaviour*. Colombia, OH: Merrill.

Spear, L. P. (2000) The adolescent brain and age related behavioral manifestations. *Neuroscience and Behavioral Reviews*, 24, 417–463.

Spielberger, C. (1973). *Manual for the State/trait Inventory for Children*. Palo Alto, CA: Consulting Psychologists Press

Spitz, R. (1965). *The First Year of life*. New York. International Universities Press.

Sroufe, L. A. (1983). Infant-caregiving attachment and patterns of adaptation and competence. In M. Perlmutter (Ed.), *Minnesota Symposia on Child Psychology*, Vol. 16. Hillsdale, NJ: Erlbaum.

Sroufe, L. A. (1985). Attachment classification from the perspective of infant-caregiver relationships and infant temperament. *Child Development*, 56, 1–14.

Sroufe, L. A. (1988). The role of infant-caregiver attachment in development. In J. Belsky & T. Nezworski (Eds), *Clinical Implications of Attachment*. Hillsdale NJ. Erlbaum, pp. 18–38.

Sroufe, L. A. (1995). *Emotional Development*. Cambridge: Cambridge University Press.

Sroufe, L. A. (2002). From infant attachment to promotion of adolescent autonomy: Prospective longitudinal data on the role of parents in development. In J. G. Borkowski, S. Landesman-Ramey & M. Bristol-Power (Eds), *Parenting and the Child's World: Influences on Academic, Intellectual and Socioemotional Development*. London: Laurence Erlbaum Associates, pp. 187–202.

Sroufe, L. A. (2009). The concept of development in developmental psychopathology. *Child Development Perspectives*, 3(3), 178–183.

Sroufe, L. A., Cooper, R. G. & DeHart, G. B. (1996). *Child Development: Its Nature and Course*. New York: McGraw-Hill.

Stattin, H. & Magnusson, D. (1990). *Pubertal Maturation in Female Development*. Hillsdale, NJ: Earlbaum.

Steinberg, L. (1990). Autonomy, conflict and harmony in the family relationship. In S. Feldman and G. Elliot (Eds), *At the Threshold: The Developing Adolescent*. Cambridge, MA: Harvard University Press.

Stern, D. N. (1990). Joy and satisfaction in infancy. In R. A. Glick & S. Bone (Eds), *Pleasure Beyond the Pleasure Principle*. New Haven, CN: Yale University Press.

Stocker, M. (1996). *Valuing Emotions*. Cambridge: Cambridge University Press.

Strongman, K. T. (1987). *The Psychology of Emotion*. New York: Wiley.

Tangney, J. F. (2002). Self-conscious emotions: The self as a moral guide. In A. Tesser & D. A. Stapel (Eds), *Self and Motivation: Emerging Psychological Perspectives*. Washington, DC: American Psychological Association

Tennes, K., Emde, R., Kisley, A. & Metcalf, D. (1972). The stimulus barrier in early infancy: An exploration of some of the formulations of John Benjamin. In R. Holt & E. Peterfreund (Eds), *Psychoanalysis and Contemporary Science*. New York: Macmillan.

Thelen, E. & Smith, L. B. (1998). Dynamic systems theory. In R. M. Lerner (Ed.), *Handbook of Child Psychology: Vol. 1. Theoretical Models of Human Development* (5th Edn). New York: Wiley.

Thomas, A. & Chess, S. (1977). *Temperament and Development*. New York. Brunner/Mazel.

Thomas, A. & Chess, S. (1984). Genesis and evolution of behavior disorders: From infancy to early adult life. *American Journal of Psychiatry*, 141, 1–9.

Thompson, R. A. (1990). Emotion and self-regulation. *Nebraska Symposium on Motivation*, 367–467. Lincoln, NE: University of Nebraska Press.

Thompson, R. A. (2011). Emotion and emotion regulation: Two sides of the developing coin. *Emotion Review*, 3(1), 53–61.

Tomkins, S. S. (1981). The quest for primary motives: Biography and autobiography of an idea. *Journal of Personality and Social Psychology*, 41, 306–329.

Tomkins, S. S. (1982). *Affect Imagery, Consciousness*. New York: Springer.

Tronick, E. Z. (2005), Why is connection with others so critical? The formation of dyadic states of consciousness and the expansion of individual states of consciousness: Coherence-governed selection and the co-creation of meaning out of messy meaning making. In J. Nadel & D. Muir (Eds), *Emotional Development*. New York: Oxford University Press, pp. 293–315.

Troy, M. & Sroufe, L. A. (1987). Victimization among pre-schoolers: Role of attachment relationship history. *Journal of the American Academy of Child and Adolescent Psychiatry*, 26, 166–172.

Tucker, D. M. (1992). Developing emotions and cortical networks. In M. R. Gunnar & C. A. Nelson (Eds), *Minnesota Symposium on Child Psychology, Vol 24, Developmental Behavioral Neuroscience*. Hillsdale, NJ. Erlbaum, 75–128.

Turner, P. J. (1991). Relations between attachment, gender, and behavior with peers in preschool. *Child Development*, 62(6), 1475–1488. doi:10.2307/1130820

Vaillant-Molina, M. & Bahrick, L. E. (2012). The role of intersensory redundancy in the emergence of social referencing in 5½-month-old infants. *Developmental Psychology*, 48(1), 1–9.

von Salisch, M. (2001). Children's emotional development: Challenges in their relationships to parents, peers and friends. *International Journal of Behavioural Development*, 25(4), 310–319.

Walker-Andrews, A. (2008). Intermodal Emotional Processes in Infancy. In M. Lewis, J. M. Haviland-Jones & L. Feldman Barrett (Eds), *Handbook of Emotions* (3rd edn). New York: The Guilford Press, pp. 364–375.

Waters, E. & Sroufe, L. A. (1983). A developmental perspective on competence. *Developmental Review*, 3, 79–97.

Weiner, B. (1986). *An Attributional Theory of Motivation and Emotion*. New York. Springer-Verlag.

Wilson, A., Passik, S. D. & Faude, J. P. (1990). Self-regulation and its failures. In J. Masling (Ed.), *Empirical Studies of Psychoanalytic Theory*, Vol. 3. Hillsdale, NJ: The Analytic Press.

Wilson, R. L. (1969) Chronological age, intellectual ability and sex as factors in the moral judgements of children. *Papers in Psychology*, 3(1), 98–127

Worobey, J. & Blajda, V. (1989). Temperament ratings at 2 weeks, 2 months, and 1 year: Differential stability of activity and emotionality. *Developmental Psychology*, 25, 663–667.

Zahn-Waxler, C., Radke-Yarrow, M., Wagner, E. & Chapman, M. (1992). Development of concern for others. *Developmental Psychology*, 28, 126–136.

Zajonc, R. B. (1984). On the primacy of affect. *American Psychologist*, 39, 117–123.

Zeman, J. & Garber, J. (1996). Display rules for anger, sadness, and pain: It depends on who is watching. *Child Development*, 67(3), 957–973.

Index

abused children *see also* adverse
    circumstances
  and anxiety 186
  in case studies 224–6
  disorganised-disoriented attachment
    119–20, 165, 212, 214
  intergenerational transmission of abuse
    140, 178, 179, 196
  physical restraint to prevent walking/
    crawling 138
  physiological effects of warm care vs
    abuse 134
  removal to new environment 167
  still seek attachment 115, 117
  in typology 214–15
acting (pretending emotions) 19, 20, 161, 213
active nature of children 50–1, 67, 126–7
adaptability
  of children in adverse circumstances 106
  and the neonatal period 60
  and temperament 125
addiction 202
adolescence
  emotional development (whole chapter)
    193–207
  brain development 49
  oppositional behaviour 173–4

adverse circumstances *see also* abused
    children; inconsistently cared-for
    children; neglected children
  and adolescence 205–7
  and children's inability to deceive with
    emotions 20
  classification of children with social/
    emotional difficulty 211–14
  and the development of morality 164
  and the development of secondary
    emotions 38–9, 148–9, 165, 214
  and egocentrism 201
  and evolutionary variation 44
  importance of understanding
    developmental variation 25
  institutional care 121
  and lack of attachment figures 121
  in middle childhood 164–8
  and play 102
  poor parenting 135–8
  reworking of emotional development
    167, 206
  and 'strange' attachments 121
  tends to start at birth 82–3
  and toddler development 105–6
  variation within adverse circumstances
    164–5

affect 3, 12–13
'ages and stages' 53
aggression
    aggressive behaviour 174–83
    and anxiety 187
    in case studies 218–22
    dealing with 182–3
    displacement of 175, 176, 177
    and frustration 174–5, 177–8
    hostile aggression 176–7
    instrumental aggression 157, 176–7
    in preschool years 157, 180
    theories of aggression 177–9
    in toddlerhood 175
Ainsworth, M. 118
alcohol 202
ambivalent attachment 119 see also
        insecure-resistant attachment
Amsel, A. 74
amygdala 16, 28, 33
anger
    and aggressive behaviour 174–5
    as basic emotion 23, 33, 38
    in case studies 228
    in early infancy 36, 66, 76, 78
    in middle childhood 166
    as negative emotion 21–2
    neglected children develop 135, 148, 214,
        215
    physiology of 24
    in preschool years 157
    and shame 99
    survival function of 23
    in toddlerhood 84, 94–6
antecedents of emotions 36
anxiety/ anxious fear
    main section 183–91
    in case studies 215, 217, 222
    desensitisation of anxiety 190
    and inconsistent care 213
    in infancy 72, 75, 78
    interference with normal development
        190–1
    in preschool years 156–8
    in toddlerhood 96–7
appraisal 35, 37
approach vs avoidance reactions 67
Arnold, M.B. 14
Aronfreed, J. 14
arousal

    in early infancy 64–5
    physiological arousal as first factor in
        emotion 16–17, 19, 32
'as if' perceptions 17, 20, 21
attachment see also disorganised-disoriented
        attachment; insecure-avoidant
        attachment; insecure-resistant
        attachment
    main section 115–21
    and anxiety 184
    attachment as the key to development
        120–1
    attachment disorders 165
    as basis for typology of children with
        emotional difficulties 211
    definitions 116–17
    and dependency/ independency 113, 115
    importance of love 104
    and infant's perception of change 72
    instinctive for child but not parent 116
    and the reciprocal relationship 84, 91–3
    secure attachment 76, 115, 118–19
    and shame/ pride 98–9
    and temperament 127–9
attention seeking 136–7, 148, 165, 206,
        213–14
attraction, of caregivers to infants 63
Augustine, Saint 2
authoritarian parenting 141–2
authoritative parenting 141–2, 173
autism
    as deficit 'theory of mind' 101
    genetic vs environmental impacts 144
autonomic arousal 17
autonomy, developing sense of 156, 200
        see also self, developing a sense of
avoidance behaviours 185, 188
avoidant attachment 165 see also
        insecure-avoidant attachment
axons and dendrites 45, 46

Bandura, A. 178–9
Bard, P. 32
Baron-Cohen, S. 91, 101
Barrett, L.F. 3
basic emotions
    basic and secondary emotions compared
        37–9
    and cognition 15
    Darwin on 31

and the Discrete Emotions Theory 33
in early infancy 66, 75
'hard-wiring' of 25, 27
and human relationships 6
and neglected children 215
in preschool years 156–7
in toddlerhood 82
Bates, J. 124, 126–7, 128, 140
Baumrind, D. 140
behaviour
    behavioural genetics 143, 146
    behaviourism 3
    challenging behaviours 8–9
    emotion related to 12, 23
    focus of psychology on 2–3
    and localisation of (brain) function 52
belonging, infants' need for 61–2
bitterness
    neglected children develop 148
    in preschool years 157
    as secondary emotion 38
    in toddlerhood 96
bodily effects of emotions 15–17
body posture, as indicators of emotion 94
bonding 116–17
boredom 51
Bowlby, J. 72, 84, 116
brain development *see also* neuroscience
    brain cell death 47–8
    brain damage and transfer of function 45
    brain structure 15, 27–9
    brain tumours 45
    early neurological development 44–50
    and emotions (overview) 6–7
    implications for child development 50–6
    moulded by early social experience 7
Bridges, K. 36, 68
'bring themselves up,' children forced to 121,
    197, 205, 214, 225–6
Bronowski, J. 42
Brown, T. 18
Brownell, C.A. 104
bullying 164
Buss, A.H. 126

Cannon-Bard theory 32
cared-for children (children in 'care') 77,
    179, 219–20, 223–7, 229
Case, R. 36
case studies

Eve 226–9
Jake Smith 215–17
Jo Lee 217–22
Michael 222–4
Nik 224–6
catharsis 177
challenging behaviours 8–9
change, perception of
    and anxiety 183–4
    and attachment 115
    infants' 70–2, 76–7
    toddlers' 97
Chess, S. 124–6, 127
childcare 120, 121
Chisholm, J. 87
Coady, T. 7
coding of mental events 67
cognition
    anxiety and intellectual performance 187
    and brain structure 15, 29
    cognitive deprivation 77–8
    cognitive growth in middle childhood
        160–1
    cognitive growth in preschoolers 154–5
    cognitive growth in toddlerhood 83
    cognitive growth rests on secure
        emotional development 84
    Cognitive Perspectives Theory 26
    'cognitive revolution' 3, 32
    'cognitive-affective structures' 33, 34, 35
    damaged development in adverse
        circumstances 39
    emotion related to 4–5, 12, 14, 19, 164
    focus of psychology on 2–3
    and grief 103
    positive thinking 160
    and the reciprocal relationship 92
    social learning/ social cognitive theory
        178–9, 182
    Structural Development Theory 36
    using cognitive approaches to help
        children with poor emotional
        development 167–8
Cole, P. 94
'collapsed' body posture 94
Colonnesi, C. 185
comparisons, dangers of 55–6
compassion, as a moral emotion 7
competitiveness, and aggression 176
confidence tricksters 20

consciousness
    in early infancy 65
    evolutionary development of 28
    and mood 12
    and the neocortex 15
    self-conscious emotions 38, 104, 156,
        174
context *see also* cultural context;
        environmental impact
    in adolescence 204–5
    and aggressive behaviour 180
    as key element in emotion 35–6, 37, 54–6
    in middle childhood 161–3
control (or lack of) of emotions
    and aggressive behaviour 181
    in preschool years 158
    in toddlerhood 89–91
    unstoppability of emotions 17–19, 25,
        29, 96, 103, 158
control, toddlers' battle for 92
control over expression of emotion
    by caregiver 89–91
    children in adverse circumstances 106
    different mechanisms for control of
        positive vs negative 106
    possibility of learning to control expression
        22
cosseting children 137–8, 147
cultural context *see also* display rules
    adolescence as a social construct 194–5
    and aggressive behaviour 180, 181
    cultural differences in attachment 117,
        120
    cultural differences in mothering 111
    culturally specific vs universal emotions 27
    emotional development has cultural
        context 54–5
    and pride 103
    and shame 99
    youth culture context 205

Damasio, A.R. 5, 17, 20
Darwin, C. 21, 31, 33
Davidson, G.W. 175
day care 120, 121
deception 23, 159
decision-making
    and anxiety 187–8
    and emotions 5
    in toddlerhood 172–3

definitions, of emotion 11–39
delayed gratification 70, 158
delinquency 196, 204, 207
dendrites and axons 45, 46
Denham, S. 100
dependency
    in adolescence 203
    and attachment 117–18
    emotional dependency 111–12
    extended adolescence 194
    financial dependency 203
    as hallmark of childhood 60, 110–15
    handling tantrums 173
    increasing independence 112–14, 137–8,
        171–2, 196–7
    instrumental dependence 111–12, 114
    meeting dependency needs 134, 137, 144,
        165. *see also* inconsistently cared-for
        children; neglected children
    over-dependency 187
depression
    and aggression 176
    in preschool years 157
deprivation *see* adverse circumstances
dermal concomitants of an emotion 15–17,
    24
Descartes, R. 19
desensitisation of anxiety 190
despair 77, 102
detachment phases 77
Diamond, J. 43
dictionary definitions of 'emotion' 12
'difficult' children (in temperament) 125
disabilities
    children with 117, 217
    parents with 217–22
Discrete Emotions Theory 26, 31, 32–5,
    37–9, 78
disdain, as secondary emotion 38
disgust
    as basic emotion 33, 38
    in early infancy 64, 66
disorganised-disoriented attachment 119–20,
    165, 212, 214
displacement, of aggression 175, 176, 177
display rules
    in adolescence 204
    and aggressive behaviour 181
    children from adverse backgrounds may
        not learn 166

cultural context 22, 161
  and peer group influence 162
  preschoolers learning 153, 159
divorce 186
Dodge, K.A. 140
Dollard, J. 178
Dozier, M. 229
drugs 202
DSM-V (Diagnostic and Statistical Manual
    of Mental Disorders, 5th edition) 13
dual coding of mental events 67, 68–9, 71, 84
Dunn, J. 94, 101, 155
duration of emotions 22

'easy' children (in temperament) 125
economics, and the assumption of
    rationality 5
Edelman, G. 14
Egeland, B. 140
egocentrism, adolescent 200–1 see also
    self-centredness
Eisenberg, N. 7
Ekman, P. 32
elements of emotions 14–20
Eliot, L. 6, 65, 66
Elster, Jon 2
embarrassment
    in preschool years 156
    in toddlerhood 103–4
emergency response function of emotions 23
emotional intelligence 6
empathy see also theory of mind
    neglected children fail to develop 148,
      167
    in preschool years 157
    as secondary emotion 38
    vs sympathy 100
    in toddlerhood 100–2, 182
environmental impact
    active nature of children 50–1
    on brain throughout life 50
    on child development 43–4, 51
    environmental differences between
      siblings 122–3
    environmental stimulus 37
    on evolution 42–3
    hard to separate from genetic 123, 143–6
    and infant brain development 48–9
    infant learns they can affect their
      environment 86

'nature vs nurture' debate 25, 43, 50, 56,
    122, 142–6
non-shared environmental impacts 123
    in preschool years 152–4
    and the role of parenting 142–6
    social learning/ social cognitive theory
      178–9
envy
    and jealousy 97–8
    as secondary emotion 38
    strong in inconsistently cared-for children
      136–7, 148
epigenetics 50, 134, 144
essential nature of children 50–1, 67
etymology of 'emotion' 12
Eve (case study) 226–9
evolution
    and dictated chance 43
    evolutionary function of emotions 22–3
    of human brain 27–9
    myth of 'simple to complex' 42, 48
exploratory function of emotions 23
expression of emotion
    in adolescence 204–5
    children from adverse backgrounds
      166–7
    control over expression of emotion 22,
      89–91, 106
    in early infancy 30
    expression of basic emotions generally
      remains for lifespan 38
    inter-family variation 155
    modified as individual matures 35
    neglected children learn to manipulate
      136
    non-verbal expressions of emotion
      19–20
    not to be confused with the emotion itself
      19–20, 204–5
    and peer group influence 162
    in preschool years 152–60
    relationship with subjective feeling/
      physiology 19–20
    and temperament 124
    theories of emotion 31
extended family, support from 128
eye contact
    blind children seek alternative 134
    importance of 134
    and the reciprocal relationship 85

Facey, A.B. 121
facial expressions
    facial feedback as causative in emotions 31
    importance of eye contact 85, 134
    as indicators of emotion 31, 33
    infant facial expressions as reflexes 34
    infant's facial expressions and existence
        of basic emotions 31, 33
    in toddlerhood 94
families *see also* environmental impact;
        parenting
    as arena for modelling 180, 181
    family (not peer) context predominant in
        middle childhood 163
    family breakdown 186
    social policies concerning 43
fathers 111, 112, 139 *see also* parenting;
        primary caregiver
fear *see also* anxiety/ anxious fear
    as basic emotion 33, 38
    in early infancy 36, 64, 66, 72, 75, 78
    Joseph LeDoux's work on 29
    neurology of 24
    phobias 188–90
    in preschool years 156–7
    in toddlerhood 94–5, 96–7
feelings *see also* subjectivity
    feeling vs emotion 18
    non-emotional (e.g cold, pain) 13, 18
fight or flight responses 16, 23, 180–1
financial dependency 203
flexibility
    and the adolescent period 202
    and the neonatal period 61
foetal development 44
Fogel, A. 86, 105
Fonagy, P. 133–4, 142, 146
foster care 219–20, 223–7, 229
'free floating' anxiety 184
Freudian psychology 3, 87, 99, 160, 176,
        177, 184
Frijda, N.H. 18
frontal neocortex 16, 24, 28
frustration
    and aggressive behaviour 174–5, 177–8
    in case studies 225
    frustration-aggression hypothesis 178
    human need for 74–5
    and inconsistent care 213
    in infancy 69–70, 74–5, 76–8

in middle childhood 166
in preschool years 157, 158–60
as secondary emotion 38
and tantrums 171
in toddlerhood 94–6, 171
fun, importance of 86–7, 90
function of emotions 22–3
Functionalist approaches to theory of
    emotions 26, 37

Galton, F. 56
gang cultures 215
Garbarino, J. 196, 204
Gardner, Howard 6
gender
    and aggressive behaviour 180, 181
    and anxiety 187
    and display rules of emotions 22
    in peer groups 162
    preschoolers learning gender roles 154
    and puberty 198–9
    and school phobia 188–9
Gendron, M. 3
generalisation of anxiety 188
genetics
    and basic emotions 25
    and brain development 50
    epigenetics 50, 134, 144
    genetic determinism 143
    'nature vs nurture' debate 25, 43, 50, 56,
        122, 142–6
    and parenting 134–5, 142–6
    polygenetic inheritance 143–4
    and temperament 122–3, 124
give and take 86, 92
Goldilocks and the Three Bears 92
Goleman, D. 6, 18, 70, 93
'good-enough' parenting 134–5, 141–2,
    144–5
'goodness of fit' model 128
Gottman, J.M. 133
Gould, Stephen J. 42–3
Greenspan, S.L. 67, 84, 86, 92
grief 103
Griffin, S. 26
guilt
    in adolescence 197
    children acquiring 43
    develops weakly in inconsistently-
        parented children 166

in middle childhood 163–4
neglected children fail to develop 148, 165, 215
and oppositional behaviour 174
over-parented children do not develop 148
in preschool years 156, 157
as secondary emotion 38
in toddlerhood 93–4, 99
guinea pigs, newborn 60

'hard-wiring' of emotions 34
Harlow's monkeys 62, 85, 120, 139
Harris, J. 142, 144–5, 146
Harris, P. 101–2, 167
hatred, in toddlerhood 96
Hebb, D. 56
Herrera, C. 155
hippocampus 134
Hoffman, M.L. 99
hormones
    and aggressive behaviour 180–1
    as mediators of response to events 16
hospital admissions, and the need for
        caregiver's presence 77
hostility vs aggression 176, 180
human genome project 143
humanity, emotions as essence of 4, 6
Hume, David 2
Hyman, S.E. 134
hyperactivity 136, 214, 215, 225, 226

identical twins
    and brain variation 52
    and the genetics/ environment debate 123
    and intelligence 145
identity see self, developing a sense of
imaginary audience 200
imaginary situations, physiological effects of
        17, 20
imaginative play 88, 102, 155, 213, 214, 215
imitation see also modelling behaviour
    in infancy 88
    in preschool years 155, 159
    in toddlerhood 87–8
impulsive action 18, 202
inconsistently cared-for children
    in adolescence 206
    and anxiety 186, 187
    and attachment 115, 119–20, 181,
        184–5, 212, 214, 228

in case studies 221
'inconsistent care group' in typology 212,
        213–14
in infancy 77
in middle childhood 165, 166
and 'not good enough' parenting 136,
        147, 148
in toddlerhood 98–9, 105–6
independence, increasing 112–14, 137–8,
        171–2, 196–7
indignation
    as a moral emotion 7
    speed of 93
    in toddlerhood 96, 103
individual development perspective 54, 55
infancy
    emotional development in infancy (whole
        chapter) 59–79
    communication of needs in infancy 63–4,
        134
    early infancy and lack of subjectivity 30
    early neurological development 44–50
    importance of warm parental care 134
    infant's facial expressions and existence
        of basic emotions 31, 33
    and the reciprocal relationship 85
inhibitions
    anxiety leads to over-development of
        inhibitions 187–8
    neglected children may fail to have
        135–6, 148, 166, 215
innateness
    of aggression 177
    of emotions 25, 34, 35–6, 37. see also
        basic emotions; genetics
    nature vs nurture debate 25, 43, 50, 56,
        122, 142–6
insecure-avoidant attachment 115, 119–20,
        181, 184–5, 212, 214, 228
insecure-resistant attachment 119–20, 165,
        184–5, 212–13, 217, 221–2
instinct
    attachment instinctive for child (but not
        parent) 116–17
    early infants' emotional expressions as 64
    instinct theory of aggression 177
instrumental competence 161
instrumental dependence 111–12, 114
intellectual disability, children with 54
intensity of emotions 22, 24

intentionality
   and aggressive behaviour 176, 179
   in infancy 7
interest
   as basic emotion 33, 38
   in early infancy 66
intergenerational influences on parenting
      138–40
intergenerational transmission of abuse 140,
      178, 179, 196
interlinked system, human as 13–14
interpersonal relationships 6–7
interpretation of emotion 21–2
introspection, and research methods 3
invulnerability, feelings of 201
Izard, C.E. 12, 17, 31, 32

Jake Smith (case study) 215–17
James, William 2
James-Lange theory 32
Janet, P. 18
jealousy
   and anxiety 222
   in preschool years 157
   as secondary emotion 38
   speed of 93
   strong in inconsistently cared-for children
      136–7, 148
   in toddlerhood 97–8
Jo Lee (case study) 217–22
joint attention 76, 83
joy
   as basic emotion 33, 38
   in early infancy 36, 64, 66, 69
   easier to control expression of 158–9
   and the reciprocal relationship 86–7
justice 7, 43, 92

Kagan, J. 12, 14
Kahneman, Daniel 5
Kochanska, G. 94
Kopp, C.B. 104
Korner, A.F. 125–6
Kozak, A. 18

Lang, P.J. 20
Lange, C. 32
language
   language context effect on development
      54–5
   in preschool years 154–5

latency period 160
Latin root of 'emotion' 12
learning see cognition
LeDoux, J. 29, 32, 33
Lee, Jo (case study) 217–22
'let's pretend'/ imaginative play 88, 102, 155,
      213, 214, 215
Levy, A. 139
Lewis, M. 36, 93, 94, 104
lies (untruths) 213, 226
limbic system 15, 16, 28–9, 33, 66, 75, 202
Livson, N. 198
localisation of function 52
Lorenz, K.Z. 177
love
   and grief 103
   importance of 104
   in infancy 74, 76
   and jealousy 97–8
   neglected children fail to develop 135,
      214, 215, 228
   and parenting styles 141–2
   and pity 100
   in preschool years 156–7
   and pride 103
   and the reciprocal relationship 85
   as secondary emotion 38
   and shame/ guilt 98, 99
   and sympathy/ empathy 100–1
   in toddlerhood 94–5

Maccoby, E. 145, 146
Magnusson, D. 199
Main, M. 119
Malatesta, C.Z. 98–9
Mascolo, M.F. 26
Maslow's hierarchy of human needs 61–2
maturation, early vs late 198
McGowan, P.O. 134
mechanistic vs organismic views of
      childhood 51
memory
   development of memory in infants 70–1
   increasing memory of preschoolers
      154–5
   involved in emotion 13
   physiological effects of emotions 'from
      memory' 17, 20, 24
mental illness, poorly developed emotional
      capabilities mistaken for 9
mentoring 207, 220, 226

mercy, rooted in childhood emotional
    experiences 7
Mesquita, B. 18
Michael (case study) 222–4
middle childhood 160–4, 173–4, 180
modelling behaviour 178–9, 180, 186
monkeys, Harlow's 62, 85, 120, 139
mood
    contrasted to 'emotion' 12
    longer duration than emotions 22
morality
    children learning through reciprocal
        relationship 92
    in middle childhood 164
    moral behaviour 7
mother as the usual primary caregiver 54,
    60–1, 118, 121 see also primary
    caregiver
motivation
    in adolescence 205
    secondary emotions have little
        motivational power in some children
        136, 166, 174
    studies of motivation and emotion 5
multiple caregivers 111, 118, 121
Munn, P. 94
'mutual hilarity' 87
myelination 30–1, 33, 49, 66, 202

nature via nurture 144
nature vs nurture debate 25, 43, 50, 56, 122,
    142–6
needs theories of childhood 51
neglected children
    and attachment 119–20, 165, 184–5,
        212–13, 217, 221–2
    case studies 228
    in infancy 63
    and (lack of) inhibitions 135–6, 148, 166,
        215
    in middle childhood 165–7
    'neglected children group' in typology
        212, 214–15
    and 'not good enough' parenting 135,
        142, 147
    surviving but not thriving 44
    in toddlerhood 84
neocortex
    in adolescence 202
    development of 15, 27–8, 33
    and self-regulation 91

and the sense of self 84
neonatal period
    early dependency 60–1
    emotional expression in 63–4
nervous system 16
neuronal level
    cognitive, emotional and social
        development interactive at 14
    growth and change in preschool years
        152–3
    left vs right brain processing of emotion 24
    neuron development in the womb 45
    neuronal growth 45–7
neuroscience
    brain changes in adolescence 201–2
    as driver for increased interest in
        emotions as topic of scientific study 4
    early neurological development 44–50
    epigenetics 50, 134, 144
    neurological concomitants of an emotion
        15
    neurological evidence for developmental
        approach 35
    neurology of emotion 27–31
    neuropsychological support for theory
        that emotional security leads to
        healthy cognitive growth 84
    role of emotions in child development
        6–7
neurotransmitters (chemical) 24, 45
NICHD Study 146
Nik (case study) 224–6
non-verbal expressions of emotion 19–20
'normal' development of an infant 72–5
normative approaches to child development
    53–4, 55
nursery care 120, 121

Oatley, K. 6
objective reality, introducing child to 135,
    137, 144, 172
ontological vs phylogenic child development
    perspectives 42–3
oppositional behaviour 170–4, 221, 222
organismic vs mechanistic views of
    childhood 51
others, awareness of see theory of mind
over-dependency 187
over-parenting 137–8, 147, 148–9
over-stimulation of children 138
over-thinking 184

'parcellation' 49
parent-child boundary 139
parenting *see also* attachment; primary
    caregiver
  authoritarian parenting 141–2
  authoritative parenting 141–2, 173
  dealing with aggressive behaviour 182–3
  demanding parents causing anxiety 185
  'good-enough' parenting 134–5, 141–2,
    144–5
  importance for child development
    (vs genetics) 142–6
  intergenerational influences on parenting
    138–40
  multiple caregivers 111, 118, 121
  nature of parenting 133–5
  'not good enough' parenting 135–8, 139,
    147–9, 181, 214
  over-parenting 137–8, 147, 148–9
  parenting situations leading to lack of
    warmth 87
  parenting styles 140–2
  permissive parenting 141–2, 186
  tantrums 172
  uninvolved parenting 142
passive reactions (of parents) to tantrums
    172–3, 182
passivity, in children 50–1
pathologisation of children 9
peer groups
  in adolescence 173, 196, 203, 204
  in middle childhood 162
  vs parenting influence 143, 148
  popularity reduced by anxiety 187, 191
  popularity reduced by oppositional
    behaviour 174
  in preschool years 153
permissive parenting 141–2, 186
personal success 6
Peskin, H. 198
phobias 188–90
physiology
  physical effects of emotions 15–17
  physical expressions of emotion 19
  physiological concomitants (elements of
    emotions) 15–17, 24, 32, 180–1
  physiological effects of warm care vs
    abuse 134
  physiological response to stimulus in
    newborns 65

puberty 194, 195
Piaget, J. 101
pituitary gland 44
pity 99–100
play
  developmental function of interactive
    play 87
  imaginative play 88, 102, 155, 213, 214,
    215
  playful interaction important in reciprocal
    relationship 86–7
pleasant-unpleasant distinction 67 *see also*
    positive vs negative emotions
pleasure principle, Freudian 87
Plomin, R. 43, 126
positive vs negative emotions
  children from adverse backgrounds tend
    to live in negative sphere 166–7
  dual coding of mental events 67
  easier to control expression of positive
    158–9
  importance of positive shared emotion
    86–7, 90
  interpretations of emotions 21–2
  neurological concomitants of an emotion
    24
  positive emotions and cognitive growth
    84
  positive secondary emotions, neglected in
    research 107
  and secondary emotional development
    68–70, 71
Posner, M.L. 123
posture, bodily, as indicators of emotion 94
poverty 87
pre-conscious emotion 19
predictability, need for 76–7, 96, 116 *see
    also* change, perception of
pre-schoolers 142–60, 180, 181
pretend play 88, 102, 155, 213, 214, 215
pretending emotions 161
pride
  and body posture 94
  develops weakly in inconsistently-
    parented children 166
  in middle childhood 164
  neglected children fail to develop 148, 165
  and oppositional behaviour 174
  over-parented children do not develop 148
  in preschool years 156, 157

as secondary emotion 38
and shame 98
in toddlerhood 93–4, 96, 103
primary caregiver
ability to put child's needs above own
135, 139, 141, 144
and attachment 76
attraction of caregivers to infants 63
child's emotional dependency on 112
conflict with parents in adolescence
197–8
dealing with oppositional behaviour 172
and development of child's sense of self
84
in early infancy 61, 63
and infant association with satisfaction
74
infants responding to change of caregiver
71
as key to advanced self-conscious
emotions 104
and mediation of child's emotional
expression 89–91
mother as the usual primary caregiver 54,
60–1, 118, 121
multiple caregivers 111, 118, 121
need not be the mother 111, 118, 121
as primary way to meet dependency needs
111
psychological unavailability 135, 147, 148
and the reciprocal relationship 84–93
and secondary emotional development
68, 69, 70
and separation anxiety (child's) 77
primary emotions *see* basic emotions
primary-school children 160–4
proactive vs reactive aggression 177
protest-despair-detachment cycle 102, 212,
223
proto-emotions 68, 75, 93, 152, 156, 158
pseudo-emotions 136, 215
psychiatry
definitions of 'affect' 13
precursor of psychology 3
and the use of 'affect' for 'emotion' 13
psychological unavailability (of parents) 135,
147, 148
psychology
dominance of physiological theories of
emotion 32, 34

and emotions (overview) 2–4
importance of recognising brain variation
52–3
and parenting 133–4, 142
psychological disorder and definitions of
'emotion' 13
reluctance to mention 'love' 104
psychopathology, and total emotional
control 19
psychopathy, and jealousy 98
puberty 194, 195
punishment
need for moderate and non-aggressive
punishments 183
severe punishment and aggressive
behaviour 178
severe punishment and anxiety 187

'quick' emotions 29, 33, 35, 37–8, 75, 82
see also basic emotions

rage 94, 174
rationalisation 19
rationality, pure rationality assumption 5
rats, newborn 60
reciprocal relationship, the 84–93
redevelopment, emotional, of children from
adverse backgrounds 167, 206
reflex actions 64
resentment
as a moral emotion 7
in toddlerhood 96
resistant attachment *see* insecure-resistant
attachment
respect 91
retaliation vs aggression 175–6
rewards and praise 5
reworking of emotional development 167,
206
right and wrong, children learning 92
risk-taking 201
Roth, T.L. 134
Rowe, D.C. 142–4, 145
'royal road' ideas 43–4, 114
Russell, J.A. 34
Rutter, M. 117, 121, 167

sadness
as basic emotion 33, 38
in early infancy 66

as a secondary emotion 102
in toddlerhood 102–3
satisfaction
in infancy 68–9, 74, 76
postponement of 70, 158
in preschool years 158
in toddlerhood 86–7, 107
Schachter-Singer two factor theory 32, 37
Scherer, K.R. 67
school context, in middle childhood 163
school phobia 188–90
Schore, A.N. 84, 91
'sculpting' (brain development) 47
secondary emotions
in adverse circumstances 38–9, 148–9,
165, 214
and aggressive behaviour 182
basic and secondary emotions compared
37–9
and cognition 17
development of 14, 24–5
and early infancy 66
effects of 'not good enough' parenting
148–9, 214
in middle childhood 164
neglected children fail to develop 135
positive secondary emotions, neglected in
research 107
in preschool years 154, 156
and social relationships 6
Structural Development Theory 36
in toddlerhood 83–107
secure attachment 76, 115, 118–19
security see also insecure-avoidant
attachment; insecure-resistant
attachment
and attachment 116
and 'bonding' 117
infants' need for 61–2, 72, 115
related to anxious fear 96–7
selection, in brain development 48
self, developing a sense of
in adolescence 196, 197, 200, 205
dislike of self 96
emotion plays integral part 7
in middle childhood 161
and peer groups 162
in preschool years 155–6
and the reciprocal relationship 84–93
in toddlerhood 83–4, 93–4, 98, 103

self-centredness 148, 197, 200–1, 228
self-confidence 106, 137, 187
self-conscious emotions 38, 104, 156,
174
self-consciousness, in adolescence 199
self-rearing children 121, 197, 205, 214,
225–6
self-regulation, development of 90–1, 159
sensations, dual coding of 67
separation anxiety 71–2, 75, 77
sexual relationships
in adolescence 195, 199, 203, 206
in case studies 223, 224
sexual impulses 13
shame
in adolescence 197
and the 'collapsed' body posture 94
develops weakly in inconsistently-
parented children 166
in middle childhood 164
neglected children fail to develop 148,
165, 215
and oppositional behaviour 174
over-parented children do not develop
148
in preschool years 156, 157
as secondary emotion 38
in toddlerhood 93–4, 98–9
Sharp, C. 133–4, 142, 146
shyness 164, 177
siblings
in case studies 217–22, 222–4
differences in emotional development
121–2
environmental differences between
siblings 122–3
sibling rivalry 98
Singer, J. 32
Skinner, B.F. 3
'slow' emotions 93 see also secondary
emotions
'slow to warm' children (in temperament) 125
smiling
development of a social smile 85
in early infancy 64
Smith, Jake (case study) 215–17
sociability 126, 127
social construct, adolescence as 194
social context for emotional development
35–6

social development, intertwined with
     cognition and emotion 14
social learning/ social cognitive theory
     178–9, 182, 186
social referencing 88, 159
social 'rules' for expression of emotion *see*
     display rules
social withdrawal 97
social/communicative function of emotions 23
society's expectations of children 8–9, 44
Sociocultural perspectives on theory of
     emotions 26, 37
socioemotional development 83, 104
sociomoral emotions 104
sociopathy, and jealousy 98
sorrow
     neglected children fail to develop 215
     as secondary emotion 38
specific state vs trait anxiety 184–5
Speilberger, C. 184–5
spinal injury 17
Spitz, R. 74
'spoilt' children *see* over-parenting
Sroufe, L.A. 23, 34, 36, 37, 39, 53, 64, 78,
     94, 135, 138, 139, 146
startle reflex 64
Stattin, H. 199
Stern, D.N. 69, 87
Stocker, M. 12
'strange situation' test 118–20
Strongman, K.T. 14
Structural Development Theory 26, 34–6,
     37, 38, 39
subconscious emotion 19, 28, 29
subjectivity
     adolescents may not divide expression
          from subjective feeling 204–5
     development of subjective awareness in
          infancy 30–1, 33, 64–6, 67, 69–70, 75
     in DSM-V definitions of diagnostic
          criteria 13
     subjective awareness can be bypassed by
          unconscious emotion 29
     subjective feeling as element of an
          emotion 17–19, 25
sulking 171, 173, 227
support for parents 128
surprise
     as basic emotion 33, 38
     in early infancy 64, 66

survival
     attachment satisfies impetus for survival
          120–1
     of children in adverse circumstances 106,
          167, 197, 207, 225, 228
     survival behaviours 8–9
     survival functions of emotions 23
Sweatt, J. 134
symbolic thought 88
sympathy
     in adolescence 197
     vs empathy 100
     as a moral emotion 7
     over-parented children do not develop 148
     in preschool years 157
     as secondary emotion 38
     in toddlerhood 88–9, 100–2

taking turns 92
Tangney, J.F. 104
tantrums 171–3
temperament 121–9, 222
'terrible twos' 91, 96, 197, 218
Thanatos (death instinct) 177
theories of emotion 26–7, 31–9
theory of mind, development of
     in adolescence 199
     and aggressive behaviour 179
     in middle childhood 161
     neglected children fail to develop 167
     and parenting 138, 173
     in preschool years 154, 155–6
     in toddlerhood 88–9, 91–3, 94, 100–1
Thomas, A. 124–6, 127
time, perceptions of 70–2, 156, 161
'time outs' 183
toddlerhood
     emotional development (whole chapter)
          81–107
     aggressive behaviour 179–80, 182
     independence in 113
     objective reality, introducing child to 137
     oppositional behaviour 171–3
Tomkins, S.S. 31, 32
trait anxiety 184–5, 187
transfer of function 45
trickery, in toddlerhood 89
trust 5
Tucker, D.M. 47, 87
two factor theory (Schachter-Singer) 32, 37

unconscious emotion
    brain structure leads to 29
    and Discrete Emotions Theory 33–4
    fear 29
uncontrollability of emotions 17–19, 25, 29,
        96, 103, 158
unexpressed emotions 161
uninvolved parenting 142
universal emotions 21, 27, 31, 66
unobservability of emotions 3

valence of an experience 67
variation
    children from adverse backgrounds are
        not the same 164–5, 211
    in emotion 21–6
    in evolution 44

in individual brain development 52–4
verbal expressions of emotion 19–20
visceral concomitants of an emotion 15–17,
        24
volition, intertwined with emotion 14
von Salisch, M. 162

wariness 71, 78, 82, 96
warmth, need for
    emotional warmth 87, 133
    physical warmth 62, 85
Waters, E. 53
'what if' scenarios 89
Winnicott, D. 134, 137
worthiness, feelings of 97, 99

Zahn-Wexler, C. 94, 207